Leany VandenBrink

INTERPERSONAL
ASPECTS
OF NURSING

INTERPERSONAL
ASPECTS
OF NURSING

JOYCE TRAVELBEE, B.S.N.Ed., M.S.N., R.N.

Hotel Dieu School of Nursing
New Orleans, Louisiana

Formerly Professor, University of Mississippi School of Nursing
Jackson, Mississippi

Second Edition

 F. A. DAVIS COMPANY, Philadelphia

LISTEN, NURSE

by Ruth Johnston

I was hungry and could not feed myself.
You left my food tray out of reach
          on my bedside table,
Then you discussed my nutritional needs
          during a nursing conference.

I was thirsty and helpless, but you forgot
          to ask the attendant to
          refill my water pitcher.
You later charted that I refused fluids.

I was lonely and afraid, but you left me alone
          because I was so cooperative
          and never asked for anything.

I was in financial difficulties
          and in your mind I became an object
          of annoyance.

I was a nursing problem and you discussed
          the theoretical basis of my illness.
And you do not even see me.

I was thought to be dying and,
          thinking I could not hear, you said you hoped
          I would not die
          before it was time to finish your day
          because you had
          an appointment at the beauty parlor
          before your evening date.

You seem so well educated, well spoken,
          and so very neat in your spotless
          unwrinkled uniform.
But when I speak you seem to listen
          but do not hear me.

Help me, care about what happens to me,
I am so tired, so lonely and so very afraid.
Talk to me—reach out to me—take my hand.
Let what happens to me matter to you.

Please, nurse, listen.

PREFACE

The purpose of this text is to assist both student and professional nurse practitioner to establish more effectively a helping relationship with hospitalized adults, and with others who may be affected by the individual and his illness.

All professional nurse practitioners strive to improve their practice and to develop more effective means of rendering care. Because nursing is always concerned with people,[1] the more knowledgeable and skillful a nurse is in the area of interpersonal relationships, the more likely it is that she will be able to meet the nursing needs of others.

In this work the term "patient" is considered a stereotype. Actually there are *no* patients. There are only individual human beings in need of the care, services and assistance of other human beings whom it is believed can render the assistance that is needed. Therefore, the term "patient" has been deleted from this book and is used only when discussing the development of the stereotype, "patient." The term "nurse" is used only for purposes of communicative economy.

A basic assumption underlying this work is that nurses should strive to establish human-to-human relationships—not "nurse-patient" relationships.

This work is divided into six sections. In Section One, the nature and purpose of nursing are discussed. The purpose of nursing set forth in this text is derived from assumptions regarding the nature of the human being. It is believed that the purpose of nursing is to assist an individual, family or community to prevent or cope with the experience of illness and suffering and, if necessary, to find meaning in these experiences.

In Section Two, three major concepts are discussed: The Human Being, The "Patient," and The Nurse. A major assumption is that the quality of care given any ill person is determined primarily by the nurse's perception of the ill individual and her beliefs concerning human beings.

In Section Three, the concepts Illness, Suffering and Hope are explored. Illness and suffering are considered as experiences undergone by human beings—not as mere theoretical concepts. A major belief is that human beings are motivated by a search for meaning in all life experiences, and meaning can be found in the

---

[1] Norris, Catherine: What insights can psychiatric nurses contribute to the development of curriculum in basic professional nursing? Concepts of the Behavioral Sciences in Basic Nursing Education. Proceedings of the 1958 Regional Conferences on Psychiatric Nursing Education. New York: National League for Nursing, 1958, p. 269.

experience of illness, suffering and pain. The importance of hope and the nurse's role in assisting ill persons to maintain hope are discussed.

In Section Four, the concept Communication is considered. Communication is viewed as a process which enables the nurse to establish a human-to-human relationship. Communication is considered a means to an end, the end being the achievement of the purpose of nursing.

Section Five consists of three chapters: The Human-to-Human Relationship, Nursing Intervention, and Surgery: A Human Experience. The human-to-human relationship is considered the means through which the purpose of nursing is achieved. In the chapter on nursing intervention, specific ways and means of assisting ill persons to find meaning in illness, suffering and pain are discussed. Psychological preparation of the individual about to undergo the stress of surgery is also discussed.

Section Six includes an Appendix and a Selected Bibliography. The Appendix, Expanding Empathic Boundaries, includes a consideration of ways and means by which teachers of nursing may assist students to expand their empathic boundaries. The Bibliography is a selected one which includes suggested reading references for each chapter. Throughout this work, if references used in the chapter are in the footnotes they are not repeated in the Suggested Reading References listed in Section Six. The Bibliography has been completely updated. References published in the first edition of this work are not repeated.

The concepts discussed in this text build and elaborate on concepts developed in preceding chapters. It is deemed important that students develop depth of understanding of concepts developed in each chapter before· proceeding any further.

It is assumed the students who use this text possess a basic knowledge and understanding of the major concepts of human physiology, biology, and chemistry. It is also assumed that students will have completed the beginning courses in the behavioral sciences and in the humanities.

The emphasis in this work is on the knowledge underlying the skills or techniques, rather than on techniques per se—although some essential techniques are discussed. It is believed essential that students in nursing develop an understanding of the knowledge underlying the skills, that is, the major emphasis must be on the *why* rather than on the *how*.

The concepts presented in this work are believed to be applicable to all clinical areas of nursing. The content is arranged in such a way that the concepts presented begin with the elementary then progress to the more complex.

ACKNOWLEDGMENTS

I wish to thank the many individuals who have assisted and encouraged me in writing this second edition.

It is with deep gratitude that I thank Miss Ruth A. Johnston, R.N., a truly "authentic" human being, who lives in pain yet walks in brightness. I am indebted to her for valuable suggestions and for her encouragement.

I owe an incalculable debt to those who cared and helped, especially Nellie Whisenhunt, Sarah Dumas, Liz and Ron Critchley, Rosalind Fernandez and Connie Ikert.

To my great and good teachers especially Dr. Teresa Ahumada, Miss Winifred A. Maher, R.N., Miss Ida Jean Orlando, R.N. (Mrs. Robert Pelletier), Miss Nellie Whisenhunt, R.N., and Miss Margaret Williams I also owe thanks.

This book is humbly dedicated to the "brotherhood of those who bear the mark of pain" and to all who strive to alleviate human suffering.

The time given by the individuals who reviewed many of the chapters is indeed appreciated. The names of these persons appear at the end of the various chapters which they reviewed.

J.T.

CONTENTS

INTRODUCTION

Every nurse can learn to establish and maintain helping relationships with others. In this work, two major requirements are stressed—first, the nurse must possess a body of knowledge with the concomitant ability to use it, i.e., she must possess and use a disciplined intellectual approach to problems. Kindness and good intentions are important in nursing care, but neither will compensate for lack of understanding of scientific concepts and principles and the lack of ability in their application. Throughout this work the operational use of concepts and principles is stressed, behavioral concepts being considered as experiences encountered and undergone by human beings—not mere dictionary definitions.

The second requirement, necessary if the nurse is to establish and maintain helping relationships, is the ability to use oneself therapeutically. In order to do this it is necessary for the nurse to possess a profound understanding of the human condition. A basic assumption of this text is that the nurse's beliefs about the nature of the human being will profoundly affect her perception of self and others, and will affect her ability to achieve relatedness. An understanding of the human condition is necessary to establish a helping relationship.

The nurse who possesses and uses a disciplined intellectual approach, combined with the therapeutic use of self, is able to establish helping relationships. It is further believed that the human-to-human relationship is the means through which the purpose of nursing is fulfilled.

The quality of nursing care given any ill person is determined by many factors. The nurse's knowledge and ability to apply it is certainly a major determinant, but an equally important determinant is the nurse's beliefs about illness, suffering and death. The nurse's philosophical beliefs about illness and suffering, or her spiritual values, will determine the extent to which she will be able to help ill persons find meaning (or no meaning) in these situations.

A nurse cannot suppose herself to be educated if she has not explored these meanings. It is as essential to discuss and formulate beliefs regarding the meaning of suffering as it is to spend time discussing ways of alleviating it! Nursing students need help in understanding and comprehending the meanings they attach to these inevitable situations of illness encountered by every human being.

Throughout this work emphasis is placed on the nurse's role as supporter and sustainer. The major assumption is: It requires far more understanding, knowledge and skill to support an individual in time of crisis than to perform any complicated technical treatment.

The ability to intervene effectively and assist an individual in a time of crisis requires study and a disciplined intellectual approach; it cannot be left to chance or intuition. The rationale of nursing intervention is stressed, and ways in which the nurse can intervene in a thoughtful, purposeful, intelligent and tactful manner are discussed.

Another major theme is that nursing is in need of a humanistic revolution—a return to focus on the "caring" function of the nurse—in the caring for the *caring* about ill persons. A professional nurse practitioner *cares* what happens to other human beings, is concerned about their physical, mental and spiritual welfare, and will act in an intelligent, knowledgeable, creative and tactful manner to assist others.

"There are numerous signs that we are beginning to lose the sympathy and compassion which have so long characterized nursing. . . . Nurses are becoming increasingly afflicted by the unrelatedness, alienation, and lack of commitment so prevalent today. . . ."[1]

Recently a physician speaking of various specialities in the medical field remarked, "But who specializes in human kindness?" The fact that such a question should be raised is a good indication of how far individuals in the health professions have strayed from the very basic goals of their profession. One has only to read the findings concerning nursing care in the Duff and Hollingshead study to discover how prevalent is this lack of caring among nurses.[2] It is the author's belief that dehumanizing tactics are being practiced increasingly in health agencies and institutions, and that there is little or *no* evidence that this trend is abating. That nurses as a group have remained silent and have done so little to protest these conditions is a sad commentary on nursing's lack of social consciousness. It is interesting to speculate how much improvement would result in nursing if nurses en masse refused to consent to, condone by omission or commission, any act which dehumanizes the human being or permits the rendering of ineffective, unconcerned and unsafe care.

If nurses do not change by becoming increasingly involved in caring *for* and *about* ill persons it is believed that the consumers of nursing and medical care will demand the services of a new and different kind of health worker. This health worker or "ombudsman" will serve as the representative, interpreter and spokesman for the ill human being and his family. His allegiance will be to the ill human being—*not* to the institution or agency which hires him. It is foreseen that progressive monolithic institutions will be among the first to hire individuals to serve as ombudsman for ill persons and their families. The functions of the ombudsman will probably be that of sustaining and supporting ill persons and their families in time of crisis. Such an individual will serve as the ill person's spokesman, clarifying and opening channels of communication between ill persons and members of the various health disciplines and in general serving as the ill person's

---

[1] Travelbee, Joyce: What's wrong with sympathy? Amer. J. Nurs. 64:71, 1964.

[2] Duff, Raymond S., and Hollingshead, August B: Sickness and Society. New York: Harper & Row, 1968.

mediator and dragoman. The ombudsman will possess an in-depth understanding of the power structure of the institution or agency as well as an understanding of the formal and informal lines of authority within the institution or agency. He will be readily available for consultation by ill persons and their families and will be the resource person to whom they can turn for assistance in solving problems created by hospitalization. The ombudsman will know which agencies or persons to contact in the hospital or community in order to solve problems with a minimum of time, effort and red tape. In general the ombudsman will render the kind of assistance not *now* provided by any single health worker.

However, there would be no need for creating the position of ombudsman if nurses assume their role as the ill person's advocate, intercessor and mediatrix. If, however, nurses do not assume their role as change and care agents, other categories of health workers may be created to assume this responsibility. Time is running out. A greater militancy on the part of nurses in effecting needed changes and in combating dehumanization is not only necessary it is *imperative*.

In the final analysis only nurses can improve nursing practice. The quality of nursing care rendered ill persons will not be improved unless nurses, individually and collectively, care enough to effect improvement. The author is hopeful and believes nurses will overcome the barriers which separate them from ill persons and their families and will increasingly band together to combat dehumanization wherever and whenever it occurs.

Nursing's professional organization must become more vocal in protesting dehumanization and in developing ways and means to assist nurse practitioners to effect changes in health care patterns and practices. The professional organization must change in order to represent nurses and the consumers of nursing care more effectively. Public opinion, citizen groups, and consumers of nursing can be mobilized to effect change. Hopefully, the symbol of the nursing organization of the future will be the outstretched hand—not the closed fist.

One wonders what the nurse historian fifty years from now will say of the nursing practiced in our particular era. Will it be said of us,

> The nurses in the twentieth century tried for a while to improve the barely minimal care given ill persons, but they gave up very easily. They compromised and because they accepted second best they became second rate. They were silent when they should have spoken and because they compromised too often there was little professional or personal integrity to them. They became cold, detached, uncaring individuals. They did not really care what happened to ill persons. Because they worshipped expediency they became expeditors. They surrendered without a fight and with hardly a skirmish.

Or will it be said of us:

> They practiced nursing under the most difficult circumstances, always trying to improve the quality of care given ill persons. They were not afraid to speak out against that which dehumanized the ill human being, and hindered them in truly caring for ill persons. They did not accept second best, neither did they compromise on important issues. Indeed there were giants on the earth in those days. . . .

How the future of nursing will be written depends on our actions today. Every nurse writes a part of this history. Each individual practicing nursing has a choice. Only she can decide how that history will be written.

SECTION ONE

The purpose of this section is to define the concept "nursing" and to suggest some appropriate roles of the professional nurse practitioner. The purpose of nursing is explored, and ways are discussed in which the purpose of nursing is achieved. The major assumption is that the purpose of nursing is achieved through the establishment of a human-to-human relationship.

First, the question "what is the unique function of professional nursing?" is considered; and second are discussed "appropriate functions of the professional nurse practitioner."

Chapter I

THE NATURE OF NURSING

What is the nature of nursing? What is the essence of nursing—its distinguishing qualities? What does nursing have to offer individuals that is not and cannot be offered by any other group of health workers?

All nurses have some ideas or assumptions about the nature of nursing, and many definitions of nursing have been written. Some writers think of nursing in relation to its aim, purpose, or reason for existing. The definitions and beliefs about the nature of nursing, found in the literature, invariably reflect the writer's orientation and belief system. A definition of nursing is important since whatever a nurse believes to be the substance or nature of nursing will determine her behavior in nursing situations and her views on nursing education and practice. A definition of nursing or a set of beliefs about nursing is the major premise from which subsequent conclusions or generalizations about nursing care develop.

PART I

NURSING: ITS DEFINITION

Nursing is an interpersonal process whereby the professional nurse practitioner assists an individual, family, or community to prevent or cope with the experience of illness and suffering and, if necessary, to find meaning in these experiences.

EXPLANATION OF DEFINITION

Nursing Is an Interpersonal Process . . .

Nursing is an "interpersonal process" because it is always concerned with people either directly or indirectly.[1] The "people" nurses are concerned with in-

---

[1] Norris, Catherine: What insights can psychiatric nurses contribute to the development of curriculum in basic professional nursing? Concepts of the Behavioral Sciences in Basic Nursing Education. Proceedings of the 1958 Regional Conferences on Psychiatric Nursing Education. New York: National League for Nursing, 1958, p. 269.

7

clude ill and healthy individuals, their families, visitors, personnel and members of the allied disciplines.

Nursing is also a "process," and by that we mean it is an "experience" or a happening, or series of happenings, between a nurse, an individual, or group of individuals in need of the assistance the nurse can offer. Nursing viewed as a process stresses the dynamic character inherent in every nursing situation. Nursing situations, being experiences in time and space, are dynamic and fluid, and are ever in the process of evolving or becoming.

Change is taking place in every nursing situation. In a single nursing encounter there is an ebb and flow of influence and counter-influence from nurse to recipient and recipient to nurse. There is continuous movement, activity, or change occurring as a result of the interaction, the nurse influencing the recipient and in turn being influenced by the recipient. Changes occur as a result of the impact of one individual on the other. *To identify and be able to bring about change in a purposeful, enlightened, thoughtful manner is a nursing activity.* A nurse is a change agent—indeed, he or she cannot be otherwise if the purpose of nursing is to be achieved. The nurse as change agent implies that the status quo is not accepted if the status quo is illness, suffering, poor nutrition, poor sanitation, poverty or a host of other problems. The nurse labors to effect a change, i.e., to assist the individual, family, or community in becoming cognizant of ways to prevent illness, disability and suffering and to act in such a way as to maintain health at the highest possible level. *The nurse is vitally concerned with change and, in a sense, it may be said that she invariably wants to change or influence others.* Nursing is, in a sense, a service which is initiated for the express purpose of effecting a change in the recipient of the service.

Assists an Individual, Family or Community . . .

A *nurse always assists others.* Who is assisted? The individual or family in need of the services of the nurse. This assisting function is held jointly by nurses and members of the other health disciplines.

Even when performing the independent functions of nursing, the nurse is in the process of assisting—as when supervising the care of an individual, observing and recording, supervising non-professional personnel, or when health teaching. The purpose of all these activities is to assist the individual to prevent, or cope with, the experience of illness and suffering or to maintain the highest level of health possible.

The assistance rendered may be direct or indirect, but assistance is what is offered. Indeed, the reason individuals or families seek the help of members of the health disciplines is precisely because they are believed to be able to render needed assistance.

Most nurses readily comprehend the nurse's role in assisting individuals and family members to prevent illness, promote health or help individuals and families to cope with the stress of illness. But how does a nurse assist a community? The nurse can fulfill a variety of functions. For example, nurses can initiate, participate in, organize and evaluate programs designed to solve community health problems. The nurse works with community members (and agencies) and members of other health disciplines in detecting potential or actual health hazards in a community and in organizing community members so that effective action can be taken. Anything which does or could interfere with the health and well being of citizens of a community is of legitimate concern of the nurse.

To Prevent Illness and Suffering . . .

Nurses are always concerned with illness and with health since both these concepts are pivotal ones in nursing practice. The concept "illness" is defined and explored in Chapter V. The concept "suffering" is explored in Chapter VI.

Concept: Health

The concept "health" is important because professional nursing is concerned with helping an individual to prevent illness or suffering and to maintain the highest possible level of health. What, then, is meant by the concept "health?"

The World Health Organization in its constitution states, "Health is a state of complete physical, mental and social well-being and not merely the absence of disease or infirmity. The enjoyment of the highest attainable standard of health is one of the fundamental rights of every human being without distinction of race, religion, political belief, economic or social condition." [2]

According to Webster's Third New International Dictionary, health is defined as "the condition of an organism or one of its parts in which it performs its vital functions normally or properly: the state of being sound in body or mind. . . ." [3]

As helpful as the above definitions may be, neither fully define the concept "health." For purpose of discussion, two different criteria of health are proposed: the subjective and objective aspects of health. *Subjective health is defined individually, i.e., in accord with each person's appraisal of his physical-emotional-spiritual status as perceived by him.* Thus subjective health is highly individualistic. In actuality, the appraisal of subjective health status implies that a person is as healthy as he perceives himself to be at any given time. An opinion regarding subjective health status is probably reached on the basis of many diverse factors. For example, an individual may believe he is "healthy" if he can perform the daily activities of living to his personal satisfaction. Some individuals equate being able to work with being healthy. It is quite possible for an individual to be diagnosed as

---

[2] Constitution of the World Health Organization. Chronicle of the World Health Organization, Annex 1, Vol. 1, No. 1-12, 1947. World Health Organization Interim Commission. New York, p. 29.

[3] By permission. From Webster's Third New International Dictionary, copyright 1961 by G. & C. Merriam Co., Publishers of the Merriam-Webster Dictionaries.

being without discernible pathology and yet perceive himself as ill. On the other hand, it is possible for an individual to be diagnosed "ill" by a physician yet perceive himself as healthy. Thus subjective and objective appraisals of health may differ. It is important for nurses to know how the individual appraises his subjective health status. If an individual believes he is ill then it behooves health workers to pay attention to the individual's perception of his health status and not rely wholly on objective appraisals of illness or health. It should always be remembered that some individuals have the ability to discern disease processes or changes in their body long before pathological changes appear in the laboratory tests. In order to understand the human being it is vitally important that the nurse ascertain from the individual *his* appraisal of his health status.

Using an objective criterion, health would be defined as an absence of discernible disease, disability, or defect as measured by physical examination, laboratory tests, assessment by a spiritual director or psychological counselor. When the physical-psychological-spiritual aspects fall within what is considered a normal range in our society the individual is judged "healthy." The person making the judgment of "objective" health may be a physician, psychiatrist, priest, rabbi or minister. The opinion of these individuals then is used to indicate that the person possesses the condition called "objective health."

Combining both criteria it would be expected that an individual who appraises himself subjectively as healthy and who is deemed healthy by individuals using an objective criterion is indeed a "healthy" person. However, when combining the subjective and objective criteria of health into a single criteria, the concept of health is not fully explained. A discussion of the concept of health raises some interesting questions. Is not health more than "just feeling good" or having negative results on laboratory tests? Are there varying degrees or levels of health? Is health a constant or does an individual's health status fluctuate within a given day? What is meant by the phrase, "promotion of health"? How does a nurse promote health? Can health promotion be taught without a clear understanding of the meaning of this most difficult concept? It is obvious that more nursing research is needed in this area in order to define operationally the concept of health.

All human beings will, at one time or another in their lives, deviate from health and become ill. It is quite possible that illness is a more common life experience than is health, especially if one uses the World Health Organization's definition as a criterion. Illness, and especially suffering, cannot always be prevented. However, it is the function of the professional nurse practitioner to assist the individual in coping with and bearing the stress of illness and suffering when he does encounter these experiences.

The process of nursing, i.e., everything the nurse does for and with the recipient, is designed to help the individual or family in coping with or bearing the stress of illness and suffering in the event the individual or family encounters these experiences.

As knowledge increases and expands in regard to the etiology of disease it is expected that prevention will become a priority area in medicine and nursing.

Within the foreseeable future it is possible that we shall see the nation-wide establishment of "well-adult" clinics. These clinics, located in accessible neighborhood
areas, will operate much in the same way that "well-baby" clinics do today. Diagnostic services will be offered to detect beginning signs of illness. Out-patient treatment services will be offered. However, emphasis will be placed on health
maintenance and disease prevention. Health teaching will be developed to a high
degree of efficiency. The clinics will be research oriented. Studies will be conducted
to identify needs, evaluate the quality and quantity of services offered, and to
assess the effectiveness of the well-adult clinic. While disease and disability probably
can never be eliminated, it is believed that many of these conditions may be
prevented. Unfortunately, it seems that when the etiology of some disease conditions becomes known and effective treatment methods are discovered, other disease
conditions emerge. Diseases of "medical progress" and iatrogenic diseases are
increasing even at this time.

With increased emphasis on prevention and out-patient treatment it is anticipated that the ever mounting hospital admission rates will decline. Other factors
should also reduce the admission rate to hospitals. It is to be expected that
eventually insurance will be available to individuals who wish to utilize the services
of "well-adult" clinics in order to prevent illness.

In the future the majority of professional nurses will work in community
health agencies, clinics and comprehensive health centers. Hospitals will probably
be reserved for ill individuals requiring intensive care for medical crises and for
persons requiring major surgical intervention. At the present time, however, the
majority of nurses work in hospital settings. There is much that the staff nurse can
accomplish in the area of prevention of disability and maintenance of health.
Health teaching is an area that has been given low priority despite lip service to the
contrary.

Health Teaching

Many nurses think of health teaching only, for instance, in relation to helping
a person with diabetes to administer insulin, or in aiding a person with a colostomy
to care for himself. But health teaching is much broader in concept. It is concerned
primarily with helping individuals and families to prevent illness, or to cope with
the experiences of illness and suffering.

Health teaching also implies more than acting in the role of interpreter to the
physician; it is more than imparting the needed information to individuals and
families, or functioning as an "information clarifier." This is not meant to negate
these vital activities or underestimate their importance. But the concept of health
teaching is more inclusive than even a total of these activities.

*The core of health teaching in nursing is (if necessary) to assist ill individuals
to find meaning in illness, as well as in the very measures they must take to
conserve health and control symptoms of illness.*

Health teaching also implies assisting ill persons to find some meaning in the acts of self-denial and sacrifice they are asked to make in order to preserve health. Without the perception of meaning in these acts it is not probable that instruction in techniques and methods will suffice (for example, how to give oneself an injection of insulin). If a person perceives his life robbed of all meaning by the measures he must take to conserve health, he may soon abandon any attempt to adhere to such a regimen. It is easy to underestimate the effect of prescribed health measures on an individual. A person used to leading a physically active life is told by his physician to walk slowly, not to carry heavy packages or walk up stairs, and to rest every afternoon. Such a person must modify and change habits established over a life time. It is no easy matter to make such an adjustment. Unless the individual perceives meaning in the measures he must take to conserve health he may, in time, decide conservation of health is not worth the effort involved. Health teaching in nursing, therefore, is primarily concerned with assisting individuals to find meaning in illness and health measures—rather than information-giving per se.

Cope with the Experience of Illness and Suffering . . .

At the present time the largest percentage of nurses work in hospital settings and are primarily concerned with assisting individuals to recover from the acute phase of illness and, in some instances, to regain health. Helping ill persons to regain health or recover from an acute phase of illness is a major satisfaction in nursing practice at the present time. One of the ways in which the nurse assists individuals to regain health is to help them cope with the experience of illness and suffering. The nurse does this by establishing relatedness with the individual, which conveys to the sick person that he is understood and is not alone. In times of great need, the realization that there is at least one warm, sensitive, knowledgeable human being to whom one can turn has sustained many ill persons and has kept many individuals from despair. The nurse demonstrates by her actions that she wants to assist the individual—not because he is ill and is expected to be cared for—but because he is himself and no one else. It is not an easy task to assist an individual to cope with illness even if there is reasonable assurance that the person will recover. It is even more difficult to assist individuals to cope with illness and suffering when there is little or no assurance the individual will ever regain his health.

Many individuals will never become well and must learn to live with a long-term illness. Aside from certain infections and communicable diseases, orthopedic conditions, and some acute surgical conditions, cure is not possible. One does not speak of cure in relation to many of the cardiovascular conditions, many of the endocrine and collagen diseases, many of the central nervous system disorders, many musculoskeletal disorders, many eye conditions, blood dyscrasias, skin conditions, pulmonary diseases, some of the cancers and so forth. Cure is not possible unless a major research breakthrough occurs in regard to the etiology and treatment of these long-term disorders. The knowledgeable nurse realizes one of the major problems will be the ill person's attitude toward his illness, because of what it may mean to him and his family.

The sick person has attitudes and feelings about his illness. In order to assist the individual it is *absolutely essential* that the nurse develop an understanding of the way in which the ill person perceives his illness. For the most part this is an area that has been grossly neglected by most nurses.

That nurses generally do not know how sick persons perceive their illness has been demonstrated in a recent study by Duff and Hollingshead. It was found that only fifteen per cent of registered nurses (working on private accomodations) had any idea about the attitude of ill persons toward their illness. Six per cent of the registered nurses working on semi-private accomodations had some knowledge of the person's perception of his illness. However, *none* of the registered nurses working on wards had any information of the individual's view of his illness.[4] It is, of course, not possible to assist an ill person to cope with illness and suffering, or to find meaning in these experiences, if the nurse has no idea about the attitude of the ill person toward his illness or disability.

To Find Meaning in Illness and Suffering . . .

What can nursing offer to the individual whose life has been irrevocably changed by the onset of a chronic, debilitating, or terminal illness? One might state that in such cases it is a function of the professional nurse to assist the individual— not in regaining his health since this is not possible, but in maintaining the highest possible level of optimal health. One cannot argue with this statement but more is required. It is evident that in many instances ill people require more than good physical care, rehabilitation, health teaching, or encouragement, although certainly these activities are important and should not be minimized. What else is required of the professional nurse practitioner? *The professional nurse practitioner must be prepared to assist individuals and families not just to cope with illness and suffering but to find meaning in these experiences. This is the difficult task of professional nursing and it cannot and must not be evaded.*

In order to accomplish the above goal it is believed that the concept of illness, as currently taught in most schools of nursing, must be drastically revised. Most nurses learn about illness by studying the common disease conditions—more specifically illness is "learned" in relation to etiology, signs and symptoms, treatment and "nursing care." Actually what is learned is that illness is an undesirable condition which must be cured or alleviated as soon as possible. This view is not undesirable, but it is not inclusive enough. There are, as has been stated, few illnesses or conditions that can be cured. Are nurses being prepared to assist ill persons, not just to cope with illness, but to find meaning in these experiences? How can nurses assist ill persons in such a manner unless the nurse herself perceives that meaning can be found under such circumstances? Illness, it is believed, should be considered as a

---

[4] Duff, Raymond S. and Hollingshead, August B.: *Sickness and Society*. New York: Harper & Row, 1968, p. 227.

natural, common life experience. This is *not* to imply that illness is a positive good, or that illness is to be preferred to health. It *does* imply that illness is a life experience which *can* be a self-actualizing one to the ill person, provided he is assisted to find meaning in this experience.

If illness is viewed as an intrinsically bad condition, it follows that the major orientation of health workers will be directed towards cure. The cure-orientation of most health workers is a major barrier in that it may hinder health workers from deriving satisfaction in helping ill persons to find meaning in illness. It is believed that nursing students need to be assisted in deriving satisfaction in helping ill persons to find meaning in illness, *as well as* in helping individuals to recover. They probably will not be able to derive this satisfaction unless the teacher in nursing believes meaning *can* be found and assists the students in arriving at this understanding.

It is believed that nurses can derive as much satisfaction from assisting ill persons to find meaning in illness as they do in helping ill persons recover. This orientation presupposes that the nurse believes illness can be a self-actualizing experience. It means a decided change in viewpoint towards the so-called "hopelessly ill" individual, especially those ill persons for whom the nurse believes she can "do nothing." Something can *always* be done to assist ill persons, no matter how gravely ill they may be; they can be assisted to find meaning in the very situation that they experience as being so meaningless. Such an approach would, it is hoped, alter beliefs about the permanently handicapped, the disabled, the bedridden, or the completely dependent so-called "unproductive individual." All such persons *can* be assisted to cope with or find meaning in illness, even though they may have no hope of recovery. This orientation may also alter prevalent beliefs about the aged ill person. It is an unspoken idea, in the minds of some health workers, that since an individual is old and has "lived his life," and since he is ill, he would therefore be better off dead; that the aged ill can still find life a great good even though he may be ill does not seem to have occurred to some health workers. Ideas about aging and long-term illness are derived from many sources. One of the most common viewpoints seems to be derived from a utilitarian, mechanistic, horribly simplistic view in which the ailing body is viewed as a machine that has broken down and cannot be fixed. The utilitarian view stresses that time should not be spent caring for an ailing body that cannot "be fixed" or overhauled. Thus it is that the human body is considered a machine by persons holding such viewpoints.

Are nurses prepared to assist the ill individuals who consider illness to be meaningless? What will the nurse say when an ill person asks, "Why did this have to happen to me"? How will the nurse respond to the anguish-laden question, "Why did this have to happen to my little girl" (or my husband, wife, son, etc.)? If the nurse cannot or does not want to discuss this problem, she has missed an opportunity that may never arise again. The ill person is thrown back on his own inner resources when he realizes that he will receive no assistance from the nurse. Unless the nurse possesses a profound understanding of the human condition, combined with a belief that illness can be a self-actualizing experience, it is unlikely that she will be able to assist the ill person in any meaningful way. She will remain mute before that which she too believes is inexplicable and senseless, or will utter cliches and platitudes.

The question, i.e., "Why did this happen to me?", can be used as a means to elicit from the ill person the meanings (if any) he has attached to the experience of illness and suffering. The nurse can explore with the individual his perception of his illness and begin to work with him in the effort to assist him in gaining some understanding of his condition. (See Chapter XI, "Nursing Intervention," for ways and means of assisting ill persons to cope with the problem of meaninglessness.)

The Individual with a Terminal Illness

Caring for an individual with a terminal illness requires great skill and understanding on the part of the nurse. How does the nurse feel about caring for a person with a terminal illness? This will depend, to a large extent, on the nurse's feelings and ideas about death and dying, her religious convictions, her philosophy of death and philosophy of life. Other determinants include the nurse's feelings about her own encounters with dying persons, i.e., relatives, friends, or ill persons for whom she has rendered care. A major determinant seems to be what the nurse, as a student, was taught or learned about caring for the dying. It is well to remember that nurses may be taught the "ideal nursing care" of the dying person and yet fail to see a high level of care actually given in practice. Nursing students are usually under the direct supervision of a faculty member and hence are directly accountable to an instructor for the quality of care given the dying person. Upon graduation, however, no such direct accountability exists in most settings. Nurses may find themselves in a position where the quality of care, as learned in school, is seldom, if ever, seen in practice. Nurses can handle this problem by persevering and rendering high quality care or by succumbing to peer pressure. It is not, easy, under the best of circumstances, to persevere in rendering the kind of care one knows should be given, but to do so in the face of group pressure requires great steadfastness of purpose on the part of the committed nurse. Research studies are urgently needed to enable us to understand what it is that enables some nurses to give high quality care despite group pressures to the contrary.

The school of nursing has a definite responsibility to assist the student to discuss ideas and beliefs about death and dying. A nurse cannot suppose she is educated if she has not explored the meaning of suffering, illness, loneliness and death. We know all human beings, at some time in life, will be confined by illness, pain, suffering, anxiety—perhaps despair, loneliness, guilt and eventually death. Nursing students need help in understanding and comprehending the meanings they attach to these inevitable situations. Is it enough to talk about pain only in relation to its origin and causes, or to think of pain in relation to narcotics and *not* inquire into the meaning of pain? Should the concept of anxiety be discussed only in relation to cause or physiological effects and inquiry *not* made concerning the meaning of anxiety? Should the student be taught ways of alleviating suffering and not given an opportunity to formulate beliefs about suffering? Should the student be taught aspects of caring for the dying patient, yet not be provided with some opportunity to explore her beliefs about death?

The student in nursing needs to develop some understanding of the meaning of these experiences in order to render professional nursing care. It is necessary for her to develop this understanding, not just because she is a student in a nursing program, but because she is a human being who will someday encounter and have to undergo the same experiences. Whether prepared or not, nurses encounter the problem of illness, pain and suffering every day of their practice in nursing. It is believed that nursing students need the assistance of the teacher in nursing in order to grow as human beings—as a result of encountering these difficult situations.

It is believed the spiritual values a person holds will determine, to a great extent, his perception of illness. The spiritual values of the nurse or her philosophical beliefs about illness and suffering will determine the extent to which she will be able to help ill persons find meaning, or no meaning, in these situations. (These problem areas are discussed in detail in Chapters V, VI, VII, and VIII. Specific ways in which the nurse may assist ill persons to find meaning in suffering and illness are discussed in Chapter XI, "Nursing Intervention.")

PART II

THE DEFINITION OF NURSING RE-STATED AS A PURPOSE

The purpose of nursing is to assist an individual, family or community to prevent or cope with the experience of illness and suffering and, if necessary, to find meaning in these experiences.

HOW IS THIS PURPOSE OF NURSING ACHIEVED?

A major assumption is that the purpose of nursing is achieved through the establishment of a human-to-human relationship. The purpose of the human-to-human relationship, in nursing, is to assist an individual, family or community to prevent or cope with the experience of illness and suffering and, if necessary, to find meaning in these experiences. The relationship is the process or means used to carry out the purpose of nursing. The reason for establishing a relationship is to achieve the purpose of nursing, and all of the nurse's activities and functions help achieve this purpose. The final measure of nursing competency is in terms of the extent to which the purpose has been achieved.

DEFINITION OF A HUMAN-TO-HUMAN RELATIONSHIP

A human-to-human relationship in nursing refers to an experience or series of experiences between the human being who is the nurse and an ill person, or an individual in need of the services of the nurse. The major characteristic of this experience (or experiences) is that the nursing needs of the individual, family or community *are* met. *These needs are met by a nurse who possesses and uses a disciplined intellectual approach to problems combined with the therapeutic use of self.* A human-to-human relationship is purposefully established and maintained by the professional nurse practitioner.

DEFINITION OF A PROFESSIONAL NURSE PRACTITIONER

A professional nurse practitioner is a graduate of a collegiate school of nursing whose aim is to assist students to learn a disciplined intellectual approach to patients' problems, and the therapeutic use of self.

In what way does the professional nurse practitioner use and possess a disciplined intellectual approach to problems? The term "possess" is defined as "to own . . . to be master of . . ., to have as an attribute."[5] In this sense, possession of a disciplined intellectual approach to problems implies that as an attribute it is a part of oneself, and as such, is inextricably woven and integrated into oneself. The term "uses" stresses the practical and utilitarian aspects of such an approach. The approach is operational, i.e., it works in practice. It is, of course, possible to use occasionally such an approach intuitively without actually possessing the underlying theoretical basis. However, the fact remains that one needs to know how to think and needs facts, concepts and principles with which to think.

A DISCIPLINED INTELLECTUAL APPROACH TO PROBLEMS

By the term "disciplined intellectual approach" is meant: (1) a logical method of approaching problems, (2) the content or theoretical aspects of nursing practice, i.e., knowledge and understanding of concepts and principles from the natural, physical, biological, behavioral, nursing and medical sciences and (3) the concomitant ability to use these concepts and principles in caring for others.

This approach represents a way of thinking, i.e., logical thinking, and focuses upon the basis of the thinking process, the use of concepts and principles, and includes the ability to translate that which is thought into creative and intelligent action, in order to meet the nursing needs of the individual, family or community.

The individual who possesses and uses a disciplined intellectual approach knows how to think logically, to reflect, to reason and to deliberate. He or she is able to ascertain and abstract meanings more readily in nursing situations and to validate these meanings. He or she has the ability to analyze and synthesize, therefore is more readily able to identify and meet the needs of individuals and families. Such an individual possesses facts, concepts and principles with which to think.

In nursing situations the use of the disciplined intellectual approach means

---

[5] By permission. From Webster's Third New International Dictionary, copyright 1961 by G. & C. Merriam Co., Publishers of the Merriam-Webster Dictionaries.

that the nurse is able to draw upon and use concepts and principles from the natural, physical, biological, medical, nursing and behavioral sciences. The nurse is able to identify concepts and principles operating in nursing situations. She is discriminating in that she is able to ascertain whether or not she needs more knowledge and understanding. The nurse knows where to go for assistance in solving health problems. Such an individual, possessing and using a disciplined intellectual approach, is able to make knowledge and understanding of concepts and principles operational—this knowledge and understanding being used to plan, implement, and evaluate nursing care.

An individual possessing and using a disciplined intellectual approach has an open mind but not an empty one. This individual is able to examine contradictory evidence with a minimum of personal bias. He or she is scholarly without being pedantic; learned, yet fully aware that learning is a life-long process and hence never ends. Such an individual has a liberal education—the basis for professional education in nursing. In short, this individual is an educated person.

In actual practice the professional nurse uses the disciplined intellectual approach in combination with the therapeutic use of self. Both abilities of the professional nurse practitioner are inseparable and are equally important, although the major emphasis inherent in these abilities differs. The disciplined intellectual approach focuses more on the theoretical (or content) aspects of nursing practice and less on process, while the therapeutic use of self is a blend of the cognitive and affective, emphasizing process more than content.

DEFINITION OF CONTENT AND PROCESS

Content is defined as the theoretical aspects of nursing, i.e., the facts, concepts and principles comprising the fund of knowledge used in nursing practice. Process is defined as the experiential aspect of nursing, or what is happening between the nurse and the ill individual.

In actuality, content and process cannot be separated since content is applied in process or emerges from process. Process also influences content since it is from nursing practice that concepts and principles are abstracted; the reverse is also true, in that concepts and principles are applied in nursing practice.

The relationship between content and process is a circular-oscillating one, each influencing and affecting the other. The disciplined intellectual approach is not the antithesis of the therapeutic use of self, but represents a perfected synthesis of intellect and affect. Such a synthesis (or a working towards it) is the hallmark of a professional nurse practitioner.

THE THERAPEUTIC USE OF SELF

The second characteristic of the professional nurse practitioner is the ability to use self therapeutically. The ability to use oneself in a therapeutic manner is enhanced in the professional school of nursing. It is assumed that students come to the nursing school with some ability to use self in a therapeutic manner. What precisely is enhanced or learned? Students are frequently helped to gain theoretical insights about their behavior through courses in the behavioral sciences and in some nursing courses. Theoretical insights are helpful, but more effective learning products accrue when learners are given the opportunity to study the effect of their behavior on others. Some imaginative faculties are experimenting in the use of sensitivity training, group dynamics sessions and videotaping of interviews between students and ill persons in an attempt to assist learners to study the effect of their behavior on others.

In order to use oneself effectively as a change-agent, or to intervene effectively in nursing situations, it is essential to know how one's behavior affects others. With gradually increasing self-knowledge the learner is able to relinquish automatic and stereotyped responses to others, and to establish newer and more effective ways of relating.

In what way is the use of self therapeutic? The term "therapeutic" is defined as "of, or relating to the treatment of disease or disorders by remedial agents or methods: curative. . . ." [6] When a nurse uses self therapeutically she consciously makes use of her personality and knowledge in order to effect a change in the ill person. This change is considered therapeutic when it alleviates the individual's distress.

By "therapeutic use of self" is meant the ability to use one's personality consciously and in full awareness in an attempt to establish relatedness and to structure nursing intervention. To use oneself therapeutically requires self insight, self understanding, an understanding of the dynamics of human behavior, ability to interpret one's own behavior as well as the behavior of others, and the ability to intervene effectively in nursing situations. To use oneself therapeutically also implies that the nurse possesses a profound understanding of the human condition. Such a nurse will have explored and can discuss her beliefs about illness, suffering, and death, and the meanings these beliefs have for her. The nurse realizes that her spiritual values, or her philosophical beliefs about human beings, illness and suffering will determine the extent to which she will be able to help others find meaning (or no meaning) in these situations.

Therapeutic use of self includes the use of reasoning and intellect, neither operating by intuition or by hit-or-miss methods. To use oneself therapeutically is an art and a science; it requires discipline as well as self insight, reasoning as well as empathy, logic as well as compassion. The emotions and feelings are guided but not suppressed by the intellect. There is an admirable balance between the two. It implies the educated heart and the educated mind—both used together and not singly but in combination for the good of the human being who is in need of the care the nurse can render.

Therapeutic use of self is not to be confused with kindly feelings. Kindness is important but it will not compensate for ignorance or lack of knowledge and understanding of scientific concepts and principles, or the ability to apply them.

---

[6] *Ibid.*

Therapeutic use of self must be combined with a disciplined intellectual approach to the ill person's problems. Since "kindness," in and of itself, is not sufficient to meet an ill person's needs, in an equal sense, it is as fallacious and one-sided to assume that all a nurse needs is to be scientifically informed, to possess a vast fund of knowledge and then to use it impersonally, treating the recipients of her care as objects and not as people.

As stated previously, the ability to use one's self therapeutically is not the antithesis of the disciplined intellectual approach but represents a perfect synthesis, or integration, of these two abilities. Such a synthesis must evolve and develop slowly over a period of time. It is a goal toward which to work realizing that a lifetime is scarcely long enough to achieve this synthesis. In the working toward this goal there is an actualization of the insight of how very little we really know as compared to what there is yet to learn. There is an alive realization of the person we could be as compared to the person we know ourselves to be. There is growing appreciation of the great debt we owe ourselves and the concomitant debt we owe others—that of increasing our ability to appreciate their utter uniqueness and irreplaceability.

It is to concretize and vividly realize the infinite value of every human being, and to expand and vitalize this realization until it permeates our every contact with others. It is to respect each individual, fully realizing that each person is a one-time-being in this world and hence is irreplaceable.

The working towards synthesis means appreciation of our beingness and the being-ness of others. Yet we are constantly in the process of becoming. It is to have the courage to continue the quest at the same time profoundly aware that the journey never ends. It is to be humble in the truest sense of the word and at the same time to derive strength from that humility. It is to expose oneself to the shocks of commitment and all that this entails. It is to care and in the caring to be vulnerable, but it is the vulnerability of the strong who are not afraid to be authentic human beings. It is the ability to face and confront reality—to face reailty not as we may wish it to be, but as it actually exists. Nurses must possess this trait if they would help others cope with the reality of illness and suffering. No one can give to another that which he does not himself possess. If nurses find no meaning in suffering how can they assist others to face the reality of it, to cope with it, to bear it, and to somehow extract some meaning or good out of such tragic experiences?

To work towards developing the disciplined intellectual approach combined with the therapeutic use of self is to realize the value of time and its implications. It is to be and to become; to live in the now of the tangible minute, to affect the future if ever so slightly by actions, and to assume responsibility for these actions. It is to learn the difficult lesson that the past is gone, the future has not arrived and that all any human being has is the present "now." It is to be able to assist others to affect the future by the way in which they cope with the "now." To sum up the therapeutic use of self in one phrase one might state that it is *commitment and affirmation.*

Summary of Parts I and II

Thus far we have explored a definition of nursing, and some appropriate activities of professional practitioners have been suggested. A purpose of nursing was explored, and the way in which the purpose of nursing is achieved has been considered. The term "professional nurse practitioner" has been defined, and the two characteristics of the professional nurse practitioner have been explored in some detail, namely, the disciplined intellectual approach to problems and the therapeutic use of self. Thus far we have not considered the question of the uniqueness of professional nursing practice or discussed what nurses can offer individuals not offered by other groups of health workers.

PART III

THE UNIQUENESS OF NURSING

Some writers believe that one unique aspect of nursing lies in the fact that the hospital staff nurse is the only health worker with the ill person over a twenty-four hour period of time. This is not actually a unique aspect of nursing since a physician might validly claim that he is always on call even though he is not with the ill person all of the time. Also various auxillary and ancillary workers might well make the same claim since they work with the ill person over a twenty-four hour period of time.

It has been stated that one unique function of nursing is that the nurse coordinates all the ill person's activities. One must ask, however, are there any instances in which coordination of activities are delegated to a less prepared group? It would seem so since properly prepared ward clerks can and do coordinate some activities.

Is the nurse unique because she possesses certain technical skills? Again one must ask: Could a less prepared group of individuals perform these same activities? Yes, because practical nurses, corpsmen in the armed forces and nursing assistants can learn them and develop a high degree of technical competence. Neither are professional nurses the only group prepared to give medications and observe for side effects—other groups have been prepared for, and are performing, this activity.

Is the professional nurse best prepared to meet the needs of the ill person? One might ask: What needs is a professional nurse prepared to meet? No health worker meets all of an ill person's needs. Only certain needs are met and not others. Here again all health workers meet some of the ill person's needs—the physician meets some needs, as does the social worker, the dietitian, the practical nurse, the nursing assistant, the physiotherapist, and the laboratory and X-ray technicians. Other groups of workers also meet needs of ill persons, for example: the minister, priest or rabbi; the ward clerk, maid, orderly, volunteer workers; the staff in the admitting department; and so forth. All health workers and other groups meet needs of ill persons, so the uniqueness of nursing cannot be established solely on the grounds that the nurse meets the needs of ill individuals.

Does nursing have a unique function that is not shared to some extent with other health workers? There is probably not a single function of nursing that is not shared to some extent or degree by other health workers. However, the professional nurse possesses an advantage in having unlimited access to ill persons (especially in hospital settings). The nurse is present when sick persons are undergoing the distress of illness and suffering, and is the only prepared health worker in a strategic position to give *immediate* assistance to the ill and suffering individual. Because of this, two major functions are identified regarding the professional nurse.

THE TWO MAJOR FUNCTIONS OF THE PROFESSIONAL NURSE

Professional nurse practitioners working in *any* setting have the opportunity to perform two major functions. These two functions are derived from the definition and purpose of nursing. The functions are:

1. *To assist individuals, families and communities to prevent or cope with the stress of illness and suffering and*
2. *To assist individuals, families and communities in finding meaning in illness and suffering (if this be necessary).*

These two functions are the guidelines used throughout this work in developing assumptions relating to the contributions of professional nurse practitioners to the health team, and in suggesting appropriate nursing activities.

It is believed that the professional nurse practitioner has the educational background and possesses the skill and understanding needed to perform these functions in an effective, competent, intelligent, tactful and creative manner. Practical nurses and nursing assistants share these functions, to a limited extent, but such groups lack the educational preparation of the professional nurse practitioner and therefore will not possess the depth of understanding, the same degree of skill, nor the ability to form the sound "on the spot" judgments as will the professional nurse practitioners.

N.B. References used in this chapter are in the footnotes. These are not repeated.

N.B. The term "human-to-human relationship" is not to be equated with the nurse-patient relationship. In this work it is assumed that the roles of nurse and patient may be barriers to establishing a human-to-human relationship. The term "nurse" is used only for purpose of communicative economy.

SECTION TWO

The purpose of this section is to examine the meaning of the concepts "Human Being," "Patient," and "Nurse"; and to explore the implications of these meanings in nursing situations.

In Chapter II the concept of the human being is discussed, a major assumption being that the quality of nursing care given any individual is determined primarily by the nurse's perception of the ill individual, and her beliefs about human beings. A major premise is that there is an utter uniqueness to every human being, each of whom is different from any other person.

In Chapter III the concept "patient" is considered as a category and a sterotype. A basic belief of this work is: there are no "patients"—the ill are individual human beings in need of the care, services, and assistance of other human beings, who, it is believed, can render the assistance that is needed. Perceiving a human being only as "the patient" or "bed 3" is a dehumanizing process. It is believed that the role of the nurse needs to be transcended in order to perceive and relate as human being to human being, instead of as nurse to patient.

In Chapter IV the concept "nurse" is discussed. "Nurse" is considered a category and a stereotype. The concept "nurse" is defined, and ways in which the human being is changed as a result of nursing education are considered. Some ways in which the role of the nurse may be transcended are also discussed.

Chapter II

CONCEPT: THE HUMAN BEING

It has been stated that nursing is an interpersonal process because it is always concerned with people either directly or indirectly.[1] The "people" nurses are concerned with include healthy and ill individuals, family members, visitors, personnel and members of the allied health disciplines. The nurse's perception of people, her concept of the nature of the human being, will profoundly affect, color and influence her behavior in all areas of life.

In order to suggest a theoretical framework of nursing practice it is necessary to consider certain basic assumptions about human beings and human behavior since any assumption relating to nursing must of necessity develop out of one's concept of the nature of the human being.

It is therefore necessary to ask the question: What is man?—and to formulate meanings which will serve as a basis of nursing action. The process continues in that it is also necessary to examine the effect on the human being of assuming the role of nurse or "patient."

Do "patients" relate differently to nurses than to other persons? If so, in what ways and to what extent? Do "patients" perceive nurses differently? What are the differences between a nurse relating with "a patient" and with a human being who is not categorized as "patient"? Does the role of "patient" affect the ability of the nurse to establish relatedness? These questions are of more than academic interest since *the quality of nursing care given any person is determined primarily by the nurse's perception of the ill person and her beliefs about human beings.*

The concept "human being" is explored in this chapter; the concept "patient" in Chapter III; and the concept "nurse" in Chapter IV.

A strangely simple yet infinitely complex question is: What is a human being? A nurse's beliefs about the nature of the human being will profoundly determine her attitude towards life and death, sickness and health, and will also determine how much value the nurse places on each human being she encounters.

---

[1] Norris, Catherine: What insights can psychiatric nurses contribute to the development of curriculum in basic professional nursing? Concepts of the Behavioral Sciences in Basic Nursing Education. Proceedings of the 1958 Regional Conferences on Psychiatric Nursing Education. New York: National League for Nursing, 1958, p. 269.

DEFINITION OF THE TERM "HUMAN BEING"

In this text a human being is defined as a unique irreplaceable individual—a-one-time-being in this world, like yet unlike any person who has ever lived or ever will live.

A biological organism affected, influenced and changed by heredity, environment, the culture and all of the experiences he encounters, confronts or runs away from.

A being possessing the innate ability to transcend the material aspect of his nature—yet imprisoned in his nature—a limited yet unlimited individual.

A creature of contradictions continually confronted by choices and conflict. Confronted by choices and the burden of choosing and deciding. Choosing one alternative rather than another and in the act of choosing to be responsible for choice and its consequences. It is to transcend the latent (but active) core of deterministic impulsion and to be free. To be a human being is to be responsible for the acts of choosing and deciding, which alter and affect the process of becoming, or transition and change in one's own life or in the lives of others. It is to act, but to act feeling the anguish of not knowing, and to make choices and decisions in full awareness of one's adequacy to do so. It is to confront the "now" with courage and freedom in order to affect, if ever in so slight a way, the to-be-future. It is to realize that life *is* conflict, and to face, confront and endure conflict which is the core of the human condition.

A human being is a thinking organism, capable of rational logical thinking, yet at times displaying irrational, illogical, "either-or," "black-white" dichotomized thinking.

A being capable of maturity yet always maintaining a soft core of immaturity.

A human being is an individual possessing the ability to know others, yet never completely being able to understand another human being. Able to communicate his individuality to others, yet always possessing a core of incommunicability that cannot be put into words and, probably if it were possible to communicate that which is incommunicable, it would not be understood by another; hence each individual possess a basic core of individuality and alone-ness that is elusive and cannot be grasped or understood by another.

A human being is a social being capable of relatedness with others—able to know, to like, to love, and to respond to and appreciate the utter uniqueness of others. At the same time capable of alienating, disliking, mistrusting and hating others. Hence a social being who is at times, and in varying degrees, pulled or pushed into unsociability or even asocial behavior.

A human being strives to transcend the self, to rise above the limitations of his human condition, or, instead of transcending, to escape, or try to forget the core of the incommunicable loneliness, longing, aloneness, restlessness and dissatisfaction that are embedded and embodied in self.

A human being is an individual who knows that one day he will die. He knows that he will die but, for the most part this knowledge remains abstract and theoretical. The human being affirms and denies, acknowledges and rejects, believes and disbelieves that life's cluminating experience will happen to him.

CAPACITIES OF HUMAN BEINGS

The human being is always in the process of becoming, evolving or changing. A distinguished feature of man is his capacity to remember the past and to antici- pate the future while living in the present. This capacity to remember and anticipate is, at one and the same time, a blessing and a burden. One can remember happy times, miserable experiences, or both. Going back in memory enables one to mentally "relive" experiences—to extract joy or pain from them, and, in some instances, to mentally "correct" them—to restructure the memory in such a way that one depicts the incident quite differently. And in the memory to behave as one would have wished to have acted. In relived experiences the individual has the tendency to blur and distort.

Memory can blur and distort experience so that the meanings extracted from remembered incidents are not useful in learning how to handle similar experiences one may encounter. Memory can, of course, have the opposite effect. Through remembering and reconstructing past experiences, i.e., when assessing the experi- ence accurately, recognizing one's true participation in it can be of immeasurable assistance in helping a person gain insight. It is important to remember that each person has the tendency to excuse his behavior and to present his action (to himself and others) in the best possible light.

Remembering may be a corrective experience, or a source of infinite regret for that which cannot be altered or changed and hence a source of guilt (whether realistic or unrealistic). In the same sense, anticipation of the future may be a source of hope or of dread. Anticipating the future, making plans, looking forward to some future time, can be powerful motivating forces enabling individuals to endure present hardships and deprivations because they know "things will be better" in the future.

However, living for a future that is yet to come is to postpone living and to be in a state of suspended animation, waiting and waiting for a time when it is believed that life will be more meaningful. Such is the genesis of hope and, at the same time, the seed of disillusionment as when the future becomes the realized concretized present and the reality of it is not as one dreamed it was to be or thought it should have been. The anticipation was more satisfying than the accomplishment and the illusion more gratifying than the realization. The satisfaction of accomplishment dies a quick or lingering death and then the cycle begins again. It is thus that becoming continues.

The human being is time-bound and time-free. He can live in the "now," remember the "what was" and anticipate, look forward to or dread the "to be future." Some individuals live in the past, others wait for a future that they believe will be more meaningful for them than the present. Others live only in the present, drifting through time, striving to forget the past and to ignore the future.

It is possible that the genesis of anxiety lies in the ability of the human being to imagine, remember and anticipate the future.

The human being's perception of time—the past, the present, and the future—probably more than any other factor, is a key to understanding, to some extent, the individual's perception of himself.

THE UNIQUENESS OF THE HUMAN BEING

A major premise of this work is that there is an utter uniqueness to every individual. Each person is different in his own unique way. This difference can be accounted for, not only on the basis of heredity and environment, but seems to be especially due to the particular life experiences each person encounters, his perception of these experiences and the manner in which he reacts to these experiences.

No two human beings are identical. Even identical twins differ in many ways. Two individuals may encounter the same experience, but each will react to this experience in his own unique way. This is true because the past experiences of the two individuals are different, and past experience invariably affects perception of present experiences. Individuals from the same family differ in many respects because each person responds differently to the psychological environment, although the physical environment has been the same for both. Each child is treated differently by his parents and others, and each child responds in his own unique way to these experiences.

It has been stated that human nature is the same the world over—that all individuals have the same basic needs and hence that people are more alike than they are different. This has resulted in the unfortunate tendency to assume that everyone is alike when the opposite is probably more valid. It is true, as far as we know today, that all human beings have the same basic needs. However, these needs may be modified by the culture of the person. Although all individuals have the same basic needs, the strength and intensity of these needs vary and they are expressed differently. There is some evidence to support the belief that differences in intensity of physiological needs may be inborn, and some to support the concept that these differences are due entirely to environment.

A guiding supposition to use in relationships with others is to assume and act on the assumption that *human beings are more different than they are alike.* Using this assumption will help one avoid the common error of assuming or supposing that others are like himself when they aren't and judging others according to what one would or would not do.

THE COMMONALITIES OF HUMAN EXPERIENCE

As there are profound differences between human beings so are there likenesses. These likenesses are not concerned with similarities between individuals but have to do with common life experiences every human being, if he lives long enough, will encounter. An understanding of the meaning of these common life experiences is essential if the professional nurse is to meet the nursing needs of people. This is not necessary because a person is a nurse, but because the nurse is a human being.

Each human being is like every human being in that all are of the family of mankind, although the differences between groups of people and individuals may be vast and profound, such as differing cultures, life experiences and language differences. Still there is one common denominator, bond, or link connecting each to the other. There is a language that can be understood by every person despite cultural, language or other barriers, and that is our capacity to comprehend the common life experiences of others, because we too will have encountered and experienced them.

The commonalities of human experiences are based on the assumption that every human being undergoes certain experiences during the process of living and reacts to these experiences in a way that can be comprehended or understood by another. It does not imply that we always understand why an individual responds as he does to these common experiences, but it does imply recognition and some degree of understanding of the experience.

What are these common life experiences? It is assumed that each individual encounters similar experiences during the process of living. All persons, at some time in their life, will be confronted by illness and pain (mental, physical or spiritual suffering), and eventually they will encounter death. Each person will, to some extent, experience anxiety, loneliness, guilt, and perhaps depression or despair. Each person will lose a loved one by death, separation or through the withdrawal of love once freely given. Hence, all will, at one time or another, grieve over the loss of a loved one. And there are probably few individuals who have not, at one time or another, asked, "Who am I?"; "Why am I here?"; "Where am I going?"; and, the all too common, "Why did this have to happen to me?"

Lest these commonalities seem morbid and depressing it must also be stressed that, although all individuals will undergo these experiences and will search for meanings in them, so it is true that most people, at one time or another, and in varying degrees, will experience such feelings as joy, happiness, contentment, wonder, love, and compassion, and they will also feel the impact of dislike, hatred, lust, anger, envy, jealousy and similar emotions.

As the common life experiences can be comprehended and understood because they transcend cultural and language barriers, as well as the barrier of the uniqueness of each individual, so too the emotions can be comprehended and understood and comprise an aspect of the language understood by all mankind.

Love, tenderness and compassion are readily comprehended and understood by individuals of all cultures and backgrounds. The language of love is universal and needs no interpreter.

VALUE AND WORTH OF THE HUMAN BEING

An understanding of the likeness and differences amongst all human beings can guide one's perception of human beings and their behavior. Another determinant of perception of others is the value of "worth" accorded each human being. There is usually a discrepancy between professed beliefs (i.e., what we say we believe) and actual beliefs as reflected in actions or dealings with others.

Many individuals profess to believe that every human being has value and worth. The professed belief is not a problem. How much value and worth accorded each person, and the criteria used by which value and worth are "accorded" others, comprise the problem that needs to be acknowledged and dealt with.

The Scale of Relative Value and Worth

In actuality there seems to exist a "scale of relative value and worth," i.e., a criterion or guide is used to assign or accord varying degrees of value and worth to others. A judgment is made and priorities are established. This scale is probably used unconsciously by most individuals, but in some instances it represents a conscious judgment. The scale seems to consist primarily of values abstracted from the culture.

In some cultures, higher value and worth are accorded a man; a child is valued more than an elderly person; a strong, healthy individual is valued above a handicapped person. Material possessions, productivity and wealth may be given high priority and those possessing them may be accorded a high degree of value. In such a culture the human being is then judged or valued in a relative way, i.e., for what he has and not for what he is.

Cultures vary in the priority listings of value and worth. All individuals are creatures of the culture in which they live and, as such, are profoundly influenced by the scale of relative value and worth prevalent in their particular culture. The individual within the culture need not ascribe to cultural belief systems, but each person needs to know what these values are, weigh their merit and act accordingly. Religious beliefs, i.e., those beliefs which are put into practice or use by the individual will, in many instances, conflict with cultural values and assignment of worth.

In this text the statement, "Every human being has value and worth," is accepted as valid and as a meaningful guide for action in the practice of nursing and in other areas of life. This assumption is also interpreted to mean that no individual can ever correctly assess the value or worth of another human being. The premise is that no one person possesses the criteria or the wisdom enabling him to assess another. Every human being has value and worth by nature of his human-ness. This human-ness is not dependent on cultural values or assessments. It *is* of itself.

N.B. Reference used in this chapter is in the footnote. It is not repeated.

Chapter III

CONCEPT: PATIENT

The concept "patient" is a pivotal one in nursing and medicine, being generally used to designate an individual under the care and treatment of a physician or other health worker. These individuals may or may not be hospitalized; however, it is common practice to dub hospitalized individuals, and those using the services of health agencies and clinics, as "patients."

The term "patient" is both a label and a category. It may also be a stereotype. The human propensity to conceptualize and generalize enables one to categorize, and to abstract meanings from perceptual phenomena. This capacity influences thinking so that a concept represents the synthesis of a mass of phenomena. It results in economy of effort and clarity in thinking. It can also result in the tendency to forget that a concept only represents, or stands for, certain aspects or facets abstracted from experience and is not the experience itself. This same human capacity to categorize and generalize can also cause an individual to apply the abstracted meanings of the concept indiscriminately.

There is a general tendency to categorize individuals. One then reacts to the category instead of the individual. As for example, the human being who is a waiter in a restaurant is generally reacted to as a "waiter" rather than a unique human being. The same situation applies in nursing when nurses perceive other human beings as representatives of a category rather than as separate, distinct, unique human beings who happen to be assuming a particular role at a particular point in time.

Once a human being has been categorized as "patient," all of the meanings a nurse attaches to this concept become a broad generalization covering "all patients," and the nurse may ignore or disregard the factor of unique differences between "patients." The nurse will then think of "all patients" as being alike and similar, and will focus on similarities to the extent that she may forget that the human being who is "patient 1" is not the human being who is "patient 2" and so on. Such is the genesis of stereotypes.

What a nurse thinks about "all patients" will then affect and influence her interactions with every individual for whom she renders care. Thus, meanings attached to categories reflect one's thinking and feeling about the individual or object to whom the term refers.

There seems to be a reciprocal oscillating type of relationship between the meaning a nurse attaches to the concept "patient" and her perception of ill individuals. *The nurse's perception of "patients" is a major factor in determining the quality and quantity of nursing care she will render ill human beings.*

How may the meanings a nurse gives to the concept "patient" be ascertained? These meanings, which guide the nurse, can best be inferred by observing and noting what the nurse says about ill persons (and to them), how she relates with them, the way or manner in which she performs her activities, and the extent to which she exhibits affective caring qualities in practice. Probably the quickest way to gain this information is to listen to statements made about ill persons during shift-change reports.

As a nurse thinks and believes so will she act. The nurse's beliefs about ill persons will be reflected in her actions and in everything she does to, or for, them. It is well to remember that it is quite possible for a nurse to "love humanity" in the abstract yet be quite unable to perceive and react to the human-ness of ill persons; in which case ill human beings are treated either as objects or as personifications of tasks to be accomplished.

DEFINITION OF "PATIENT"

A basic assumption of this work is that the term "patient" is a stereotype and a category. The term is useful only because it provides for communicative economy. Actually there are *no* patients. There are only individual human beings in need of the care, services and assistance of other human beings, whom, it is believed, can render the assistance that is needed.

All of the assumptions about human beings (see Chapter II: Concept, The Human Being) therefore apply to every individual categorized as "patient." As a human being "the patient" possesses the assets and liabilities of the human condition; in this he does not differ from any other human being. How then does he differ? The difference is in requesting the assistance of other human beings believed capable of helping him solve health problems. There are, of course, exceptions to this as in the case of some mentally ill persons, in which instance such individuals may not seek or request help or even desire it; such individuals have assistance thrust upon them and have no choice in the matter. However, generally speaking, most "patients" request assistance which means that the individual has made a choice and believes that he has a health problem (or will have one). A decision is made to seek assistance and then to request it or apply for it. The individual may or may not decide to accept the assistance offered. Refusal to accept assistance from health workers is of multiple causation, however, it is probable that a major factor has to do not with the assistance offered per se, but with the way or manner in which the assistance is offered.

If nurses, physicians and other health workers do not perceive and relate to human beings *as* human beings, do not exhibit a caring quality, do not communicate to the ill person that he matters to them as an individual, then it ill behooves them to throw up their hands in horror when ill persons discharge themselves from hospitals and clinics and seek the assistance of quacks and others of that ilk.

Perceptions of others always have a reciprocal influence on both the perceiver and the person perceived. In the process of dehumanizing a human being, not only will the health worker fail to assist the ill person and may be directly responsible for causing him to seek assistance from quacks, but the very process of dehumanizing will affect the health worker doing the dehumanizing so that he will find little satisfaction in working with or for the "objects" or non-human things he created. It matters very much, to both ill person and health worker, as to whether the human being is perceived and related to as an object, personification of a chore, or as a "patient."

PERCEPTION OF THE HUMAN BEING AS "PATIENT"

In what way does perceiving a human being as "a patient" affect the nurse and the nursing process? It requires little thought, effort or emotional involvement on the part of "the nurse" to view human beings as "patients." The "patient" is an abstraction, a set of expectations personified by tasks to be performed, treatments to carry out, an illness, or a room number. No one likes or feels warm towards a patient but towards a human being whose personality and uniqueness is perceived and experienced. It therefore matters a great deal whether an individual is perceived as "a patient" or as a unique human being. A nurse never sympathizes, understands, or has compassion for a patient but for a particular human being. It is probable that once an individual is designated "a patient" that a dehumanization process begins if ever so subtly. It well may be that once an individual assumes the role of "nurse" or the role "patient" a wall goes up between these two human beings until, unless this process is interfered with, both perceive the other as an abstraction or a set of abstractions.[1]

The role of "nurse" needs to be transcended in order to perceive and relate as human being to human being, instead of "nurse" to "patient." The individual uniqueness of the "nurse" is perceived by the "patient" as is the uniqueness of "the patient" by "the nurse." *It is only in human to human relatedness, which means transcending roles, that a relationship is established.*

It is quite possible for a nurse who begins to practice nursing to perceive the human being in every ill person she encounters. But it is also possible that as time goes by she may lose this quality and begin to perceive only the task to be accomplished and ignore the human being to whom or for whom the task is to be performed. She may perceive an illness instead of the human being who is ill, or she may stereotype "all patients" and endow them with a cluster of characteristics they do not possess—such as assuming that "all patients are dependent" and acting on

---

[1] Adapted from Travelbee, Joyce: What's wrong with sympathy? Amer. J. Nurs. 64:71, 1964.

this assumption without further reflection. The human being is not perceived, only his endowed characteristics. Such a process is termed "the process of human reduction."

The Process of Human Reduction

The process of human reduction refers to the diminishing capacity to perceive ill persons as human beings accompanied by an increasing proclivity to perceive ill persons as an illness, or as a task to be performed, instead of as human beings. Stereotyping "all patients" and endowing them with a cluster of characteristics they do not possess is another way of dehumanizing individuals. All of these perceptions have one common characteristic—they all ignore truth. The terms "process of human reduction" and "dehumanization" are used synonymously.

THE HUMAN BEING PERCEIVED AS "ILLNESS"

The process of human reduction or dehumanization takes place when an individual is perceived as "an illness" instead of as a human being with an illness. In some instances even the individual's illness is not accorded to him, and he is referred to as "Dr. Smith's appendicitis." One might say that being perceived as "Dr. Smith's appendicitis" is dehumanization raised to the second power.

An individual does not "equate" himself with his illness. If this were so then treating or caring for "the illness" would satisfy the human being. However, in reality, it does not work this way since illness is generally perceived as "a something" one has, and not "something" one is. To perceive an individual as an illness is to ignore his humanity, and individuals so perceived are well aware that they have been dehumanized. Such individuals may be "grateful" of the attention given their illness; however, they will also feel resentment towards those who have so dehumanized them.

THE HUMAN BEING PERCEIVED AS "TASK"

Why do some nurses perceive "patients" as tasks? What has happened to the nurse who has lost her capacity to perceive the human being in every ill person she encounters? A nurse beginning to practice may possess the capacity to perceive and respond to the human-ness of each patient to a high degree. But as time goes by her perception may change and she may begin to categorize and stereotype, eventually proceeding to the point where human beings are perceived not as unique individuals but as personifications of "all patients." As one nurse stated, "Only their faces change—but after awhile they all look alike to me."

The process of human reduction can occur to any nurse in any setting. However, it probably develops more rapidly in those nurses working in situations where there is a great deal of work to be accomplished, too few people to accomplish the work and too little time in which to accomplish it. Such a process probably is a protective energy-saving device. In order to meet institutional expectations, the nurse sets up a system of priorities and strives to accomplish that which is absolutely necessary and to do this in the shortest possible period of time. With time at a minimum the ill person is translated into a "demand," representing innumerable tasks requiring expenditure of energy that is already at a low ebb. The ill person is perceived as a "doctor's order" to carry out, a chore possessing a pulling quality, or a task one must perform in the midst of innumerable tasks. Ill persons may be perceived as treatments to be performed, objects to be manipulated or as bodies to be processed by means of a conveyer belt type of "nursing" approach.

As the ill person gradually becomes a chore, a task, or an object, the nurse withdraws and directs her energy towards meeting only institutional expectations. The uniqueness of the individual human being for whom she renders care is not perceived. Her perception is of the tasks she must perform because they are "expected" of her. Such nurses may be regarded as "good nurses" by the institution; however, they are *never* regarded as "good nurses" by the human being who happens to be the "patient."

Many nurses undergoing this process are aware that their perception of the ill human being is changing and are concerned about it. It bothers them that they cannot spend more time "getting to know the ill person as an individual"; however, as time goes on this nagging remnant of a "nursing conscience" fades away. Expediency gains ascendance over excellence in nursing care. Some nurses remain in such situations trying desperately to make full use of every available minute of time in order to give ill persons individual attention. Many nurses, unable to tolerate the frustration involved in such a situation, resign, go to a position in another institution hoping that conditions will be better. Others leave nursing. Thus are some effects of the process of human reduction.

THE HUMAN BEING PERCEIVED AS "A SET OF STEREOTYPED CHARACTERISTICS"

Besides the process of human reduction where the individual is perceived as non-human, i.e., as a task to be performed, or an illness, there are other ways of dehumanizing ill people and one of these is to perceive them in terms of specific characteristics believed true of "all patients." For example, "all patients" may be considered helpless, dependent creatures who must be cajoled and coaxed lest they retreat into a solidified, ossified permanent stage of helplessness and utter dependency on the all-knowing, all-giving mother figure of a nurse. If a nurse believes "all patients" are helpless and dependent she will act on this belief and will probably infantilize the person to such an extent that he will soon exhibit the expected behavior. Infantilizing individuals is a way of manipulating and controlling them thus rendering them non-threatening to the nurse who seems to possess a stronger need to be omnipotent than does the average person. Nurses who operate in terms of this belief do not perceive ill persons as unique human beings, neither do such nurses assist individuals to grow toward maturity.

Another way of perceiving ill persons is to view them as not-too-bright, child-like creatures who must never, under any circumstances, be told anything about their condition. Thus a temperature reading becomes an incommunicable esoteric secret known only to the elect few or the in-group. It is deemed better to let the individual become anxious and worried about his temperature than to tell him what it is and thereby cause him to worry. Nurses become masters of the art of "waffling"—a British term meaning to talk a great deal while saying nothing.

Perception of the ill person as a human being who is unique is the only way of avoiding stereotyping the individual as "helpless and dependent" or as "not-so-bright." Of course, some human beings may seem "helpless and dependent" and some may "not be too bright." But this is not true of all ill persons; neither is it true of all nurses. It is a label or a stereotype.

Labels are useful in "identifying the contents or giving other appropriate information as to the destination of a parcel, the use of a medicine or the title of a book."[2] Labels serve no purpose when applied to people. An ill person is a unique, different human being whose individuality and uniqueness can be experienced but not labeled or stereotyped. How does the individual react or respond when he is perceived as and treated as "a patient"?

EFFECT ON THE HUMAN BEING WHEN PERCEIVED AS "PATIENT"

In what way does being treated as "patient," i.e., as a task or non-human object, affect the individual who has been perceived in this manner? There are many different ways individuals can respond to the process of human reduction. The particular response seems to be based on many factors, one of which is the individual's perception of the threat and the habitual techniques he uses to cope with threat.

The most common emotional response an individual feels when subjected to the frustration of dehumanization is anger. The engendered anger may be expressed openly and directly to the provocative agent or subtly and indirectly, especially if the individual does not feel safe in expressing anger because he fears retaliation. The anger engendered by the provoker may be displaced onto another person with whom the person feels safe.

The anger may not be directed towards any particular person; however, the individual may experience feelings of irritability, tension and restlessness or may develop transient somatic symptoms. Instead of anger, an individual may experience sadness, depression, hopelessness and apathy.

Besides the factors already mentioned, an individual's response to dehumanization is also determined by his perception of himself and others, and the resources

---

[2] By permission. From Webster's Third New International Dictionary, copyright 1961 by G. & C. Merriam Co., Publishers of the Merriam-Webster Dictionaries.

he possesses. It is quite possible that an individual's social class, position and financial status determine the extent to which he will be subjected to the process of human reduction. However, if subjected to dehumanization, he will, if his position and financial status are above average, be better equipped to deal with the problem if it occurs. If complaints are not effective he can simply leave and seek assistance elsewhere.

Individuals, especially those in the lowest socioeconomic group, are not as well equipped with resources to deal with dehumanization. Many of these individuals accept dehumanization, many times without even publicly protesting, because they realize that there is no other place to go to obtain health assistance. Their human dignity is given as payment for health care.

Many nurses who work in large general hospitals where the "patient" population is composed primarily of individuals from the lowest socioeconomic category are very much aware of the dehumanizing tactics practiced by personnel working in these institutions. That nurses, as a group, have done so little to protest these conditions is a sorry commentary on nursing's lack of social consciousness.

In these institutions policies and practices are designed to meet the needs of personnel, not the needs of the ill human being. One has only to spend some time observing the way in which ill persons are "treated" in admitting rooms, clinics and emergency rooms of these monolithic institutions to realize the extent to which ill persons are dehumanized.

It is not unusual for the ill human being to travel many miles by bus to arrive in time for an eight o'clock clinic appointment and then have to wait anywhere from four to six hours in order to receive a few minutes of medical assistance. One has only to observe ill persons sitting on uncomfortable hard-backed chairs in large disorderly admitting rooms—rooms devoid of comfort and ordinary human amenities—to begin to gain an understanding of the impact of the dehumanized treatment "rendered" these individuals.

That ill human beings should be "treated" in such a manner by health workers and professional people whose function is to help and heal is indeed incomprehensible and indefensible. Unfortunately some personnel working in charity hospitals lack any vestige of human charity.

And how humbling an experience it is to observe the incredible patience as they wait interminable hours to receive "free" medical attention. And how humiliating it must be to be perceived by health workers as clinic numbers, cases to be seen or as bodies to be processed.

Many factors, of course, affect the individual's reaction to dehumanization. One factor seems to be related to the number of people perceiving him as "patient" or "case" as compared to "human being." A little humanization seems to go a long way. Generally speaking, if an individual is related to as "human being" by at least one health worker he may be able to draw enough strength from the relationship to cope with ten other health workers perceiving him as "patient."

Whenever a human being is given the label or title "patient" he is subject to being stereotyped in accordance with health workers' beliefs about "all patients."

"Patient" is a title or label and any title given an individual seems to have an obscuring effect in that the title or label may be given precedence over the human being having the title. An individual may be perceived on the basis of his title and not in terms of his human-ness. When ill persons say, "I want to be treated as a human being," they are communicating their resentment at being stereotyped and dehumanized. The resentment is valid and realistic since in invalidating, negating and obliterating the human-ness of others we deny their very nature and thereby subject them to an unforgettable, humiliating and almost unreconcilable affront.

It can be stated categorically that in order to establish relatedness with others it is necessary to perceive and respond to the human-ness of others. In order to perceive and respond to the human-ness of others the facades of title, position or status must be transcended. Therefore the role of nurse and the role of patient are barriers to relatedness and only when these barriers are overcome is relatedness possible.

It is one of the tasks of the professional nurse to perceive and respond to the human being in "the patient" and to assist the ill human being in responding to the human being who is "the nurse."

N.B. References used in this chapter are in the footnotes. These are not repeated.

CHAPTER NOTE:

The term "patient" is not used in this text except as an example of a label applied to ill human beings. The term "nurse" is used in this text for purposes of economy in communication, and when used, refers to a human being who is a graduate of a collegiate school of nursing whose aim is to teach students to learn a disciplined intellectual approach to problems, and the therapeutic use of self.

Chapter IV

CONCEPT: THE NURSE

It has been stated previously that a professional nurse practitioner is a graduate of a collegiate school of nursing whose aim is to assist students to learn a disciplined intellectual approach to problems, and the therapeutic use of self. This statement lists qualifications, or criteria, for a particular type of nurse practitioner, i.e., a professional nurse practitioner. It does not explain or elaborate on the concept "nurse," neither does it explain what being a nurse means, or what this may signify to others.

It is necessary to elaborate on the concept "nurse" because it is believed that one of the tasks of the nurse is to perceive and respond to the human being who is "the patient," and to assist the ill individual in responding to the human being who is the nurse. Only when each perceives the other as a unique individual does a relationship become possible. A corollary assumption is that the role of nurse must be transcended in order to establish relatedness with ill persons and others. It is therefore essential to elaborate on the "role of the nurse," to know what is meant when we say this role must be transcended.

Some fundamental questions about the concept nurse are: Who is a nurse? What is a nurse? What meanings may be attached to the concept "nurse"? Of what significance are these meanings? Who attaches such meanings? Under what circumstances? Why? Can it be said that an individual is in the role of nurse? Is the "role of nurse" a "something" that is assumed or enacted at certain times and not others? Is the role of nurse a hinderance in establishing human-to-human relatedness with others? Is an individual a nurse only when she works or assumes the responsibilities of nurse? Is "nurse" an accretion—a something that can be put on and taken off as though it were a garment? Who is a nurse?

DEFINITION OF THE TERM "NURSE"

A nurse is a human being, and all of the assumptions about human beings (see Chapter II, Concept: The Human Being) therefore applies to every human being categorized as nurse.

A nurse, then, is a human being sharing in common the human condition of all peoples. How then is a nurse differentiated? The major deviance is that the nurse possesses a body of specialized knowledge and the ability to use it for the purpose of assisting other human beings to prevent illness, regain health, find meaning in illness, or to maintain the highest maximal degree of health. A nurse, however, practices only within circumscribed areas that have been defined, and is legally accountable for deviance. Thus a nurse is responsible legally for nursing actions.

A nurse is an individual who has been irrevocably and profoundly changed as a result of her specialized knowledge and education. She has learned a body of scientific knowledge and has the ability to use it, has developed new skills; but more important she has been confronted with the vulnerability of the human being in a way that an adolescent or young adult entering another occupational field has not.

The most profound changes are brought about by exposure to illness, suffering, and death, in that these experiences are irrevocably removed from the status of comfortable abstractions, becoming instead profound realities. Illness and suffering become incarnate (i.e., they are given bodily form and substance); their effects are observable, or inferable, in a human being.

Illness becomes a "something" that can and does happen to human beings. The comfortable consideration of illness as an abstraction is no longer possible when a nurse is confronted with an ill individual who requires her assistance. Illness becomes a thuddingly real phenomenon to a nurse who sees, feels, touches or smells its effects in the human body.

Suffering also ceases to be a theoretical concept when perceived as a crying, moaning, screaming human being, and dying becomes an undeniably shattering reality to the nurse caring for the moribund individual.

THE CRISIS OF PERSONAL VULNERABILITY

No human being can be repeatedly exposed to illness, suffering and death without being changed as a result of these encounters. So too, the nurse is changed because, in being confronted with the vulnerability of others, she comes face to face with the compelling force of her own vulnerability in a way that it cannot be disregarded. The manner in which the nurse deals with this crisis will determine her ability to perceive, respond to and care for the human being in the ill, suffering or dying "patient."

It is essential that the young student in nursing be given an opportunity to discuss her thoughts and feelings regarding these experiences with a knowledgeable nursing teacher; with this help she will be assisted in resolving the crisis in such a way that it will have desirable effects, both for the student and the ill persons she will encounter in the future.

Without assistance a student is likely to respond by attempting the impossibility of trying to deny or control her feelings. There is an imperativeness to these feelings. The student, without assistance, is thrown back on her own resources and will tend to handle these feelings in the same manner in which she has dealt with trauma in the past.

One common outcome is to withdraw from the individual or situation producing the feeling with indifference or detachment. Indifference and detachment become protective mechanisms in that they prevent the nurse from experiencing the full impact of the anxiety that is engendered in the situation.

Another outcome of the unresolved crisis of personal vulnerability is to handle one's feelings by denying their import. The anxiety engendered by the feeling is reduced by levity, jokes, jesting, and reacting in a casual facetious manner. Such a nurse has been so overwhelmed by her feelings that she deflects them to the ill person who then becomes the object of the nurse's jests, jokes, crudeness and levity. One has only to listen to the manner in which some nurses discuss a dying person to realize the prevelence of this response.

What can the detached or facetious nurse offer the ill, suffering or dying human being? Such a nurse may perform the necessary nursing procedures conscientiously and faithfully, and it cannot be said that she will not give of herself to ill persons. She will give that which she possesses, namely, fear, indifference, callousness and emptiness.

How are such nurses perceived by others? Generally speaking, nurses who exhibit detachment, as well as those exhibiting facetious behavior, give rise to the image of the nurse as hardened or "hard-boiled." The "hard-boiled" nurse is not a nurse who has little feeling but an individual who has felt too much too long, and has had to deny or control her feelings thus rendering her impotent to truly care for others. She will not be able to meet the needs of ill persons because her own needs have not been met. If this pattern is not interfered with, such nurses will repeatedly exhibit the same indifferent or facetious behavior. Instead of being able to use the crisis of personal vulnerability to help her realize her humanity and the human-ness of others, it has made the nurse an emptier, unhappier, more frightened human being. The tragedy is that this pattern could have been prevented.

In place of detachment, or a type of facetious response, the crisis of personal vulnerability may be handled selectively, i.e., a nurse is able to respond to and truly care for only certain ill, suffering and dying human beings and not others. Such a nurse may be able to develop a relationship and be warm and supporting when caring for a young person, but not an older one; a male, but not a female, and so forth. Cultural values, of course, are a factor in influencing the selection of the ill person with whom the nurse can respond, but it is most probable that a nurse is better able to care for those ill persons who are not constant reminders of her own vulnerability. Hence it is not uncommon to see nurses who can respond warmly (and somewhat emotionally) to a dying child but not to the dying elderly individual. The probable reason (aside from the cultural factor) is that it is more difficult to "see oneself" in a dying child than in an older person.

Thus far only the non-useful, non-productive ways of dealing with the crisis of personal vulnerability have been explored. What is considered to be a desirable resolution of this crisis? With assistance it is hoped that this experience of vulnerability can be used to deepen the nurse's understanding of the human condition, specifically of the common bond uniting her with mankind and thereby increasing her compassion and other fellow feelings.

Through discussing her thoughts and feelings about the ill, suffering or dying individual, the nurse can begin to clarify her feelings and realize that these feelings represent her beliefs about illness, suffering and death. Through such discussions she begins to realize what it means to be a human being and gradually is able to accept her own humanity.

This acceptance of human-ness of self precedes acceptance of others as human beings. This acceptance, or realization, is a felt, profound permeating type of understanding—an understanding rooted in oneself and becomes as much a part of oneself as is the bloodstream. It is oneself. Once such a type of understanding occurs the individual is irrevocably changed. The resolution of the crisis of personal vulnerability results in the nurse's increased capacity to reach out to others in a way that was not possible before. She is more readily able to transcend self. *Transcendence in nursing means the ability to get beyond and outside of self in order to perceive and respond to human-ness of the ill, suffering, or dying individual.* It means the ability to cut through the facades of role, title, position or status, in order to relate with another human being. It is the ability to focus on others and in the process of focusing to realize fully one's own being. It is to vitalize and realize self, not to annihilate it.

Thus the crisis of vulnerability can determine the nurse's capacity to realize her own humanity as well as her capacity to respond to, and care for the ill, suffering or dying human being.

CONSCIENCE AND THE NURSE

Another important way the nurse has been changed as a result of her specialized knowledge and education is that she has absorbed certain beliefs and value systems, and will have developed a "nursing conscience." This "nursing conscience" is that aspect of conscience wherein the nurse experiences guilt when realizing that she has not fulfilled her responsibilities. It is not separate and distinct from conscience per se, but represents one aspect of it. As in the case of conscience in general, the nurse may or may not heed, act or not act on the promptings of this conscience. She may ignore her feeling of guilt—expiate it by removing (if possible) its cause or "absolve" herself through using rationalization, projection, or other mechanisms. A nurse, then, is subject to a particular type of guilt by virtue of being a nurse.

There are few nurses who have not experienced some feeling of guilt when an ill person dies and who do not wonder if there was something more that could have been done to save the individual's life. Even the most detached or facetious nurse experiences this nagging doubt. Even when the nurse intellectually knows that she has fulfilled all of her nursing responsibilities she may still experience this goading guilt. The death of an ill person represents many different things, but many nurses experience this event as a reflection on their professional and personal adequacy. An event of this type may also revive the experience of personal vulnerability, at least momentarily, for those nurses who have resolved this crisis previously. It will reinforce the detached or facetious nurse's responses. Thus it is that being a nurse subjects the individual to certain profound experiences and demands not encountered by individuals in other occupations.

THE HUMAN BEING PERCEIVED AS "NURSE"

A nurse is a human being, but by virtue of her specialized education she may be perceived, not as a unique human being, but as a category or stereotype. The term "nurse" is as much a label as is the term "patient" and nurses are dehumanized in the same way that patients are. Instead of being perceived as an utterly unique human being, the nurse may be perceived as a servant or as a means of assistance, i.e., as a pair of untiring hands and feet. She may be "appreciated," but if she is it will be for her utilitarian value, not for her uniqueness.

Nurses, like ill persons, are also subject to generalizations. As in the case of certain nurses who believe "all patients are alike," nurses also may be endowed with certain attributes or characteristics believed true of all nurses and reacted to on the basis of these beliefs. Ill persons and their families, physicians and other health workers will ignore individual differences amongst nurses and fail to perceive and respond to the human being who is the nurse.

The human being who is nurse reacts to dehumanization as does any human being. What differences does it make if an individual is perceived and related to as "nurse" instead of as human being? Are the two incompatible since a nurse is a human being? It is true that a nurse is a human being, but if she is not actually perceived as such, instead being perceived as a stereotype, then it is obvious that human-to-human relatedness can never develop.

It is not possible to develop relatedness with a stereotype, a category or a label—only with another human being whose uniqueness is apprehended and to whom we respond. It has been stated that it is one of the tasks of the professional nurse to perceive and respond to the human-ness of the ill person, and to assist the ill person (and others) in responding to the human being who is the nurse. The stereotype is the greatest barrier to such relatedness.

A nurse may be subject to generalizations (often erroneous) about what she does, as well as what she is. Ill persons and health workers, as a rule, know only in very general ways what a nurse does or can do. They do not usually understand the nature of the assistance the professional nurse is prepared to offer. Hence the "role" of the nurse is as subject to distortion as the nurse is stereotyped.

THE ROLE OF THE NURSE

It has been stated that the role of the nurse must be transcended in order to relate as human being to human being instead of "nurse" to "patient." Further, that it is only in human-to-human related-ness, which means transcending roles, that a relationship is established.

What is meant by the statement, "the role of nurse must be transcended?" A basic assumption underlying this statement is that ill persons and others tend to perceive and interact with the nurse on the basis of their stereotypes about nurses. What must be transcended is the barrier of the stereotype of "nurse" and all of the meanings attached by ill persons and others to this stereotype. The nurse, in turn, must transcend the barrier of the stereotype "patient" and all of the meanings she attaches to this stereotype.

The "role of the nurse" has its own meaning to nurses and may (and usually does have) a quite different meaning to the recipients of nurses' care. Generally speaking ill persons and their families, as well as health workers, interpret the role of the nurse in two ways—first, in accord with what they actually see a nurse do, as well as the manner in which a nurse performs these activities; and second, in terms of their particular beliefs and stereotypes about nurses and nursing practice.

The "role of the nurse" may be a barrier to human-to-human relatedness in the same way that the role of "patient" is a barrier. "Nurse" is a title or label and any title or label given an individual seems to have an obscuring effect in that the title or label is given precedence over the human being having the title. An individual may be perceived on the basis of his title and not in terms of his humanity. In the case of the nurses it seems that a nurse is more often perceived (and judged by others) on the basis of not only what she does, i.e., her activities, but more important on *how* she performs these activities.

Lacking prior experience with nurses, ill persons may rely on hearsay, knowledge gained through reading or from television or radio; lacking these the ill person will supply in fantasy what has not been experienced in actuality.

Stereotypes about others are changed only when the individual holding such beliefs receives evidence to the contrary and undergoes an experience which convinces him that his former belief is invalid. He then undergoes a change in perception. *The task of the professional nurse is clear; it is to purposefully change (or revise if necessary) the beliefs others have about nurses or nursing.* This change is accomplished through the actions of the professional nurse. The desired result is that the nurse will be perceived as a helping human being eminently qualified to assist because of what she knows, what she does and can do.

It is believed that nurses are often stereotyped because they have not allowed themselves to be known as human beings by ill persons. A probable reason for this is the old nursing exhortation about "not getting involved with patients." This shibboleth has probably done more harm over a longer period of time to more people than any other "nurse-ism" has done or is likely to do.

HOW THE ROLE OF THE NURSE IS TRANSCENDED

How is the role of the nurse transcended? The role of the nurse is transcended when the nurse perceives each individual for whom she renders care as a unique human being, and when the nurse allows herself to be known as a human being by each of these individuals.

Nursing activities are transcended when they are considered as a means to an end but not as the end itself. They are transcended when all of the nurse's activities are directed toward the recipient of her care. The primary object or goal of all nursing activities is to assist the ill human being who is the recipient of the nurses' care. Activities are a means to an end, not the end itself.

There are probably few nurses who would not agree that the purpose of nursing activities is to assist the ill person, and that all of a nurse's actions are designed with this aim or object in mind. However, it is apparent that all too often nursing activities become an end within themselves and the reason for these activities is overlooked. The nurse caught up in a vortex of activities is not likely to focus on the human being for whom these activities are performed. She will focus on what needs to be done, not on the human being for whom the activities are designed. The activity-oriented nurse cannot perceive and respond to the ill human being; neither will she be able to transcend the role of nurse. Nursing activities then do not help her to perceive and respond to the recipient of her care; instead the focus on activities separates her even further from establishing human-to-human relatedness.

Why are so many nurses activity-oriented? There are no research findings to validate this assumption; however, it is believed that instructors in schools of nursing place too much emphasis on teaching students to learn techniques and develop psychomotor skills *before* helping them to learn how to interact on a human-to-human level with ill persons and others. This is not to deny that nurses need to know *how* to perform nursing techniques, measures and procedures. However, the ability to use oneself therapeutically in order to assist ill persons to cope with or bear the stress of illness is *as* important a nursing function as is the ability to perform various techniques.

Nursing activities can, however, be used as a vehicle through which the nurse responds to the humanity of the ill person and assists the ill person to respond to the humanity of the nurse. When two human beings interact with each other they will establish relatedness to the extent that they perceive each other as separate unique human beings, not as labels, categories, titles or stereotypes. The role of nurse must be transcended because it is not possible to establish human-to-human relatedness if the barriers of role, title, status or position are present. (For more specific ways in which the role of the nurse is transcended, see Chapter X, "The Human-to-Human Relationship.")

N.B. See Suggested Reading References for Chapter IV, in Section VI, for references which amplify the content in this chapter.

SECTION THREE

The purpose of this section is to explore the concepts "illness" and "suffering."

The concept "illness" is discussed in Chapter V. Illness is considered as a category and a classification. The factors which influence an individual's perception of illness and his response to a diagnosis of illness are explored.

The concept "suffering" is considered in Chapter VI. The nature of suffering is discussed in terms of its phases, effects and possible meanings to the ill individual and others.

In Chapter VII the concept "hope" is discussed. The genesis and characteristics of hope are discussed and the nurse's role in assisting the ill person to maintain hope are considered.

In Chapter VIII the meaning of illness and suffering as human experiences encountered and undergone by human beings is discussed.

Chapter V

CONCEPT: ILLNESS

It has been stated previously that each human being is unique, but as there are profound differences between human beings, so are there likenesses. These likenesses are not concerned with similarities between individuals but have to do with common life experiences that every human being, if he lives long enough, will encounter. One of these common life experiences is that all persons will be confronted by illness and pain (mental, physical or spiritual suffering), at some time in their life, and eventually with death.

Every human being needs to think through and come to some understanding of the meaning of these common life experiences. It is doubly necessary that the nurse do so. A nurse encounters the ill, the suffering or the dying individual every day of her practice.

It has been stated that the quality of nursing care given any ill person is determined primarily by the nurse's perception of ill persons and her beliefs about human beings. This statement is too understated since *the quality of nursing care given any ill person is determined by the nurse's beliefs about illness, suffering and death. The spiritual values of the nurse or her philosophical beliefs about illness and suffering will determine the extent to which she will be able to help ill persons find meaning (or no meaning) in these situations.*

In this chapter, illness is considered as a category and a classification. The meaning of the nature of illness (or the concept of illness) and ways in which an individual may respond to illness are discussed.

DEFINITIONS OF THE TERMS "ILL" AND "ILLNESS"

Webster's Third New International Dictionary defines the term "ill" as "... that causes or is accompanied by pain or discomfort or inconvenience or that is otherwise disagreeable ..." [1] The term "illness" is defined as "... an unhealthy condition of the body or mind: MALADY ..." [2]

---

[1] By permission. From Webster's Third New International Dictionary, copyright 1961 by G. & C. Merriam Co., Publishers of the Merriam-Webster Dictionaries.
[2] *Ibid.*

The above definitions are criteria of illness; however, the experience of illness itself is not explored. The experience of illness is influenced by cultural beliefs about illness.

CULTURAL BELIEFS ABOUT ILLNESS

All individuals are creatures of the culture in which they live, and reactions to illness are always colored and influenced by cultural beliefs about illness. One current cultural belief about illness is that it is a condition to be prevented or avoided if at all possible. If an individual becomes ill he is expected to seek medical assistance, to "cooperate" with the physican and to get well as soon as possible. Failure to cooperate with a physician's instructions or to "do as he is told" is often interpreted as a desire to remain ill and such an individual may be stigmatized as a person who "enjoys" the attention that his illness gains for him. That anyone could enjoy the secondary gains or prerogatives of illness is viewed as reprehensible, and such an individual is often considered "weak and dependent."

In a culture which considers health, strength, youth and productivity as life's greatest good, anyone deviating from these conditions is viewed as pitiable, especially if the individual becomes ill through "no fault of his own" and if he strives to recover. If he becomes increasingly unproductive, bedridden and completely dependent on others, an unspoken thought is that the individual would "be better off dead." In a culture that stresses independence, it is not unusual to hear individuals express the fear of becoming "a burden" to others. To be dependent and "a burden" seems to be feared more than death.

Every culture seems to have certain criteria of "manliness and womanliness." Men and women are expected to behave in certain ways and not in others. These definitions and cultural expectations may encourage individuals to seek and follow medical advice, or may have the opposite effect. In our particular society where women are viewed as "the weaker sex" (despite research studies to the contrary) it is almost expected that women will more often be ill than men. Some men seem to have a tendency to equate illness with weakness and to view illness as a threat to their masculinity.

Illness is a social as well as a human problem. The way in which the culture considers these problems in general, effects, or may create, certain attitudes towards the human problem of illness. In an activity-oriented society taking great pride in its ability to solve complicated technological problems, there may emerge a belief that *all* problems (whether technological or not) can be solved, or, if not solved, at least something can be done about them.

A concomitant belief is that questions can be answered if one but searches and strives long enough, and that difficulties surrounding problems can be surmounted. While this attitude has resulted in numerous technological advances, it has also left the impression that the problems of illness and suffering are equally amenable to solution.

The ill individual in our society (especially one suffering from an incurable malady) may find it difficult to believe that he cannot be cured. Resignation is not a highly prized virtue in an activity-oriented society. Acceptance of the inevitable comes slowly, if at all.

It may be that we lack the fatalism and stoicism of individuals of some of the Eastern cultures, or that our philosophy of life does not include the ability to accept the fact that not all of life's problems can be solved.

Most nurses have encountered individuals suffering from incurable maladies who visit every well-known medical center in the country expending time and energy, trying to find a cure for that which has no cure. Who has not encountered the mother of a mentally retarded child—a mother who refuses to accept the fact that her child will never be normal? So much time, energy and money are wasted in the realization of the impossible. Perhaps one could say in rebuttal that a searching for a cure is, in and of itself, a demonstration of hope. In and of itself the belief in the possibility of obtaining a cure (or amelioration of symptoms) cannot be criticized. Hope probably enables more individuals to bear the burden of illness and disability than does any other factor. But the searching for an improbable cure precludes acceptance, and hope is killed and revived, only to be killed again.

Which is the better way? To assist the individual (or his family) to accept that which is inevitable, or to encourage the search for a cure which does not exist? When hope is killed (even if it is revived and killed again) what is the individual left with but an anxious desperation akin to despair? Yet how very human it is to seek assistance and cure of an incurable malady or disability. And who among us is really wise enough to answer these questions with any degree of certainty? It is well that we should remember to walk in humility when confronted with the human anguish engendered by such problems.

It is the role of the physician to discuss with the ill person the nature of his illness and the rehabilitative and curative measures which will be taken. It is also his role to interpret to the ill person (or his family) the individual's probable prognosis. Nurses also share in this responsibility. Nurses have not always acknowledged or accepted their responsibility in assisting individuals to accept their illness or in aiding them to live with the knowledge of their prognosis. (For specific ways in which the nurse can assist ill persons in such situations see Chapter XI, "Nursing Intervention.")

Our culture also influences attitudes about illness in the various age groups. Thus it seems to be expected that as an individual grows older he will be more subject to illness. It is considered "natural" that old age, illness and disability "go together." It is quite possible within the foreseeable future that the belief that "illness and aging go together" will be irrevocably disproved or at least considerably altered. Research on illness and the aging process, as well as increased emphasis on the prevention of disease and disability, may dramatically alter this belief.

Because it is believed that illness and aging go together it is not unusual to hear nurses and other health workers state that they are not "too disturbed" when an older person dies because he has "lived his life" but they are disturbed if the individual is young and has "his whole life before him." One somehow wonders if nurses and other health workers do not communicate this belief to the elderly ill individual. That an elderly ill person can find meaning in living, although very ill and suffering, does not seem to occur to many health workers.

All health workers, being subjected to their culture, are influenced by cultural beliefs about illness, as are all ill persons in that particular culture. Health workers (as well as ill persons) attach their own meanings to the concept of illness. Some of the general and specific meanings of the concept of illness are discussed from the standpoint of health workers and ill persons.

THE CONCEPT OF ILLNESS

The term "illness" is a classification. An individual must fulfill certain criteria in order to be classified as ill. The most usual way an individual becomes classified as ill is by the diagnosis of illness made by a physician who corroborates the individual's belief that he is, in fact, ill. This is not to say that an individual is *not* ill when a physician fails to make the diagnosis of illness. It does mean, however, that, in our society, diagnosis made by a physician is a more bona fide certification of illness. An individual diagnosed as ill by a physician is more readily accorded the prerogatives of the ill than is an individual who believes himself to be ill (and may in fact be so) without such corroboration. Like health, illness is also defined subjectively; i.e., an individual is as "sick" as he perceives himself to be at any particular time.

The term "illness" is also a category. Physicians and other health workers tend to place illnesses into two categories: major and minor. A major illness, being considered a "serious" illness, has a poor or dubious prognosis. The term "minor illness" usually refers to an illness with a "good" prognosis and hence is classified as "non-serious."

These descriptive categories used for the purpose of communicative economy indicate, in a rough manner, the extent to which a person's life is threatened by a disease process or injury. While these categories may be useful it should be remembered that, although the physician or other health workers may consider an illness as a "minor one," it in no way follows that the individual suffering from the illness will perceive it as such. There is no such condition as a "minor illness" to the individual with the illness and there is probably no such surgery as "minor surgery" to the individual undergoing this experience.

Every illness or injury is a threat to the self, and the way in which the ill person perceives his illness is more important than any health worker's categorization system. *A health worker cannot know in advance how the individual perceives his illness until the health worker explores this with the individual and elicits from him the meanings he attaches to his condition.*

Illness is a very nebulous concept since illness is not observable; only its effects or results can be noted. Some of the results of illness can be readily observed or inferred; others are discernible through means of laboratory tests. X-ray examination, and other means. In other instances the effects or results of illness can only be inferred but not validated. Individuals may seek the assistance of health workers because they "don't feel well" or "believe somethings is the matter" with them. In other instances, overt signs of illness motivate the person, but, probably more than any other factors, pain and discomfort motivate individuals to seek assistance. The assistance is sought in order to alleviate pain and discomfort, to prevent further development of the illness, to corroborate the individual's belief that he is, in fact, ill and to procure ameloriation of symptoms and cure. Inability to work or adequately perform the activities of daily living are other factors motivating individuals to seek medical attention.

Of course, not all ill persons seek the assistance of a physician in order to corroborate (or discount) the presence of illness since an individual may be ill without knowing it and without ever having had the diagnosis of illness made by a physican. And, as previously stated, an individual may be ill although diagnostic tests and examinations fail to confirm or corroborate his illness. Some individuals seem to possess the ability to sense or "feel" the beginning symptoms of illness (during its earliest stages) before such findings are manifest through physical examinations or other diagnostic means. Such individuals may become very frustrated in their attempts to convince physicians and others that they are in fact ill. A diagnosis of illness *may* be accorded them, but the illness is apt to be considered that of a psychological nature. One such patient said:

> I've been to four doctors and none of them can find anything wrong with me. I don't want to be sick—it's just that I know I am and no one listens. The last doctor I went to told me that I was just nervous and he gave me a tranquilizer. Of course, I'm nervous and he'd be nervous too if no one believed him. Well, I've had it—this is the last doctor I'm going to . . . I just hope and pray that this time my lab tests are positive. (Incidentally, the results of the tests were positive.)

It is not for the purpose of criticizing physicians that this situation is discussed. Nurses will encounter such persons and it is utterly necessary that they refrain from labeling and reacting to them as "courters of ill health." If a person perceives himself to be ill (whether he is, or is not), then for all practical purposes he is ill. It is not within a nurse's province to diagnose, or to come to a decision as to whether or not an individual is ill. It is, however, the task of the professional nurse to perceive and relate, as human being to human being, with all of the recipients of her care. Whether or not the individual is or is not ill in no way negates this obligation.

Besides cultural beliefs about illness and health workers' concepts about illness, many other factors affect the way in which an individual will respond to illness or a diagnosis of illness. How does an individual arrive at the decision that he is ill? Generally this belief is arrived at through the individual experiencing some symptom of his illness. The way in which the individual will respond to a diagnosis of illness has to do with what the individual believes his symptoms may represent. The term "symptom" is defined as "subjective evidence of disease or physical disturbance observed by the patient . . ."[3]

---

[3] By permission. From Webster's Third New International Dictionary, copyright 1961 by G. & C. Merriam Co., Publishers of the Merriam-Webster Dictionaries.

Symptoms and Their Meaning to the Ill Individual

What the individual knows or has heard (whether true or not) about the meaning of his symptoms will influence or affect his readiness to seek medical assistance. Many individuals (or their relatives) before consulting (or bringing their relatives to consult) a physician will ask friends, relatives, neighbors and acquaintances all kinds of questions about the possible meaning of the presenting symptoms. The symptoms may or may not be recognized as being indicative of an underlying disease process. For example, "growing pains" in children may be considered as normal. The possibility that children with such symptoms may be suffering from rheumatic fever may not even be realized.

On the other hand the symptoms may be recognized as an indication that "something is the matter." As a rule at least one friend or neighbor has had (or thinks he has had) similar symptoms and makes a "diagnosis." Such informants are usually not in the least bit reluctant to suggest various remedies (which may or may not be efficacious). Various suggested patent medicines may be taken in an attempt to "cure the illness." If these remedies fail, or pain and discomfort become too severe, most (but not all) individuals will seek medical assistance. There are, of course, many exceptions to this generality.

The ill individual is indeed fortunate if he is not subjected by at least one "friend" to an account of someone having the same symptoms as the ill person who suffered terribly and died a horribly gory death. Such "friends" are usually as descriptive and graphic as they are sadistic and it is a rare individual who has not encountered at least one of these persons.

Unrecognized Symptoms

Some symptoms of illness develop slowly and insidiously; when this happens it may be difficult for the individual to realize that he is ill. For example, an individual with a thyroid deficiency may, over a period of time, develop marked feelings of fatigue. If he becomes too exhausted he may assign all sorts of meanings to his symptoms such as "overwork," vitamin deficiency and the like. In some instances he may even believe that most people suffer from the same degree of fatigue that he experiences. One has only to listen to frequent comments made by others about "being tired" to understand how it is possible to arrive at the conclusion that such fatigue is "normal."

Delay in Seeking Medical Assistance

Before an individual consults a physician he generally has some beliefs (whether erroneous or not) as to the meaning of his symptoms or, in some instances, has either "diagnosed" himself or been "diagnosed" by a friend or relative. The meanings he has attached to his symptoms may motivate or hinder an individual from seeking medical assistance. Why do some persons delay so long in seeking medical assistance especially when they have every reason to believe that they are ill and need medical help? One prevalent reason is that the individual is afraid of what the diagnosis may be. He may be afraid that he has cancer or some other malignant disease and thus will not seek verification from a physician. Such an individual would rather live in fear than face such a probability. Of course, he may have cancer and will delay seeking attention until nothing can be done to save him from that which he dreads.

Individuals (especially women) having symptoms related to the rectal, genital or mammary areas of the body may be reluctant to consult a physician because of a false sense of modesty. Individuals who have, or think they have, a venereal disease may hesitate to seek medical assistance because of a fear of censure, or because they are afraid that the nature of their illness may become known to their relatives or to others.

Some individuals refuse to seek or delay seeking medical assistance because they do not have the money to pay a physician and refuse to "accept charity." Others fail to seek medical advice because they mistrust physicians; such individuals usually have had an unfortunate experience with a physician in the past and generalize their distrust from one physician to include *all* physicians and health workers.

Some individuals do not consult physicians because of religious prohibitions. Religious groups prohibiting such consultation usually have certain designated church members who pray for, or in some other way assist, the ill person.

The most common reason given by individuals who delay seeking medical advice is that they "do not have the time." Another reason is that they "do not want to lose a day's pay." A third prevalent reason given is that the person "hasn't the time to pamper himself." Such individuals usually "don't think much of people who run to the doctor with every little ache and pain." These "stoics" are usually well supplied with stories about friends or relatives in whom a diagnosis of serious illness had been made and who had been given five years to live but instead of dying within the five years had outlived the physician who had made the prognostication and died at the venerable age of 90 or 100 years.

The reasons listed above may or may not be valid and realistic. However, they are in effect a denial that the symptoms of illness possibly could be serious. One wonders if such persons are motivated out of fear or if they have a larger degree of omnipotence in their character than does the "average" person. Illness is a threat to the self and individuals will tend to deal with the threat of illness in the same manner in which they characteristically dealt with other stress situations in life. If characteristically they withdrew, refused to face problems or ignored them, then generally speaking the stress of illness will be dealt with in the same manner.

This is not always true, but usually individuals tend to meet present stress situations by using those defense mechanisms which helped them to avoid or circumvent anxiety in the past.

Reactions to a Diagnosis of Illness

Some individuals go to physicians for routine physical examinations in order to prevent illness. Generally, however, the individual consults a physician because he believes himself to be ill. Most ill persons wish to be cured of their illness and to be freed of pain and discomfort. The ill person usually comes to the physician with at least some vague preconceived idea about the nature of his illness and the meaning (whether accurate or not) of his symptoms. The ill person also brings with him his cultural beliefs about illness and his preconceptions, or assumptions, about physicians and the nature of the assistance that they can offer. Since illness is a threat to the self, probably every individual experiences some degree of anxiety when consulting a physician.

Reactions to a corroborated diagnosis are highly variable and depend on many factors. The individual's habitual manner of coping with stress and the degree to which the self is threatened influence any reaction to a diagnosis of illness.

An individual's reaction to a diagnosis of illness is influenced by the physician's interpretation of the nature of the illness, its duration and the probable prognosis, i.e., whether the illness is long or short term, the extent to which the person will be handicapped or inconvenienced by his illness and the degree to which the person's life is threatened (or robbed of its meaning) by the illness. The measures which must be taken to control the symptoms of the illness or cure the individual, i.e., whether or not hospitalization, surgery, or other procedures are necessary, are other factors influencing an individual's reaction to a diagnosis of illness.

How the physician interprets this information to the ill person is probably a major determinant motivating the way in which the individual will respond to the physician's directions and suggestions. The amount of personal interest shown by the physician is probably another major determining factor in assisting the ill person to decide whether or not to heed the physician's advice, or believe or trust the physician.

Not all individuals are threatened by illness. There may be many reasons for welcoming a diagnosis of illness. For example, the individual who "knew" she was ill despite the fact that four physicians did not corroborate her belief. A diagnosis of illness in such a situation is welcomed and the person is "relieved."

Other individuals, while not exactly welcoming a diagnosis of illness, may not find it too disheartening (especially if the symptoms of the illness are not too distressing). Some may use illness as an excuse to avoid disagreeable tasks or stressful situations, to manipulate others, or to gain sympathy and attention. These persons, while not at first welcoming a diagnosis of illness, may learn to enjoy the secondary gains or prerogatives of illness. This is not necessarily neurotic behavior although it can be. There are probably few persons who have not, at one time or another, "resorted" to a headache or some other physical symptom in order to avoid some disagreeable situation or to gain attention. There is nothing wrong with wanting attention per se. The desire for attention seems to be a natural human need however questionable one's method of obtaining attention may be.

It has been stated that most ill individuals experience some degree of anxiety when consulting a physician. The individual may experience various emotional reactions when the physician interprets to the ill person his diagnosis, the nature of the illness and the probable course, prognosis and the measures which must be taken to control the symptoms or cure the illness. These emotional reactions may include a lessening of anxiety and a feeling of relief, especially if the illness is not of a serious nature.

Not all individuals suffering from a "minor illness" react with a lessening of anxiety when the nature of their illness is interpreted to them. Any emotional reaction to illness is always dependent on the individual's perception of the illness, the degree to which the self is threatened and especially the extent to which the individual believes his illness will interfere with his ordinary daily activities. Some persons exhibit a more profound emotional response to the measures which must be taken to control the symptoms of their illness than to the illness itself. As one person commented:

> "I'm 55 years old and never had anything wrong with me in my whole life except a cold once in a while. Now they tell me I've got diabetes. I've got to stick myself with a needle every day. I don't know if I'll ever be able to stick myself. He wants me to go on a diet—I can't eat this and I can't eat that . . . I don't have many pleasures in life and eating is one of them . . . somehow it doesn't seem fair. Oh, I want to get to feeling good again but I just wonder if it's worth it . . ."

This particular individual at first exhibited a "stunned response" when told the nature of her illness and the measures which had to be taken to control the illness. Following the initial "stunned response" she became increasingly depressed. Over a period of time with the assistance of the physician and the office nurse she was able to accept, to some extent, the nature of her disability.

Emotional responses to a diagnosis of illness are highly variable and individualistic and are not easily discernible by an observer. A health worker can never assume that because he (the health worker) thinks he would react in a certain way to a particular illness or disability, that the ill person he encounters with this condition will react in the same way. The only way a health worker can understand how an ill person perceives his illness, or the measures which must be taken to combat the symptoms or cure the illness, is to explore this with the individual and to elicit from the individual the meaning *he* attaches to his condition.

Thus far illness has been discussed only from the standpoint of the afflicted individual. In actuality the illness of one person affects many others.

THE RAMIFICATIONS OF ILLNESS

As a pebble thrown into a still pool disturbs all of the water within the pool, so it is that the effects of one person's illness reach out beyond that individual affecting, to some extent, every person with whom the ill individual comes in contact with or knows. The ill person's immediate family, his relatives, friends, acquaintances, associates and co-workers are all affected, to some extent, by the individual's illness.

Illness can be a threat to the ill person's family depending on the nature, course, and prognosis of the illness. It can generate worry, concern, guilt, fear and deep anxiety amongst family members. The way in which members of the family and friends react to the illness undoubtedly affects the ill peron's perception of his illness. Illness of one family member especially if it be a long-term disabling illness, affects the relationships of family members to each other. The ill man's wife may have to take on added responsibility and take a job in order to support her husband and children. Children are also profoundly affected by the change in family relationships. Plans for the future may have to be altered, especially since the economic effects of long-term illness may cause a drastic change in the standard of living previously enjoyed by the family.

Illness may also affect the family's pattern of everyday living. Consider the effects on a family when the wife can no longer attend to her household duties or care for her young children. Many families do not have the money to hire a full-time maid, and, in many communities, homemaker services are not available. Children may help raise each other, be cared for by relatives, neighbors or family friends or be placed in foster homes. It is not usually recognized that the illness of a wife and mother can be as devastating economically and psychologically as the illness of the husband or father of the family.

There are also other less obvious ramifications of illness. The ill person may no longer be able to engage in activities which once brought enjoyment and pleasure to family members. Husbands and wives may be deprived of the companionship of their spouses. In concrete terms this means the husband or wife must either attend social functions alone or not attend at all. This lack of companionship may severely curtail all social activities within the family circle and frequently the spouse who is not ill experiences a deep sense of aloneness, loneliness and abandonment.

These are only a few of the ramifications of illness; there are many more since the illness of one person affects the lives of many others. The society in which the person lives is affected by his illness, since society is composed of individuals. The illness or death of one person affects all others in that society even those who do not know and will probably never hear of the ill person or of his death—all are affected if ever so remotely by the illness or death of that individual. We are all bound each to the other by the common links of our humanity and that which affects one ultimately affects all others. It is as written by John Donne in 1624 in "Devotions upon Emergent Occasions":

"No man is an island, entire of itself; every man is a piece of the continent, a part of the main. If a clod be washed away by the sea, Europe is the less, as well as if a promontory were, as well as if a manor of thy friend's or of thine own were; any man's death diminishes me, because I am involved in Mankind, and therefore never send to know for whom the bell tolls; it tolls for thee."[4]

---

[4] Donne, John: Devotions upon Emergent Occasions, (1624) as quoted in English Literature and Its Background. Bernard D. Grenbanier, et al., Ed. Vol. 1. New York: The Dryden Press, 1949, p. 537.

Illness as a human experience will be discussed in Chapter VIII. Following is a summary of salient factors which tend to influence an individual's perception of his illness, and an individual's response to a diagnosis of illness. Some of these factors have been discussed in some detail in the text; others are new inclusions.

FACTORS WHICH INFLUENCE AN INDIVIDUAL'S PERCEPTION OF ILLNESS AND HIS RESPONSE TO A DIAGNOSIS OF ILLNESS:

1. Cultural beliefs about illness.
2. Symptoms and their meaning to the ill individual.
   a. What the individual "knows" or has heard (whether true or not) about the meaning of his symptoms.
   b. The amount of pain, discomfort or inconvenience caused by the symptoms of the illness.
   c. The extent to which symptoms interfere with or prevent the individual from pursuing his customary way of life.
   d. The ease with which symptoms can be controlled.
3. The area of the body involved and the symbolic meaning to the individual.
4. The extent to which the signs or effects of illness are visible to others (as, for example, skin disorders, deformities, etc.). The reaction of other persons to the visible manifestations of the illness.
5. The individual's habitual manner of coping with stress and the degree to which the self is threatened.
6. Preconceptions and assumptions about physicians (and other health workers) and the nature of the assistance they can offer.
7. An individual's reaction to a diagnosis of illness is influenced by the physician's interpretation of:
   a. the nature of the illness
   b. its duration and probable cause
   c. symptoms
      (1)-extent to which the person will be handicapped or inconvenienced by his illness
      (2)-amount of pain and discomfort caused by symptoms
   d. measures which must be taken to control the symptoms or cure the illness, i.e., whether hospitalization, surgery or other procedures are necessary
      (1)-the ill person's perception of the measures which must be taken
   e. probable prognosis
      (1)-degree to which the individual's life is threatened by his illness
      (2)-degree to which the patient feels that life is robbed of all meaning by his illness
8. How the physician interprets the information in #7 and the amount of personal concern or interest shown by the physician for the ill person.

9. The way in which family, friends and others react towards the ill individual.
   a. Reaction to the family and others to the signs and effects of illness.
   b. Amount of concern or interest shown the ill individual by relatives, friends and others.
10. The way in which health workers perceive the ill individual, i.e., whether as an illness, room number, category, stereotype or as a human being.

N.B. References used in this chapter are in the footnotes. These are not repeated.

Chapter VI

CONCEPT: SUFFERING

Suffering, like illness, is a common life experience encountered by every human being. All persons, at some time in their life, will be confronted by illness, pain (mental, physical or spiritual suffering) and eventually will experience death.

Suffering is an experience that is perceived and undergone by the individual. Each individual perceives the experience of suffering in his own unique way. The manner in which an individual perceives suffering is highly dependent on the significance that the person attaches to this experience. The meanings the individual attaches to suffering also determine, to a great extent, the individual's ability to endure or undergo this experience.

A basic assumption is that illness and suffering are spiritual encounters as well as emotional-physical experiences. In Part I of this chapter the concept "suffering" is defined and explored in terms of its nature, phases, effects and possible meanings to the ill individual and others. The problem of physical pain is explored in Part II.

PART I

THE NATURE OF SUFFERING

Every human being suffers because he *is* a human being, and suffering is an intrinsic aspect of the human condition. At one time or another and in varying degrees, every human being encounters distressing difficulties which are, for the most part, unavoidable and unforeseeable. In order to experience suffering an individual must perceive a situation as distressing and he must have a conscious awareness of the distress. Usually, but not always, the individual desires alleviation of the distress. An individual who does not wish alleviation of suffering is not necessarily motivated by neurotic masochism. Some individuals who do not seek alleviation of suffering, although they may not object to it, are motivated by religious convictions, i.e., they believe suffering has merit.

DEFINITIONS OF THE TERMS "SUFFER" AND "SUFFERING"

The term "suffer" is defined as ". . . to be subjected to physical or mental pain . . . endure with distress: to feel keenly or acutely: labor under . . . to submit to or endure death, affliction, penalty, or pain or distress . . . to be the one acted upon as distinguished from the one acting . . . to be in a state of disability . . . be subject to something disabling . . ." [1]

The term "suffering" is defined as "the state or experience of one who suffers: the endurance of or submission to affliction, pain, loss. A pain endured or a distress, loss, or injury incurred." [2]

As described in Webster's Third New International Dictionary, suffering is a term having various shades of meaning. Generally, suffering is a term used to describe the human experience of mental and/or physical pain. More specifically the term is also used to describe the human experience of affliction, loss, distress or injury. In everyday conversation the term "suffering" is frequently used in a restricted sense, i.e., it refers almost exclusively to the experience of physical pain. In this text, "suffering" is considered in its general as well as its specific meaning. Emphasis is placed on suffering in illness. The definition of suffering used in this book follows.

DEFINITION OF SUFFERING

In this text, suffering is considered as an experience which varies in intensity, duration and depth. Basically, suffering is a feeling of displeasure which ranges from simple transitory mental, physical or spiritual discomfort to extreme anguish, and to those phases beyond anguish, namely, the malignant phase of despairful "not caring," and the terminal phase of apathetic indifference.

The Malignant Phase: Despairful "Not-Caring"

Despairful "not-caring" is experienced when the individual has suffered mentally, physically or spiritually too intensely, over too long a period of time, without assistance and without surcease of suffering. Such a person is usually dominated by angry feelings of hopelessness which are bitterly expressed. The individual protests bitterly that he does not care and the vehemence of his protesting is an indication of how deeply he truly cares—how very much he has suffered and how needful he is. It is not necessary for an individual to have a terminal illness in order to experience despairful "not-caring." Usually, however, such a person has suffered intense physical or mental pain over a prolonged period of time. The illness may be a "minor" one from the standpoint of prognosis, but it is not experienced as "minor" by the individual who experiences the full impact of

---

[1] By permission. From Webster's Third New International Dictionary, copyright 1961 by G. & C. Merriam Co., Publishers of the Merriam-Webster Dictionaries.
[2] *Ibid.*

the effects of his illness. If not assisted an individual may progress to a terminal phase of suffering, i.e., apathetic indifference.

The Terminal Phase: Apathetic Indifference

Apathetic indifference occurs when the individual progresses beyond the stage of despairful "not-caring." Such an individual seems impervious and imperturbable. He does not complain; neither does he bitterly express the angry feelings of hopelessness so typical during the phase of despair. In despair, even though an individual tries to convey that he does not care, it is apparent his not-caring is a superficial facade, and such behavior is a desperate plea for help. But in the phase of apathetic indifference the cry for help is stilled, probably because the individual believes no one can or will help him. Nurses generally describe such individuals as having "lost their will to live." The individual seems as if he is beyond being touched or bothered by anything that can happen to him. Such an individual is not calm and serene; rather one gets the impression that he is dominated by an all-pervasive feeling of utter hopelessness. He is beyond caring. As in the phase of despair, an individual may not necessarily be suffering from a "serious" illness from the standpoint of prognosis in order to suffer this intensely. He may have a "minor" illness; the physician may expect he will recover and to all outward signs and indications he "should" recover, but he doesn't because he has lost the desire to live.

It is probable that if the individual's plea for help is not met during the phase of despair that apathetic indifference may be a logical next phase. An individual who displays behaviors as described in the phase of despairful not-caring is in desperate need of assistance. The behaviors as described in despair are signs of a malignant condition, which, while reversible in this phase, may progress to apathetic indifference. It is possible for nurses to assist ill persons in this phase, but it is far more difficult to do so since such a condition may be irreversible. It is the role of the professional nurse to intervene and attempt to assist the person *before* he progresses to the phase of despairful not-caring. In the event he does progress to this phase every possible attempt must be made to help him while his condition is still reversible. As there are medical and surgical emergencies demanding immediate action, so are there interpersonal emergencies. *Despairful not-caring is an interpersonal emergency and calls for immediate concerted action.* For specific suggestions in assisting ill persons in the malignant and terminal phase of suffering see Chapter XI, "Nursing Intervention."

CAUSES OF SUFFERING

Suffering is experienced when the individual encounters various types of distressing difficulties. A distressing difficulty may include any of the following experiences which can happen to oneself or to a loved one: illness, physical pain, mental pain, losses of all kinds—i.e., of a loved one through death, divorce, desertion or separation; of a love object such as a beloved pet or material possessions; of position, status or prestige; of one's integrity—and various types of real or imagined injuries to pride and self-esteem. An individual may also suffer because he feels cut off from others—that he remains on life's periphery and is uninvolved, uncommitted, uncared for and uncaring. To be locked in the prison of self and care only for self is also to suffer, especially if this be combined with an inability to reach out to others and to establish a meaningful relationship with at least one other human being. An individual may also suffer if he believes he has transgressed his religious convictions when he has strong feelings regarding these convictions.

THE RELATIONSHIP BETWEEN CARING AND SUFFERING

The relation between caring and suffering is paradoxical—that (with the possible exception of physical pain) suffering is usually always contingent on caring, although it is possible to suffer because one does not, or cannot, care. To care is to experience some degree of attachment towards the object of one's care and concern.

Generally an individual must care for that which he loses, or is in danger of losing, in order to experience suffering. Usually an individual does not feel any suffering about that which he is not concerned. However, it is possible to suffer intensely if an individual has no one to care for, or no one who cares for him. Such a person may have a great capacity to love and to care, but lacking a recipient suffers from intense and severe loneliness.

The degree of vulnerability to suffering is usually always related to the extent, or depth, of the capacity to care. However, the inability to care can also generate intense suffering; not to care is to experience life as a vacuum and the desolateness and emptiness of this type of not-caring can be the genesis of profound anguish.

Since suffering is an inherent aspect of the human condition the individual will experience suffering at one time or another in life. It is probable that the more an individual cares for, and about, others the wider the range or the greater the possibilities for suffering. Although caring is, in a sense, the cause of suffering in that the more an individual cares the more vulnerable he is, it is also true that an individual is able to enrich his experience (in terms of deepening the meaningfulness of his life) and to realize his humanity to the extent that he cares for and about others.

An individual who cares for or about very few persons is probably not as exposed to as many possibilities for suffering, but neither will his life be enriched by meaningful contacts with others.

When an individual cares for or about only a very small number of persons, he will suffer the loss of these objects of his concern. Persons of this type generally do not add to the range and depth of their caring and as a result become increasingly driven inward towards self. The gravest danger such persons face is the loss of objects of care, and increasing non-involvement with others. With increasing non-involvement and turning towards self, such persons become increasingly vulnerable to the experience of the anguish of not caring.

It is probably an act of courage to care because in caring one exposes himself to the chance of being hurt by the objects of his care. Suffering cannot be avoided because it is an intrinsic aspect of the human condition. The meanings an individual derives from and through the experience of suffering can enrich his life, or cause him to think of living as a meaningless experience. What possible meaning can be found in suffering? Since this work is designed to assist nurse practitioners, meaning attached to suffering as a result of illness will be stressed.

SOME DETERMINANTS OF MEANING OF SUFFERING IN ILLNESS

The meanings an individual attaches to the experience of suffering in illness are derived from many sources. Cultural beliefs about suffering and illness undoubtedly influence the individual. For example, if a society asserts that the pursuit of pleasure and "happiness" is the sole or chief good in life then it is understandable that suffering will be viewed as an experience to be avoided if at all possible.

An individual's religious convictions (i.e., his actual beliefs, not those he professes to believe) will strongly influence his ability to cope with suffering when he is undergoing this experience. The individual's actual beliefs are stressed (as opposed to his professed beliefs) since it is quite one matter to be philosophical about suffering, when one is not suffering, and quite another to accept and find meaning in this experience when one is feeling its full impact. The way in which the individual has dealt with the experience of suffering in the past will also determine his ability to cope with present suffering.

REACTIONS TO SUFFERING AND ILLNESS

There are many ways of reacting to suffering and illness. These reactions are multi-determined and are produced in part by a combination of all of the factors discussed in the section in this chapter entitled "Some Determinants of the Meaning of Suffering in Illness" and in Chapter V, "Concept: Illness." All reactions to suffering in illness are highly individualistic. It is difficult to develop generalizations about so unique an experience. However, it is probable that most individuals attempt to arrive at a reason or cause of illness and suffering. They want to know *what* has caused this illness to occur to themselves (or to loved ones). The second most prevalent question is *why* has this happened to themselves (or to loved ones). It is probable that most reactions to suffering and illness can be classified into two broad categories: the "why me?" reaction; and the "acceptance reaction" or the "why not me?" type of reaction.

The "Why Me?" Reaction

The "why me?" reaction is probably the most common of all responses to suffering and illness. The source of the "why me?" reaction is probably non-acceptance of the experience of illness and suffering. In turn, non-acceptance engenders other emotional responses which vary in degree, intensity and duration. The most common emotional responses and behaviors which may be engendered by non-acceptance are anger (which may range from annoyance to vehement bitter rebellion), self pity, depression, anguish, despairful not-caring and apathetic indifference. All of the above responses, with the possible exception of the terminal phase of apathetic indifference have some degree of fear and anxiety blended in them. One manifestation of the "why me?" reaction is the tendency to want to hold someone, or something, responsible for what has happened.

Blaming

An individual may blame himself or his loved one for causing or being exposed to illness. For example, if an individual who is obese develops a heart condition he may be "blamed" for his illness, especially if he had been advised to lose weight and did not. An individual who does not dress appropriately on a cold day and subsequently develops a severe upper respiratory illness may be blamed because it is believed that his actions brought about the illness. Similarly, individuals who are heavy smokers and develop lung cancer may be blamed for causing their illness. Individuals who are under the care of a physician and do not cooperate with medical advice and therefore suffer an exacerbation of symptoms may blame themselves, or be blamed by others, for indirectly "causing" their own illness. This type of blaming response can be carried to an extreme, as for example, an individual who has fallen down and broken a leg is blamed because "he is careless and didn't watch where he was going."

Blaming as a response to illness and suffering is being stressed because it is a fairly common reaction, and because health workers are not immune from responding to blaming an ill person for directly, or indirectly, causing his own illness.

In other instances an outside object or other persons are blamed for one's illness. Instead of being ill because an individual "brought it on himself," the person may blame his illness on the fact that he "worked too hard," "had too much to do," "had to do two people's work," etc. Other individuals blame illness on circumstances, bad luck, or fate. In other instances, individuals may believe that illness was caused because they transgressed their religious convictions, and illness consequently was sent as punishment.

Bafflement

Another type of behavior frequently seen in conjunction with blaming is bafflement. Even though the individual has affixed blame on himself or others for his dilemma, he may still wonder why this illness or suffering has happened to him. He may wonder why he was singled out or "picked out." The perennial question is: *Why did this have to happen to me?* This type of question is frequently combined with various reasons as to why the person feels he should be exempt from misfortune. A case history in point is that of a twenty year old married woman recovering from a hysterectomy. This woman states:

"I keep asking myself why this had to happen. I'm a good woman and I've always loved children. I've always wanted to have as many children as I could and now I know I won't ever be able to have any. Look at all of the women who have children and don't love them or don't want them—or who try to get rid of them. Oh, I know I'll have to learn to accept it but somehow it doesn't seem fair . . ."

Such individuals display a hurt perplexity and bafflement, combined with a feeling of having been unjustly or unfairly treated. The individual frequently cannot even direct his anger towards a "blame object" at this point. There is only a permeating, all-pervasive feeling of being ill-treated, and the person finds little or no meaning in such "unjust" and unwarranted suffering. These feelings soon solidify into a depressive episode or a self-pitying attitude.

Depression

Varying degrees of sadness, discouragement and depression are frequently engendered by illness. Depression is defined as anger turned inward toward the self. Any loss of self-esteem, status, prestige, body function or body part may induce depression. In a sense the ill person may be said to go through a process of grieving the loss of bodily function or a body part.

To be helpless and dependent on others for care can produce deep feelings of worthlessness in some individuals. It may be quite depressing for an individual to realize he is becoming increasingly debilitated. To observe the wasting process in one's body, to experience unrelenting pain and to realize that recovery is not possible, is frightening as well as depressing. To know that nothing can be done to reverse the disease process, that there is literally no hope of recovery, comes as a crushing realization. Mere words in a book cannot describe the feelings of helplessness and powerlessness experienced by an individual who realizes that he is unable to alter his destiny.

Besides depression there is the discouragement engendered by relationships with others. When an individual first becomes ill or is hospitalized, friends and relatives may call, visit or write very frequently. But as time goes by, visits from friends and relatives may gradually decrease. It is a fortunate individual indeed who has at least one relative or friend who will maintain interest and continue to visit him if he is hospitalized over an extended period of time. The same withdrawal pattern seems to operate if the ill person is at home. Contacts with friends and relatives other than the person(s) caring for the ill individual tend to diminish as time goes by and the ill person does not recover. The effect of withdrawal of other people from the ill person can lead to a kind of sensory restriction. This is especially true if the ill person is homebound, cannot ambulate or seek the companionship of others. One effect of sensory restriction is to increase the ill person's feelings of loneliness and boredom. The belief that one's relatives and friends have forgotten or do not care enough to phone or visit can further deepen the individual's sense of depression, loss and worthlessness.

The ill person's world becomes increasingly restricted and loneliness can become almost unbearable. To be bedridden and in pain and to have no hope of recovery is difficult enough to bear—how much more difficult it is when the ill person realizes that his friends and relatives have lost interest in him.

Ill persons have the same needs as do healthy individuals, as for example, the need to be appreciated, needed and loved. It is especially when one is ill that small acts of kindness and thoughtfulness by others are so deeply appreciated. A get well card may be treasured by an ill person as a tangible reminder that he has not been abandoned and that someone *does* care. The old saying, "little things mean a lot" is especially true when applied to an individual with a long-term illness.

Some authorities recommend the ill individual develop a hobby in order to keep himself occupied. Having a hobby can be helpful to the homebound person but *hobbies do not take the place of contact with people.*

As one homebound ill woman said:

> "I watch television sometimes and if I feel up to it I sew a little. Joe doesn't get home until four-thirty . . . it makes the days seem so long. He phones every day to find out how I'm feeling but no one else calls. I used to phone my friends but I know they are busy and have housework to do. I always seem to phone at the wrong time. Well, Mary (a friend) used to phone but she doesn't any more. The last time I talked to her she said she'd call me more often but she was afraid I might be sleeping and she didn't want to wake me up. I told her to call anyway . . . I can sleep anytime . . . But I know she is busy. I used to have a lot of company . . . I don't know . . . maybe I've been sick too long . . ."

There are, of course, many reasons why friends and relatives may not wish to phone or visit an individual who has been ill over a long period of time. An ill person who complains too much, or who makes the visitor feel guilty for not coming to visit more often, may cause friends and relatives to withdraw. Another reason why friends and relatives may withdraw is that the ill person reminds them of their own vulnerability to illness and suffering. A more prevalent reason for withdrawal is that it requires time and effort to disrupt one's daily routine in order to visit or phone an ill person.

The ill person is, at times, at a marked disadvantage in that he may find himself in the position of having to "cheer up" his visitors and reassure them. A person who has been ill over a period of time knows from experience that if his visitors feel threatened, uneasy or uncomfortable relating with him they will not return. An individaul with a long-term illness who *wants* company soon learns that he must spend some time reassuring his visitors and making them feel comfortable. If the ill person lacks insight regarding this problem he may soon find himself almost completely abandoned by others. Depression is then increased when the individual feels "cut off" from friends and relatives. Besides depression many ill persons experience longing.

Longing

There are times when an ill person may feel a deep, surging, almost over-whelming desire to be well again. The desire to feel strong, to participate in activities denied one may almost inundate the individual with strong feelings of inexpressible longing and yearning. Longing can be a deeply painful experience especially when such feelings are accompanied by the inescapable knowledge that no matter how much one wishes, yearns, or hopes nothing will be changed. An ill person, who, prior to the development of his illness, enjoyed hiking or other outdoor activities may, especially on a beautiful spring day, become overwhelmed with a longing to engage just one more time in these activities. As one bedridden paralyzed man said:

"Oh, do you know what I really wish for? If I could just walk again in the sunshine—just one more time—to feel the sun on my face . . ."

All human beings long for that which they strongly desire. The ill, however, are thrown back on their own resources and have fewer outlets for their emotions than does the well individual. Deep longing may induce despair in individuals who are striving to begin the difficult task of accepting their illness. This longing may be so intense that the individual mourns missed experiences and undergoes a grief reaction.

Depression and the frustrations resulting from unfulfilled longing may also induce self-pitying behavior in the ill person.

Self-pity

Self-pity is engendered and a general "I-feel-sorry-for-myself" attitude is displayed. Such self-pity is probably anger turned inward toward the self. Angry feelings vary in intensity and duration and, as stated, may range from annoyance to bitterly expressed rebellious feelings—a precursor to the phase of despairful not-caring. To feel sorry for oneself is an intense suffering. The individual is imprisoned within himself and enveloped in leaden, heavy feelings of self-pity. He may dislike feeling as he does, may be ashamed of himself; he may wish he could change, but may be unable to take any positive steps towards diminishing this feeling. If any individual views illness as an injustice, an unnecessary affliction, or as an affliction from which he somehow should be exempt, it is not surprising if the consequent feelings of anger and rage follow. It is a shattering experience to realize how very vulnerable one is and it is never easy to accept this understanding. It is even more difficult, and sometimes an impossible feat, if the person has never prepared himself mentally or spiritually for such a situation and has always assumed he somehow would be exempt from all of life's suffering because he is who he is.

There is another manifestation of the "why me?" reaction that has not been explicitly explored—anguish. Anguish is experienced in both the acceptance response and the "why me?" The difference in experience between these two reactions is: in the "why me?" reaction the individual cannot accept the experience or use it to enable him to find meaning in his suffering whereas for the individual who accepts suffering it is possible to do so.

The nurse can assist individuals with the "why me?" reaction, and indeed is obliged to do so in order to prevent the person from progressing to the malignant phase of despairful not-caring, and into the terminal phase of apathetic indifference characterized by a loss of the desire to live. Specific ways in which the nurse may assist such individuals are discussed in Chapter XI, "Nursing Intervention." The "why me?" reaction has been discussed at some length because it is the most common response to the experiences of illness and suffering. A less common response is the "acceptance reaction."

The "Acceptance Reaction"

The acceptance reaction is the least common of all responses to suffering and illness. Although this reaction is uncommon, nurses will encounter such individuals and it is necessary for them to understand the nature of this reaction. Although such individuals react to suffering and illness with acceptance, they still need assistance from the professional nurse practitioner. The nature of this assistance is not the same as in the "why me?" reaction, but nevertheless help is still required. Specific ways in which the nurse may assist individuals displaying the acceptance reaction is discussed in Chapter XI, "Nursing Intervention."

An individual who displays acceptance as a reaction to illness and suffering is able to receive these conditions without protest (i.e., in the sense that an injustice is being done), and in some rarer instances is able to make an affirmative response to these conditions. By an affirmative response is meant the individual is able to view his illness or suffering as a channel through which good may be derived, and in so viewing his illness in this manner experiences a type of resignation that is akin to deep serenity. That an individual is able to view illness as a channel through which good may be derived is not to imply a pollyannaish attitude. An individual with overdetermined false optimism is not able to cope with suffering over any prolonged period of time. The attitude of optimism soon crumbles under the onslaught of pain and the myriad sufferings of illness. An individual who accepts illness is a person who is able to cope with whatever suffering he encounters. This is not to say that such a person never wavers, is never anxious, or never needs reassurance or encouragement. It does mean, however, that such a person is able to bear the weight of these sufferings over a long period of time with patience and a type of serene resignation unknown to a Pollyanna.

There are some individuals who are able to cope with major stress, but quite incapable of coping with what one patient calls "those horrid small inconveniences of being ill which are harder to accept than anything else." An individual who accepts illness usually is able to cope with these "horrid small inconveniences" without undue stress.

The individual who displays an acceptance reaction does not desire to be ill, he does not like to suffer; neither does he seek suffering for its own sake nor does he desire the secondary gains of illness. Suffering and illness are received without protest by a person whose philosophy of life has always included the belief that he is human and vulnerable and that illness and suffering are an intrinsic aspect of the human condition.

What is it that assists individuals to accept suffering and illness? There are many paths to acceptance and many levels of acceptance. An individual may demonstrate acceptance because his philosophy of life has been built around his beliefs about the human condition. He realizes what it means to be a human being and never exempts himself from all of the vulnerabilities of his humanity, i.e., he never believes that death, suffering and illness are experiences that should happen to others but never to himself. Such a person is able to realize that what is inevitable will happen to him. He is also able to accept, what is in some ways a far more difficult truth, the fact that those he loves will suffer and die. This realization is an accepted belief so embedded in the self that it governs the individual's thoughts, feelings and actions. Only a profoundly humble, brave, and probably stoical person can confront and face the fact that he is human and will suffer and die, as will his loved ones. Only such a person can grasp such truths without the need to deny or negate them. By understanding these truths the individual is enabled to accept his own sufferings and sufferings of those he loves. This is not to imply that such a person will never murmur or doubt even the validity of his own beliefs; rebellion may flare—the individual may display feelings of fear and anger, but these feelings will be transitory. He accepts because he has prepared himself for the occurrence of the inevitable, as it will invariably happen to every human being and he is able to cope with it. He is attuned to life in that he has accepted his humanity unconditionally, never expecting to be exempt from all of the manifold frailties of the human condition. Such a person comprehends what is meant by:

"There is an appointed time for everything, and a time for every affair under the heavens. A time to be born, and a time to die, a time to plant, and a time to uproot the plant. A time to weep, and a time to laugh; a time to mourn, and a time to dance."[3]

Other individuals are able to accept illness and suffering because of their religious convictions. Their acceptance is based on a realization of the human condition combined with a profound belief in the tenets of their creed. In order to demonstrate this type of acceptance an individual must have firmly believed, as well as followed his religious convictions. It is improbable (but not impossible) that an individual who has never practiced any of his religious beliefs will gain the strength he needs to cope with distress. It is true that some individuals may "all of a sudden" display an interest in religious matters and seem to derive much strength from these beliefs, but if the individual's "interest" is not sincere the force of these convictions will probably diminish, especially if the individual recovers or if he undergoes extreme suffering.

---

[3] "Ecclesiastes," *The Holy Bible*. Vol. III, Job to Sirach. Paterson, N. J. St. Anthony's Guild Press, 1955, Chapter 3, Verses 1-2 and 4, p. 443.

The individual who is able to cope with suffering because of his religious convictions does not talk as much about his convictions as he lives them. His behavior is a demonstration of beliefs he holds. Such is acceptance based on religious convictions.

Such is the nature of the "why me?" and the "acceptance" reaction. These reactions are best inferred through observing the behavior of the persons involved.

There are many other factors which may affect one in his perception of suffering in illness that have not been explored. One area that has not as yet been considered is the effect of physical pain in illness.

PART II—THE PROBLEM OF PAIN

Mental and physical pain or distress are common human experiences which each individual encounters during the process of living. Pain is a problem to the individual undergoing this experience, to the physician attempting to alleviate the distress, and to the nurse who works with the ill and suffering human being.

THE NATURE OF PAIN

The term "pain" is a concept used to designate a particular type of human experience. Like illness, pain is a nebulous concept since pain itself is not observable—only its effects are noted.

Pain and suffering are intensely lonely experiences; even when the individual is feeling their full impact it is very difficult (if not impossible) to communicate the experience of pain to another in such a way that the other fully comprehends what is being experienced. Because it is difficult to communicate the experience of pain it is also difficult to assess the degree or intensity of pain which another is experiencing. Health workers frequently develop inferences as to the intensity of pain they surmise a person is experiencing, but no health worker can be absolutely certain that he is accurately assessing the actual intensity of pain being experienced. It is not possible; any inferences developed are, at best, a guess.

DEFINITION OF "PAIN"

According to Webster's Third New International Dictionary pain is ". . . state of physical or mental lack of well-being or physical or mental uneasiness that ranges from mild discomfort or dull distress to acute often unbearable agony, may be generalized or localized, and is the consequence of being injured or hurt physically or mentally . . . and that usually produces a reaction of wanting to avoid, escape, or destroy the causative factor and its effects . . ." [4]

---

[4] By permission. From Webster's Third New International Dictionary, copyright 19 by G. & C. Merriam Co., Publishers of the Merriam-Webster Dictionaries.

Physical pain is one form or type of suffering. However, in everyday conversation the term "suffering" is used to refer almost exclusively to the experience of physical pain. Usually mental distress is seldom referred to as "mental pain" except in a colloquial sense of having "hurt feelings" or "wounded pride." However, pain cannot be neatly categorized as being either mental or physical since pain affects the entire person. Mental pain, or distress, certainly affects the person physically; but the converse is true in that physical pain affects the individual emotionally as well. One aspect of the human organism can never be separated from the whole. Even though physical pain can be localized in one part of the body, in actuality the individual as a whole suffers, not just the body part.

What factors tend to influence the way in which an individual will respond to pain?

FACTORS INFLUENCING AN INDIVIDUAL'S REACTION TO PAIN

Any individual's reaction to pain is multi-determined. *An obvious determinant is the cause, duration and intensity of pain and the amount of relief afforded the individual by means of various medications.* The person who knows he has a malignant disease may tend to react to pain in a different manner than an individual recovering from an appendectomy. The person who has every assurance that his pain will quickly diminish and that he will soon be cured of his illness is apt to respond somewhat differently than the person who realizes that he must live in pain the rest of his life. Very intense pain may cause an individual to lose consciousness; however, an individual can live for years experiencing the remorseless tenacity of chronic pain. The effects of pain can have effects on the human being long after pain itself has been relieved. Fatigue and lassitude are residuals or frequent after-effects of pain, and time is required for the individual to recuperate from the devastating effects of such experiences. Besides fatigue and lassitude, anxiety is often a residual. An individual may fear the reccurrence of severe pain. Even the individual who lives with pain may, in an interval of respite, become anxious while awaiting the onslaught of pain, pain he *knows* will return. Such individuals may request narcotics to *prevent* pain—not to relieve it. Whether pain is sporadic or chronic, the intensity of the pain suffered is a major determinant which will affect any individual's reactions. Stoicism is not a strong defense against pain, for even the most stoical person can be reduced to a screaming human being when experiencing the agony of kidney colic or trigeminal neuralgia. An individual who is never given enough medication to relieve his pain will respond quite differently from the person who obtains complete relief from pain by taking drugs. A frequently overlooked fact is that an individual who has had a prolonged painful illness in his recent past, especially one requiring fairly large amounts of narcotics, will probably require larger amounts of narcotics for a present, less painful illness.

Other major factors influencing an individual's reaction to pain are: the cultural background of the person, his philosophical beliefs, and religious convic-

tions. The culture proscribes certain behavioral responses to pain, some of which are deemed acceptable, others unacceptable. For example, in some groups it is an acceptable behavioral response for a male to cry when in pain; in other groups such behavior is viewed not only as unacceptable but as rephrensible. In such groups, crying is acceptable behavior only for women and children.

An individual's philosophical beliefs and religious convictions will affect reactions to pain. These determinants have already been discussed in the sections in this chapter entitled "Some Determinants of the Meaning of Suffering in Illness" and "Reaction to Suffering and Illness."

Other major factors influencing an individual's reaction to pain are: the degree of anxiety and fear engendered by pain, and the manner in which others respond to the afflicted individual.

Pain is one of the symptoms of illness, and all symptoms engender some degree of anxiety and fear in the afflicted individual. A major determinant seems to be the location of the pain. For example, it has been repeatedly observed that individuals suffering from coronary thrombosis are prone to be very fearful and anxious. In some instances, individuals are highly anxious prior to the development of a painful illness and are apt to over-react to the experience of pain. This "over-reaction" seems to be contingent on the degree of fear and anxiety, because anxiety and fear seem to potentiate pain; the converse is probably equally true in that pain may potentiate anxiety and fear.

The manner in which nurses, physicians, relatives, friends and others respond or react to the individual in pain is probably a major determinant in either assisting or hindering the person in coping with his distress. Some salient questions are: Is the afflicted person offered compassionate care? Are others interested in him and interested in relieving his distress? Does he sense that he is being given narcotics only to "shut him up"? Does he perceive that others do not even believe he is in pain? Some individuals in pain are acutely aware when others do not believe that they are really in pain.

In such cases the afflicted person has no alternative but to keep trying to convince others that he is in pain. It is difficult enough to experience pain but it is even more exasperating when the person realizes that neither the doctor nor nurse believes him and thinks that he is exaggerating or "just putting on."

What causes nurses to develop the opinion that a person is "just putting on"? It is quite probable the individual's manner and the number of times that complaints are made are major factors which influence others towards the distressed person. An individual who calmly requests "something for pain" (and doesn't ask too often) is treated quite differently from the whining, crying individual who asks the nurse for narcotics every four hours on a permitted schedule.

Another probable reason why nurses develop the inference that a person is "putting on" is that health workers seem to develop a "mental yardstick" [5] by

[5] Adapted from Laughlin, Henry P.: Concept of the personal yardstick. The Neuroses in Clinical Practice. Philadelphia: W. B. Saunders Co., 1956, p. 112.

means of which they make decisions about the amount of pain they believe an individual recovering from a particular type of surgery, or suffering from a particular illness, should have.

For example, consider pain as ranging on a continuum from 0 to 100 percent. An individual recovering from a tonsillectomy and adenoidectomy is "allowed" 5 percent of pain; from an appendectomy 15 percent, a hemorrhoidectomy 60 percent; a person with trigeminal neuralgia or kidney colic is "allowed" 90 to 100 percent of pain. All of these percentages are also modified by a time factor; individuals with certain conditions are only "supposed to have" a certain percentage of pain for a given period of time and then it is expected (by the health worker) that pain will gradually diminish. The patient who exceeds the percentage or time limit devised by health workers will probably be labeled as "someone who is putting on," "who can't take it," "a crock," "neurotic," or "potential drug addict."

Such a crude mental yardstick may have some utilitarian value, but it should be remembered that each human being is unique; each will respond to pain in his own unique way. If a person says he is in pain, whether or not there appears to be an organic basis for his complaint, the nurse must accept the person's statement as being his perception of the experience. Since it is the person's perception the nurse has no choice but to accept it as valid and attempt to find ways to assist the person. (For specific ways in which the professional nurse practitioner can assist the person in pain see Chapter XI, "Nursing Intervention.")

N. B. References used in this chapter are in the footnotes. These are not repeated.

The author wishes to thank Thomas Kelly, O.M.I., who reviewed this chapter.

Chapter VII

CONCEPT: HOPE

Hope has long been recognized by health workers and lay people alike as a factor motivating human behavior. Hope enables human beings to cope with difficult and stressful situations, deprivation, tragedy, failure, boredom, loneliness and suffering. It is probably the motivating thrust of hope which energizes the ill human being and enables him to overcome obstacles and to engage in the difficult tasks inherent in the recuperative process. Many ill persons will never regain health and must learn to live with the effects of a lifelong illness. How relevant is it to speak of hope in relation to such persons? *A basic assumption of this work is that it is the role of the professional nurse practitioner to assist the ill person to experience hope in order to cope with the stress of illness and suffering.*

PART I—DEFINITION OF HOPE

Hope is a mental state characterized by the desire to gain an end or accomplish a goal combined with some degree of expectation that what is desired or sought is attainable. According to Lynch, "hope . . . is a sense of the possible."[1] The hoping person believes that if he obtains the object of his desires, life will be changed in some way, i.e., will be more comfortable, meaningful or enjoyable. Although the hoping individual may expect to obtain the object of his desire, the probability of attaining the goal may vary. For example, an incurably ill individual may hope for recovery, even though there is little or no possibility that he will be cured. In such an instance one can say the process of hope is operative; however, the goals of the individual are, barring a miracle, unrealistic and probably unobtainable. The individual who lacks hope perceives no prospect of change or improvement in his life, neither does he perceive a solution to problems or a way out of his difficulties.

---

[1] Lynch, William F.: Images of Hope. Imagination as Healer of the Hopeless. New York: The New American Library, 1965, p. 24.

GENESIS OF HOPE

What are the origins of hope? Why is it that some individuals habitually experience hope during difficult life situations while others quickly become despondent and hopeless? Hope in any situation must spring from reason and does not exist without a foundation.

According to Erikson, hope emanates from a favorable ratio of trust to mistrust; the individual learns to hope provided his environment is suitable to the development of this virtue.[2] The child first learns to trust the world in the personification of the mothering figure. The probable basis of trust is the knowledge that help will be forthcoming when needed. Hope then probably emanates from the knowledge that help from outside one's self is available in times of need and distress. The person learns to trust himself and to trust others to help when help is required. The act of hoping is not secret and solitary. Hope is invariably related to the expectation of assistance from other people and subjective knowledge gained from personal experience.

Differentiation and Characteristics of Hope

Hope is strongly related to dependence on others. Help, or the cooperation of others, is required in order to survive. As individuals, we are dependent on other people—on farmers to grow food, on workers in canning factories, manufacturers, grocers, etc., to supply us with goods and services needed to maintain life. We depend on workers in the transportation field to convey us to and from work, or we depend on an automobile (made, sold, and serviced by other people). In the civilized world each individual is highly dependent on the help or cooperation of others merely to live through each day. The ill and suffering human being, also, depends on others and hopes for their assistance even though he may not wish to ask for help. Many ill persons do not seek assistance because independence, a deeply engrained American trait, has been throughly embedded in their character structure. Having to receive assistance or depend on others is deeply distressing to some people. Why? Is it that the individual really does not trust—that he lacks hope—or that he does not believe others will assist him? Is refraining from asking for help a defense against being rejected by others? Is the individual too proud to ask others for help believing that it is demeaning to request assistance, that others will think him inadequate? In our culture, dependence, in the sense of being "a burden" to others, seems to be feared by many individuals more than death. And yet we do not recognize the fact that we are dependent on others in order to survive. Perhaps it is time to acknowledge that independence, in the sense of a human being not needing other people, is simply a myth. Hope, then, is invariably related to the expectation of assistance from others, especially when one's inner

---

[2] Evans, Richard I.: Dialogue with Erik Erikson. (Vol. III in the series, Dialogues with Notable Contributors to Personality Theory.) New York: Harper & Row, 1967, pp. 12–18.

resources are not sufficient. Therefore, the hoping person is placed in a dependent position when help from others is accepted.

Hope is future-oriented. The individual who hopes desires a change in his present life situation. He is, in effect, dissatisfied and finds little comfort in living in the now of the present moment. However, all any individual has is "the now" of the present moment. The task of the hoping individual therefore is to use the "now" in such a way as to build and structure the future in order to attain that which he desires.

Hope is related to choice. The hoping individual believes he has some choices available to him. When a person hopes he perceives some alternatives or avenues of escape in the situation. Having some choice in a difficult situation, being free to choose one alternative over another, probably more than any other factor, is a major source of the human being's sense of freedom and autonomy. Even though the choices available are not palatable, there still remains the freedom to choose and to decide for oneself. This fact, in and of itself, can engender in an individual the feeling of being in control, at least to some extent, of his own destiny.

Hope is related to wishing. In this text the term "wishing" is defined as the act of desiring to possess some thing or condition, accomplish a task or undergo an experience. Wishing is a component of hoping but is differentiated from hope only on the basis of the probability of attaining the object of one's wish. The wish is closely related to "magic hope." The individual who utilizes magic hope realizes that the possibility of his obtaining the object of his wish is very slight; as for example, an individual wishes he had a million dollars. The individual *knows* he is not likely ever to have a million dollars but the fantasy is a pleasant one. Other daydreams may be concerned with fantasies regarding engaging in heroic behavior, rescuing someone from danger, being highly competent in some endeavor, winning a championship in some sporting event, or possessing the power to control others, or magically cure them of illness. The list is endless. The contents of the daydream are highly individualistic to each person. Knowledge of the *kind* of daydreams an individual engages in would probably provide useful data upon which to base nursing intervention. Daydreams spring from yearnings within the person—to know a person's daydreams is, in a sense, to gain an awareness of his deepest longings.

To wish, then, is to desire the improbable or impossible and to have knowledge of the low degree of probability of ever gaining the object of one's wishes. The individual who hopes, on the other hand, possesses, as Lynch states, "a sense of the possible" [3] and the individual strongly believes that that which is hoped for can, and will be, obtained. The hoping person may require the cooperation and assistance of others to gain what is desired or he may obtain it through his own efforts. Usually, however, the hoping individual requires the assistance of others to gain what is needed.

The individual who wishes does not make any concrete plans to obtain the object of his wish (for example, the one million dollars) because he realizes it is

---

[3] Lynch, *op. cit.*, p. 24.

highly improbable that he will ever be able to gain that which is desired. The individual who hopes, however, thinks of ways and means to reach his goal.

Hope is closely related to trust and perserverence. By trust is meant the assured belief that other individuals are capable of assisting in times of distress and will probably do so. There are, however, as has been stated, individuals who will not request help because they do not wish to be "dependent" on others. The individual may trust; however, he may be incapable of requesting assistance. Some individuals, having requested assistance from another person and having been ignored or denied help, may lose trust in others and depend solely on themselves. This situation can be a devastating one for the ill person who realizes that no one will help and that he must proceed alone.

Perseverance is the ability to keep trying, to continue to work towards solving one's problems, ameliorate one's distress, or change one's status or condition. Perseverance is a quality which enables an individual to confront difficult experiences over a fairly long period of time and to do so without losing courage and giving up, and probably requires a strong act of the will. Without perseverance it is not likely that any ill person would be able to accomplish the work of recovery or rehabilitation.

Hope is related to courage. The hopeful person possesses courage. What is courage but the ability to realize one's inadequacies and fears and yet to persevere towards one's goals, even though there may be little or no certainty that the individual will be able to attain the object of his hope. The courageous person *is* afraid but he is able to transcend his fear for the sake of achieving his goal. The courageous person is one who, while feeling afraid and unsure, makes a conscious choice to act and acts knowing only too well that his resolve may weaken, or his course of action may be wrong. The courageous person, in a sense, rises to the occasion and attempts to gain some degree of mastery or control over it. He is an active individual and does not passively allow situations to overwhelm him without fighting back. Though he may be unsuccessful in his endeavor, it is still a source of comfort to the person that he did not deny his difficulty or run from his problems.

It is probable that most individuals do not realize how much courage they possess, since it is very difficult to predict one's own behavior in an unforeseen situation. Who amongst us *really* knows with any degree of certainty how he will react? Many times it is only in retrospect, i.e., after the stressful situation has occurred, that the individual can truly judge whether or not he behaved courageously. If one has been able to confront and not run away from problems and difficulties, then it is highly probable that courage will not be lacking when the person sorely needs the sustaining grace of this quality.

Many individuals think of courageous behavior only in relation to an individual being able to face desperate life situations or extreme emergencies. But there is also a need for courage in confronting the less dramatic—but no less real—problems an ill person may encounter. Courage is needed to deliberately inflict pain on oneself, for example, injecting oneself with insulin three times a day. The person with a long-term illness who experiences chronic pain over a period of years (or decades) needs courage just to face each day and to live through it without giving way to despair.

Courage is not an automatic process. An individual does not become courageous simply because he wishes to be. Courage is a quality which must be produced with each individual experience—by confronting *each* problem and difficulty as it occurs in one's life and doing one's best to cope with such a situation. The individual who is courageous does not deny or run away from problems and difficulties. What has been stated about not running away from one's problems and difficulties may seem to be very simple. However, it is by no means as easy as it sounds. It is not easy to face each of life's small problems or difficulties without succumbing to the very human propensity to "forget it" or "ignore it," hoping magically that the problem or difficulty will disappear by itself. Granted if one ignores problems long enough some problems may disappear or someone else may solve them. But what is the effect on the individual who knows he has shirked his responsibility—who knows that he could have helped himself or others and chose not to do so? An individual who habitually reacts to problems and difficulties in this manner is not likely to display courage during those times when courage is needed.

Thus far the characteristics of hope have been described. Actually, any thing, condition or state within the realm of human imagination can become the object of a wish, but not everything can be hoped for in the sense that "all things are possible." That which is hoped for *is* within the range of possibility. The mental outlook of the hopeless person is very different from that of the individual who experiences hope.

PART II—HOPELESSNESS

The hopeless individual is devoid of hope, i.e., he does not strive to solve problems, or cope with difficulties of life, because he does not really believe that any change can be effected. This type of individual usually does not envisage choices or alternatives which are available to him; those individuals who do perceive choice at their disposal usually lack the initiative, or the motivating power, which would enable them to become involved actively in changing their life. The hopeless person, even when presented with alternatives or possible solutions, will frequently express such opinions as, "I don't see any way out," or "There is nothing I can do." An overwhelming sense of the futility of even *trying* to cope with problems pervades the hopeless person. The individual experiencing hopelessness does not really believe others will help him in times of distress. If other individuals do strive to assist him, he usually believes their efforts will be futile. The hopeless are oriented to the present—not the future; they are overwhelmed by difficulty and find it difficult even to think about the future.

Generally, the individual feels caught in a trap, enmeshed in a problem or difficulty for which there is no way out. The frustration of experiencing such helplessness may engender such behavioral reactions as pessimism, apathy, despondency, hostility, the "despairful not-caring" or "apathetic-indifference" kinds of behavioral reactions previously described in Chapter VI, "Concept: Suffering."

GENESIS OF HOPELESSNESS

No one is born "hopeless." To experience hopelessness an individual has to have, at least at one time or another in his life, experienced hope then lost it. What engenders hopelessness in the ill person? Hopelessness probably occurs when an individual has suffered mentally, physically or spiritually, too intensely, over too long a period of time, without assistance or without surcease of suffering.

It has been stated that hope is dependent, to some extent, to some extent, on the assurance of help from others. One would then expect that ill persons would receive the required assistance from nurses and other health workers in order to maintain hope and avoid hopelessness. However, one finding of the Duff and Hollingshead study was that physicians and nurses are not interested in the anguish and fears of ill persons. The efforts of ill persons to discuss their fears were largely ignored by nurses and other health workers.[4] Perhaps by way of rebuttal to these findings one could argue that the Duff and Hollingshead study was concerned with only one hospital and that nurses and health workers generally do not behave in this manner in other hospitals or in other sections of the country. One would like to believe this is true; however, there are other reported studies which lead one to believe that this situation *does* exist in various sections of the country.

PART III

THE NURSE'S ROLE

It is the task of the professional nurse practitioner to assist the ill person to maintain hope and avoid hopelessness. Conversely, it is also the professional nurse's task to assist the individual experiencing hopelessness to regain hope.

Some ways and means of assisting ill persons to maintain hope and avoid hopelessness are considered in Chapter XI, "Nursing Intervention." Generally, the professional practitioner assists individuals to maintain hope and avoid hopelessness first by being *available* and *willing to help,* for example, by being available and willing to listen to the ill person's anxieties and fears. There is simply no way to assist the ill human being unless the nurse is available, is approachable and willing to talk with the ill person about his concerns and difficulties as he (the ill person) perceives them to be. The nurse renders expert and compassionate nursing care and is alert and astute in observing signs of psychological distress, as in observing signs of physical distress. Let there be no mistake about it—ill persons need expert physical care; the stress on psychological aspects in no way should be construed as

---

[4] Duff, Raymond S., and Hollingshead, August B.: *Sickness and Society.* New York: Harper & Row, 1968, p. 277.

meaning physical care can be neglected. Actually, one way to *induce* hopelessness in an ill person is through paying little attention to his comfort or physical needs. It should be emphasized that some ill persons will not request anything from a nurse because they believe "the nurse is too busy." *It is the role of the professional nurse practitioner to render the needed assistance without being asked.* If the nurse is not certain what it is the individual requires she then asks the ill person. If it is a need the nurse can meet she proceeds to do so. It cannot be overly stressed that the burden of offering and rendering assistance is that of the nurse, not the ill person. Ill persons should not *have* to ask nurses to meet many of their needs; the professional nurse practitioner should be able to anticipate these needs.

There is no substitute for talking with ill persons and getting to know them. The nurse, through observing and communicating with the ill human being, should be particularly alert to statements made by the ill person which give some indication of the manner in which he perceives his illness, his perception of the measures he must take to conserve health or recover, and his beliefs regarding his probable prognosis.

Since hope is related to choice the nurse allows the ill person to make choices regarding his care whenever this is possible. Although the range of choice available to an ill person may be restricted by virtue of his illness, there are still areas of choice and the ill human being can, and should, be allowed to choose or state his preferences. For example, an ill person may prefer one comfort measure above another. The nurse, however, is not likely to be aware that the ill person even has preferences unless he tells her or she elicits this data from him.

Since hope is related to trust, the nurse attempts to demonstrate by her behavior that she is capable and willing to assist the ill person in times of need. Trust must be earned by the nurse. There are few ill persons who automatically trust a nurse they do not know.

The nurse cannot "give" hope to another person; she can, however, strive to provide some ways and means for an ill person to experience hope. At the present our knowledge is very limited. Research is urgently needed to investigate the nature of hope and find ways to assist individuals to maintain hope or overcome hopelessness. This lack of knowledge, however, should not be used by professional nurses as an excuse for failure to try to assist ill persons and their families. The professional nurse tries to help; she does not always succeed; but she *always* tries to help and to comfort.

N.B. References used in this chapter are in the footnotes. These are not repeated.

The author wishes to thank Ruth A. Johnston, R.N. who reviewed this chapter.

Chapter VIII

ILLNESS AND SUFFERING AS HUMAN EXPERIENCES

Illness and suffering are experiences. Webster's Third New International Dictionary defines experience as ". . . participation in events; an encountering, undergoing or living through of things in general as they take place in the course of time . . ."[1]

It is essential that the professional nurse practitioner comprehend illness as a human experience. It *is not* sufficient to learn about illness from the standpoint of etiology, signs and symptoms, treatment, nursing care and prognosis, while ignoring inquiries concerning the *meaning* of illness. In order to render thoughtful, intelligent care to individuals, there is a need for nurses to understand the profoundly real yet more intangible concept of illness as an experience that is undergone by a human being. Without this understanding a nurse can never relate as human being to human being; and those for whom she renders care will not be helped in any meaningful way.

The perceptions of illness, suffering and pain presented in this chapter are derived from comments made by ill persons (or their families). These perceptions range from the mundane to the dramatic, but do, nevertheless, record perceptions of illness and suffering *as* experienced and are not fictionalized.

It has been stated that a person realizes that he is ill by contrasting his present condition with a previous time when he did not have the present illness. All individuals have a tendency to take for granted the ability to see, hear, speak, touch, taste, smell, write, and to reach and pick up objects. The ability to dress ourselves and to care for our personal needs is also taken for granted, until such time should arrive that we are unable to perform such simple yet infinitely intricate tasks. Our strength, energy and vitality are not noticed until through illness we begin to experience their loss. In a like manner, freedom from physical pain, discomfort and

---

[1] By permission. From Webster's Third New International Dictionary, copyright 1961 by G. & C. Merriam Co., Publishers of the Merriam-Webster Dictionaries.

mental distress are taken for granted. Many persons cannot even envisage that those they love will become ill, suffer and die. All know that these experiences will come to pass, but it is an uncomfortable reality that we would rather put off by not thinking about it. But these experiences are inevitable. It is essential that nurses comprehend illness as a human experience. This understanding is necessary, not just because an individual is a nurse, but because she is a human being who will someday encounter and have to undergo these same experiences. Illness, pain, suffering and death are not simply abstractions; they are experiences undergone by flesh-and-blood human beings. What is the human experience of illness and suffering?

THE HUMAN EXPERIENCE OF ILLNESS AND SUFFERING

To be ill and to suffer may be to experience any or all of the following:

To be ill is to encounter and endure the symptoms of one's illness and to experience the myriad and varying emotional responses that accompany the threat of illness. It is to experience, in a profound way, one's utter vulnerability and to realize how very frail a human being one actually is.

It is to change one's perspective, to some extent, and to view life somewhat differently—to readjust one's scale of values. To rearrange one's hierarchy of relative importance so that what was once considered unimportant, or taken for granted, is now of great significance. It is to realize that what one previously considered so important is really of minor significance.

To be ill is to be lonely and to be unable to assuage or even communicate the basic core of one's loneliness. It is to try to reach out to others and to fail. It is to try to communicate "how it is" or "how one feels," and to realize how little others grasp, and how inadequate words really are.

To be ill is to be afraid. It is to fear the known and the unknown, to fear the present and the future. It is to experience the profound fear that one does not have a future. It is to fear that one will be proved incapable of coping with the present and all its trials. It is to fear displaying one's inadequacies and lack of courage to others. It is to realize that not only "doth conscience make cowards of us all" but that fear has an equal impact and effect.

To be ill is to worry about what will happen because one is elderly and lives alone in a furnished room and has no living relatives or friends. It is to fear disability, dependency, and what will happen should one have to be hospitalized. It is to worry about who will pay the rent and care for the few material possessions one has left. It is to wonder who will care for the mementoes of a long dead past. It is to worry about who will care for the pet—the dog, the cat, the canary or the goldfish—if one is hospitalized and there is no one to go to for help. It is to realize that there is no one to notify in case of death when the young woman in the admitting office asks this question. It is fear engendered by this complete and utter loneliness.

To be ill is to worry about getting the money to pay the hospital bill, the doctor's fees, the rent or the mortgage, and the note on the car. It is to wonder whether one's job has been lost because one has been ill too frequently and too long.

To be ill is to worry about one's spouse or dependents, to worry what will happen to them should one's illness progress and one becomes incapacitated and a burden, or dies.

To be ill and hospitalized is to have one's daily life drastically altered and to have to adapt to institutional needs and expectations. It is to be awakened at six a.m. to have one's temperature taken or to be awakened at night to be given a sleeping pill.

It is to experience the boredom and monotony of hospitalization. To experience the desperation of waiting. It is to want something, or someone, and to push a buzzer and wait for someone to answer. It is to push a button and to respond to a voice coming from a box on the wall asking, "What do you want?" and to experience the humiliation of telling the voice coming from the box on the wall that one needs a bedpan. It is to wait for the morphine or demerol injection because it isn't four hours since the last one was received. It is to wait for the bedpan or a glass of water or for someone to pick up something that fell to the floor. It is to wait for visitors, and to be glad when they leave and one can rest.

To be ill and in pain is to believe that everyone without pain must be happy or at least content.

To be ill is to experience the fatigue engendered by chronic pain that does not cease. It is to become aware that although others experience pain the fact that others suffer is of no comfort when one is undergoing the relentless thrust of pain.

To be ill is to comprehend what it means to live in pain and await the benediction of sleep or to long for death to relieve the unremitting discomfort.

It is to become easily depressed and discouraged or to find one's eyes well up with tears at an imagined affront, a kindness, an old memory, or a loved one's face.

To be ill is to experience fatigue, malaise, or utter and complete weariness of body, mind and spirit.

To be ill is not to care, to be beyond caring, to feel too tired; so weary that nothing matters and nothing is real but the weight of one's weariness and inertia.

To be ill is to experience the shame of being overwhelmed by self-pity. It is to weep at one's helplessness and to experience the sorrow when observing one's own body weakened and wasted.

To be ill is to comprehend that it is impossible to truly communicate the experience of illness to another human being. It is to realize that distress cannot really be shared and that each of us is alone in his distress.

To be ill is to observe the effects of one's illness on others; to observe the studied cheerfulness of one's visitors who talk about everything but one's illness, or the friends who discuss their own complaints and come with their burdens ready to pile on anyone who will listen and cannot run away. It is to listen to the relatives and friends who insist that one looks fine and that they wish *they* could take a nice long rest.

It is to respond to the physician's manner and to be more sensitive how one is treated by him. It is to sense or infer that the physician cares or understands or to bear the crushing realization that the physician may not care and does not understand.

To be ill is to observe the nurse's facial expression when she takes one's temperature or blood pressure or dressing one's wound and to wonder what her facial expression means.

To be ill is to keep telling oneself that everything is all right, that the physician said there was nothing to worry about, to want to believe but to be haunted by the nagging doubt of disbelief.

To be ill is to be unable to sleep and to lie awake at night and worry because tomorrow one will learn the results of the X-rays and the laboratory tests. It is to try to sleep and yet be caught up in a relentless vortex of memories and haunting fears. It is to escape into sleep but to dread awakening because there is another day to be lived through, somehow. It is to lie awake at night in a hospital room listening to all of the magnified sounds one never hears during the day. It is to sleep fitfully and awaken tired and exhausted.

It is to experience the frustration of trying to walk (or talk, or move, or care for oneself) when one has lost this ability. It is to reach for an object on the bedside table and to miss it and send it clattering to the floor.

To be ill is to be afraid of death and of the long loneliness of dying. It is to realize profoundly that one can die and that death is not just an experience that happens to someone else. It is also to wonder what will happen after death.

To be ill is also not to be afraid of death—to welcome it as a friend and to look forward to life's culminating experience. It is to view death as the beginning of a newer, happier time—a life where no one is tired, unhappy, or in pain: a place of comfort, light and peace. It is to view death as a means of coming home and leaving the land of one's exile if these are the beliefs one has always held.

To be ill is also to feel one's strength slowly returning and to be allowed out of bed and to be astonished at how long a distance it is from the bed to the door and how very tired one becomes.

It is to endure the effects of an illness when one never really feels well and to somehow keep on working. It is to work when one doesn't know how he will get through the day. It is to somehow hold on, and keep going; to try to smile so that others will not realize how tired one is and how very ill one feels.

It is to pace oneself in order to conserve waning strength and energy—to have to make decisions on the basis of one's symptoms. To have to refuse an invitation to a friend's apartment for dinner because the friend lives on the second floor and the steps are too long and steep.

To suffer is to be immersed in a black ocean of pain.

To suffer is to wait while a loved one is in surgery and to watch the clock and to be astonished that a minute can last so very long.

To suffer is to see a loved one in great pain and anguish and to be unable to help him. It is to experience the anguish of impotence and to live with the knowledge that there is nothing one can humanly do to assist a loved one.

To suffer is to learn of a loved one's fatal illness—to live with this knowledge day after day and to keep up a pretense of cheerful hopefulness.

To suffer is to wait two hours between the five minute periods one is given to visit a loved one in the intensive care unit. It is to spend much of the time listening to the sounds of the respirator and watching the spiking lines on the monitor.

It is to leave the hospital and go home because one has been told that there is nothing one can do and that the hospital will call in case there's a change. It is to go home and dread the phone call that says to hurry because there's not much time left.

To suffer is to experience the impact of so much stress that one doesn't feel anything anymore. It is to experience numbness of body, mind and spirit and to bear the impact of a tiredness that eludes rest.

To suffer is to realize that one's relative is unconscious and is dying, and to wish one had told the relative how much he was loved and appreciated but to realize that it is much, much too late.

To suffer is to listen to the physician when he explains that if one's relative lives he will probably be "a vegetable." It is to be placed in the position of having to decide whether or not the extraordinary means being used to keep one's relative alive should be continued or to recommend that they be discontinued. It is to know that whatever the decision may be that one must live with the effects of this decision the rest of one's life.

To be ill and to suffer is to encounter some, or all, of these experiences and in the encountering to be changed by that which one has encountered. Illness and suffering are lonely experiences in that it is difficult to express or explain to others that which one has experienced. But as experiences they become a part of oneself in that a type of knowledge or understanding is gained. Individuals invariably attempt to explain illness and suffering to themselves. These explanations are gropings for reasons as to why the person was afflicted. Such explanations, as has been stated, frequently emerge out of one's philosophy of life as well as his religious convictions.

It is the task of the professional nurse practitioner to attempt to grasp the meaning of illness and suffering as human experiences. This is not an easy task since the afflicted person frequently has difficulty in communicating his perception of illness and suffering. Neither can the nurse "put herself in the ill person's place." The only possible way in which the nurse can truly grasp some insight into a world so different from her own is to elicit from each ill person his perception of his illness. Nurses *can*, however, gain some insight into the world of the ill person by reading some of the many personal accounts of illness written by individuals who have undergone these experiences. (See "Suggested Reading References" for Chapter VIII in Section VI.)

N. B. Reference used in this chapter is in the footnote. This is not repeated.

SECTION FOUR

The purpose of this section is to explore the concept "communication" and to examine the implications of the communication process in nursing situations.

In Chapter IX the term "communication" is defined and discussed. The communication skills needed by the professional nurse practitioner are discussed as are the communication techniques. The major causes of communication breakdown are explored.

In this chapter, communication is viewed as a process which enables the nurse to establish a human-to-human relationship.

SECTION FOUR

Chapter IX

CONCEPT: COMMUNICATION

Communication takes place during every encounter the nurse has with the recipients of her care. It occurs when nurse and ill person converse with each other, as well as when each is silent. The ill individual communicates something to the nurse by his appearance, behavior, posture, facial expression, mannerisms and gesture, as does the nurse to the ill individual. Both nurse and ill person communicate, whether or not they are aware that it is happening.

Every interaction, with an ill person affords an opportunity for the nurse to get to know the individual and to ascertain and meet the ill person's nursing needs, thereby establishing a human-to-human relationship and achieving the purpose of nursing. Whether or not these goals will be achieved depends on the nurse's behavior in the interactive process, and the extent to which the nurse's actions are purposeful and helpful to the recipients of her care.

A major belief of this work is that it is the task of the professional nurse practitioner to plan, direct and guide purposefully the interaction with the ill person in such a way as to fulfill the purpose of nursing.

The nurse must also be able to (1) understand the meaning of the ill person's communication and (2) use this information in order to plan nursing intervention. The professional nurse needs to know *if* communication is taking place and *what* is being communicated in the nursing situation. The nurse also assesses and evaluates the extent to which the purpose of nursing is being achieved in the interaction.

A major assumption of this work, then, is that communication is a process which can enable the nurse to establish a human-to-human relationship and thereby fulfill the purpose of nursing, namely, to assist individuals and families to prevent and to cope with the experience of illness and suffering and, if necessary, to assist them to find meaning in these experiences.

It has been stated that communication is a process which can enable a nurse to establish a human-to-human relationship. The term, human-to-human relationship, in nursing, refers to an experience or series of experiences between the human being who is the nurse and an ill person, or an individual in need of the services of the nurse. The major characteristic of this experience (or experiences) is that the nursing needs ·of the individual are met. These needs are met by a nurse who possesses and uses a disciplined intellectual approach to problems combined with the therapeutic use of self. The human-to-human relationship is established and maintained purposefully by the professional nurse practitioner.

It should be stressed that it is quite possible for a nurse and an ill person to communicate effectively and yet never establish a human-to-human relationship. The ability to establish relatedness seems to be dependent on the extent to which the nurse possesses and uses the disciplined intellectual approach combined with the therapeutic use of self.

Part I of this chapter contains introductory content relating to the communication process. The tasks of the professional nurse practitioner and the unchanging goals of the interaction are discussed in Part II. The content of communication is considered in Part III and the communication abilities are discussed in Part IV. The use and misuse of communication techniques are considered in Part V and causes of communication breakdown are explored in Part VI.

PART I—THE COMMUNICATION PROCESS

DEFINITION AND DISCUSSION OF THE CONCEPT "COMMUNICATION"

Webster's Third New International Dictionary defines communication as "the act or action of imparting or transmitting . . . interchange of thoughts or opinions: a process by which meanings are exchanged between individuals through a common system of symbols (as language, signs or gestures) . . ." [1]

According to Webster's Third New International Dictionary communication is an act (or behavior) and a process. Communication is behavior since it always involves physical and mental activity on the part of the sender and receiver of the message. Communication is also a process through which meanings are exchanged, so that in order to communicate there must be a sender (or source), a recipient (or receiver), and the meanings (or messages) must be understood by the individuals involved.

Communication is an oscillating reciprocal process as discussed in the introduction to this chapter. In a single interaction there is an ebb and flow of influence and counter-influence as the nurse and ill person observe each other and communicate thoughts, feelings and attitudes. Communication, then, may be considered as a process of sharing or transmitting thoughts and feelings. However, individuals will

---

[1] By permission. From Webster's Third New International Dictionary, copyright 1961 by G. & C. Merriam Co., Publishers of the Merriam-Webster Dictionaries.

N.B. The term "human-to-human relationship" is not to be equated with the "nurse-patient relationship." In this work it is assumed that the roles of nurse and patient are barriers to establishing a human-to-human relationship. The term "nurse" is used in this text only for purposes of economy in communication.

not share anything meaningful with another until they are relatively certain that that which they share will be accepted—not ignored, discounted, devalued or ridiculed.

Communication is a reciprocal process. It is the process the nurse uses to elicit and give information as well as the means through which ill individuals and their families seek assistance. The nurse communicates in order to motivate and influence ill persons and is, in turn, influenced by them. It is also through communication that the nurse conveys (usually non-verbally, i.e., by a look, a glance, or the manner in which she performs her ministrations) the extent to which she cares for those persons for whom she is responsible. In turn, the ill person communicates his perception of the nurse, i.e., the extent to which he views her as a helping human being.

Communication is also an experience in which one participates. Depending on *what* is conveyed in the interaction it can be a mutually significant experience, a meaningless one, or a frustrating experience.

Communication is a dynamic force capable of profoundly influencing and affecting the degree of interpersonal closeness in nursing situations; it can be used to draw others closer, to repel, to help, or to hurt them. The nurse's basic intentions and the way she perceives human beings is invariably communicated in nursing situations. Despite lip service to the contrary, if the nurse is not interested in ill people as human beings the disinterest will be communicated, and the ill person will respond accordingly.

It is through perception and communication that the uniqueness of others may be revealed or concealed.

Communication is the instrument through which changes are effected in nursing situations. The nurse invariably wishes to influence the recipients of her care; she is ever alert to opportunities and ways to influence others. The professional nurse deliberately speaks and acts in such a way so as to initiate and induce change. Communication, therefore, can be a creative process.

Each interaction is alike, yet unlike and different from any other, hence it is not possible to develop or adhere to rigid rules and procedures in interacting with people. This is not to say that the development of the skills and abilities of communication is unimportant. A craftsman must be skilled in using the tools and techniques of his craft, he must have mastered them and be in command of them in order to focus his attention on the end to be achieved, and not on the means to the end. Thus it is that the nurse must develop the necessary communication skills and abilities. A nurse is a craftsman in the truest sense of the word, and every interaction offers an unlimited opportunity for creatively influencing others. The more creative, knowledgeable and skillful, the more able will the nurse be to tap the unrealized force and latent power contained in communication.

It has been stated that communication is a continuous process—an experience during which meanings or messages are transmitted between individuals. These meanings are transmitted through verbal and non-verbal modes of expression.

VERBAL AND NON-VERBAL COMMUNICATION

Verbal communication is communication by means of words—written or spoken. Non-verbal communication refers to the transmission of messages without using words; in an interaction, individuals communicate non-verbally by gesture, facial expression and body movement. Communication without words includes sounds such as those associated with crying, groaning or screaming. Meanings are also transmitted non-verbally by touch or smell. Other examples of non-verbal communication include transmission of meaning by signs and symbols—by pictures, music, dance and pantomime. Non-verbal communication is a continuous process in every face-to-face encounter. Non-verbal communication invariably accompanies verbal communication as when two individuals are conversing. It is the underlying theme which adds dimensions of meaning to that which is said. For example, gestures are used to emphasize and illustrate comments. Non-verbal communication also occurs when each person is silent. Each person, through observation of cues from the other, perceives and/or communicates feelings or impressions to the other.

Depending on the sensitivity and receptiveness of the individuals involved, it would seem that this perception and interpretation of the thoughts and feelings transmitted during an interaction also include the ability to sense, or perceive, the basic intentions of the other person, which leads to inferences as to whether or not the individual is sincere and means what he says. Whatever is transmitted during an interaction (i.e., thoughts, ideas, impressions, feelings, intentions) is first perceived, then interpreted. If the message is perceived and correctly interpreted, communication is said to have taken place.

PART II—COMMUNICATION AND THE INTERACTIVE PROCESS

GOALS IN THE INTERACTION

The goals to be achieved in the interaction—(1) *to know persons,* (2) *ascertain and meet the nursing needs of ill persons,* and (3) *fulfill the purpose of nursing*—are continuous and unchanging. These goals are achieved only on a temporary basis, they are never permanently achieved in the sense that they will not have to be achieved again. For example, the purpose of nursing is an unchanging goal and guide in nursing situations, since many ill persons require continuous assistance in coping with the stress of illness and suffering. Although an ill person's need for assistance may be met temporarily, such needs are not met on a permanent basis because when one need is met another set of needs then emerges. Hence the purpose of nursing is an unchanging over-all objective and the terminus of all nursing endeavor. The goal "to know ill persons" (or the recipients of one's care) is unchanging; no individual can be completely known and every interaction provides an opportunity to enhance the process of knowing.

In order to achieve these goals, certain prerequisties are needed by the nurse:

1. Understand *what* is to be accomplished in the interaction (i.e., the establishment of a human-to-human relationship in order to achieve the purpose of nursing).

2. Understand *why* the purpose of nursing is to be achieved (i.e., understand the underlying theoretical basis of the purpose of nursing, namely, the nature of the human being, the meaning of illness, suffering, health).

3. Understand *how* to interact and communicate in such a way as to achieve the purpose of nursing (i.e., possess the required communication skills and abilities and the competencies needed to establish a human-to-human relationship, and the knowledge underlying these skills).

It is to be noted that communication is not an end within itself—only a means to an end, namely, achievement of the goals of the interactive process in order to fulfill the purpose of nursing. Communication is considered a process which enables and assists the nurse to accomplish these goals.

Each goal is discussed individually. Ways of using the communication process in order to achieve these goals are stressed.

The Goal: "To Know III Persons"

Nurses are continually urged to "get to know patients as individuals." What is meant by this phrase? What is the value of "knowing patients?" Actually the phrase is a misnomer since only human beings are known—not patients. The nurse who is the human being perceives and responds to the uniqueness of the human being who is the recipient of her care and is, in turn, responded to in the same manner. To know someone, then, it is necessary to encounter, perceive, respond to, and respect his uniqueness. In order to do this the nurse must be able to focus on others and be perceptually receptive. This implies an ability to perceive the human being who is concealed or hidden by the label "patient." It is the ability to "see with fresh eyes" without the need to categorize, classify, label or pigeon-hole others.

It is obvious that ill human beings cannot be known if the nurse presupposes that all ill persons are similar.

The professional nurse is able to separate her needs and desires from that of the recipient of her care. The nurse, therefore, does not assume that ill persons will wish to be treated as she (the nurse) would wish to be treated if she were ill. Through communicating the nurse attempts to identify the individual's needs and does not superimpose her needs on others. Neither does the nurse attempt the impossible, i.e., to try to "put herself in the ill person's place." Instead of attempting the impossible, the nurse strives to understand the meaning of experience as interpreted by the individual undergoing the experience. Therefore, the nurse elicits this information from each individual.

There is a difference between having information about an individual and the experience of knowing the individual. A nurse may have information about an ill person, i.e., may know his age, religion, where he lives, what he does, and may have read his chart thoroughly and may understand the nature of his illness and the measures to be taken to alleviate his distress, and still not know the ill person. *Knowing is the process of experiencing and responding to the uniqueness of others.*

Why should nurses know the recipients of their care? Nurses need to experience and respond to the uniqueness of ill persons to assist them in coping with the stress of illness and suffering. Every human being is different and will respond to stress in his own unique way. Unless the nurse understands each person's habitual manner of coping with stress and the behavior he demonstrates when in distress, she is not apt to be able to assist him in any meaningful way. The nurse may not recognize the individual's need for help since not every ill person will request assistance from the nurse. However, even an individual who cannot readily seek assistance from others is more likely to request help if he *knows* the nurse, and perceives her intent to help. Ill persons and their families are much more apt to tell nurses of their fears and anxieties when they know and are known by the nurse, and when they trust her.

Nurses who know ill persons are more apt to be able to detect not only obvious changes in an individual's condition but are enabled to recognize the more subtle changes that may be occurring.

It is probably through knowing ill persons individually that nurses develop a sense of timing in nursing situations, i.e., when to speak and when to be silent, when to urge the other person to speak and when to refrain from urging. Nurses need to know *when* to communicate or intervene as well as *what* to communicate in nursing situations.

It is believed that getting to know the ill human being is as valid and necessary a nursing activity as is performing procedures or rendering physical care. Every interaction can enhance the process of knowing. Unless the interaction is consciously perceived as a medium through which the goals are to be achieved, there is a great danger that the activities nurses perform may take precedence over the human being for whom the activity is performed.

Some nurses instead of being "activity-oriented" are "sign and symptom centered" because their education has overly stressed the importance of observing signs and eliciting information about symptoms. Such nurses tend to concentrate on the sign to be observed or symptom to be studied and never take time to know the human being *with* the sign or symptom. This is not to say that the observation of signs and recording of symptoms is unimportant. It is a *vital* nursing activity. But if the observation of signs and ascertaining of symptoms are the sole reasons for an interaction, then the establishment of a human-to-human relationship is not possible.

The process involved in knowing ill persons is discussed in detail in Chapter X, "The Human-to-Human Relationship."

There are many other reasons why nurses should know the recipients of their care. A major reason is that the nurse is better able to ascertain and meet the needs of the ill human being.

The Goal: "To Ascertain and Meet the Nursing Needs of the Ill Human Being"

The human-to-human relationship is the means through which the purpose of nursing is achieved. A characteristic of the human-to-human relationship is that the nursing needs of the individual or family are met. In order to meet needs, these needs must first be identified. *It is through observation and communication that nurses ascertain the needs of ill persons—the first necessary step in planning nursing intervention.*

Observation

The nursing process consists of overlapping stages: observation, interpretation, decision-making, action (nursing intervention) and appraisal (or evaluation) of one's actions. These stages are also considered to be basic skills needed by all nurses.

Observation is the first step leading to nursing intervention. It is also an inherent aspect of the communication process. It is possible for a nurse to be a skilled observer without necessarily being able to purposefully use the communication process, but it is practically impossible to communicate meaningfully and purposefully without being a skilled observer.

Definition of Observation

"Observation . . . refers to the collection of raw sensory data prior to interpretation. Observation includes the content of the data, i.e., what is seen, heard, smelled, etc. To observe is to notice, be mindful of, or focus on what is happening in a situation; it implies intentional scrutiny or concentrated attention. Observation is an active process, a meaningful as well as a purposeful process." [2]

Purposes of Observation

From a survey of basic nursing textbooks in various clinical areas the purposes of observation may be grouped broadly as follows: to infer "patients' " needs and problems in order to plan appropriate nursing action, to assist the physician in diagnosing the individual's illness, to assess the efficacy of therapies prescribed by the physician, to gather information about the ill person in order to share these findings with other members of the health team, to prevent complications and sequelae, and to observe signs of illness. As can be inferred, the importance of separating sensory data from interpretation of the data is *not* stressed or implied.

---

[2] Travelbee, Joyce: Intervention in Psychiatric Nursing. Process in the One-to-One Relationship. Philadelphia: F. A. Davis Company, 1969, p. 28.

It cannot be denied that the purposes of observation as stated in the texts surveyed *are* important and therefore should be given priority; however, one gets the impression that the ill human being is not viewed in his totality during the search for signs and symptoms of illness.

The professional nurse practitioner does not "observe signs of illness," the nurse observes an ill human being who may (or may not) be experiencing symptoms of a particular illness, and validates (with the ill person if at all possible) the subjective experience he is undergoing.

The purposes of observation are many and varied; however, it is *always* the ill human being who is observed, not signs of illness.

Observation is a process used to get to know the ill individual as a unique human being. This is a necessary first step to develop a human-to-human relationship. A more specific purpose is to collect raw data in order to interpret and validate its meaning (whenever possible with the ill person), and decide on a course of nursing action. Collecting raw data is a necessary prerequisite in planning, structuring, giving, and evaluating nursing care for an individual or group. Whatever reasons a nurse may have for observing an ill person—whether to assess the effect of a particular drug, to watch for signs of illness, or to detect signs of anxiety or depression—the process is the same and the nurse invariably begins by collecting raw data.

Data Collection

The data the nurse collects consist of what is seen, heard, smelled, touched, i.e., everything taken in via the sense organs. It is important to identify and collect raw data prior to interpreting their meaning. For example, a person frowns. The raw data, "wrinkling of the brows" or "frowning," may be interpreted as indicating pain, anger, worry, preoccupation, depression, etc. The nurse has no way of knowing whether or not the interpretation of the data is correct unless the interpretation is validated with the individual involved. What *is* important is that the nurse is able to notice and report what was *actually seen and heard* prior to interpretation.

In addition to the purposeful collection of raw data there is another important aspect of observation: experiencing.

Experiencing as an Aspect of Observation

Experiencing means focusing on the individual within the total context of his setting and environment, not parts or aspects of the whole. One reacts as human-to-human and allows the other's personality and uniqueness to become real, on a level other than what is *known about* him. There is a sense of confronting a *real* person.

A nurse intent upon taking an individual's blood pressure may focus almost exclusively on the dial on the sphygmomanometer and never perceive, much less experience, the uniqueness of the individual whose blood pressure she is taking.

Using the same example, when a nurse experiences another individual, she focuses on and perceives the uniqueness of the individual before focusing on one aspect of the whole. In a sense the *entire* person is perceived and responded to before attention is focused on a portion of the individual. The nurse may narrow the focus of her attention to the dial of the sphygmomanometer; however, at the same time, she strives to experience the personality of the other individual.

Experiencing is not an esoteric art; it is in operation whenever one individual consciously focuses attention on, and strives to know, another person.

Decision-Making and Interpretation

Observation is also an inherent part of the process of decision-making in nursing situations. The sequence is as follows:

1. Observation
2. The development of interpretations (based on past knowledge)
3. The decision to act or not to act on the basis of one's interpretations and inferences

This decision-making has tremendous implications in nursing situations. The decisions to be made range from the selection of comfort measures to decisions which may mean the difference between life or death for an ill individual.

An example of the process of observation as it relates to interpretation and decision-making follows. The nurse observes that an individual has small red spots on his arm. She interprets the raw data and may infer any of the following: the red spots are (1) caused by a drug reaction, (2) the result of "heat rash," (3) caused by the individual rubbing his arm on the sheet or (4) the beginning signs of a communicable disease.

If the nurse decides that the red spots are caused by the individual rubbing his arm on the sheet she will obviously act in a different manner than if she decides the individual is showing signs of a communicable disease or the results of a drug reaction.

The nurse's interpretations may be valid or invalid. The nurse therefore checks the interpretations with the ill person (if possible) in order to validate her assumption.

Nursing intervention, then, is planned on the basis of validated interpretations as elicited during the interaction. The appropriate measures are then initiated to meet the need. The required assistance may be given by the nurse or another health worker. However, it is through purposeful use of the observation and communication process that needs are ascertained.

Nursing Actions and Appraisal

Following interpretation and decision-making the nurse acts or intervenes. Not only are needs ascertained through the communication process, they are also met. For example, an ill person may require health teaching or may need information. The individual may be in need of encouragement to assist him in coping with the stress of illness. Such needs for assistance are met through *what* the nurse communicates to the individual in the nursing situation.

The nurse appraises or judges the quality or efficacy of her nursing actions. Criteria are established, by the nurse practitioner, before appraisal, if this is possible. Appraisal centers about the achievement of particular objectives of care. The extent to which the nurse is able to achieve these objectives is the criterion used to evaluate nursing actions.

Summary of Part II

The professional nurse practitioner *intentionally* strives to interact and communicate in such a way as to achieve the following goals: (1) to know ill persons, (2) to ascertain and meet nursing needs and (3) to achieve the purpose of nursing.

Whether or not the goals of the interaction will be achieved depends on many factors. Certainly the nurse needs to know *why* goals are to be achieved, *what* it is she must strive to accomplish in nursing situations, and *how* to accomplish these goals.

However, the nurse may have an understanding of all of these factors and yet fail to accomplish these goals if she lacks a conscious awareness of *what* is being communicated between herself and the ill human being. *What* is transmitted in nursing situations is also known as "the content of communication."

PART III—THE CONTENT OF COMMUNICATION

A major premise of this work is that nurses need to know if communication is taking place in nursing situations; if the exchanged messages have been understood by all concerned. But it is equally as important to develop an understanding of what each participant is communicating.

It is quite possible for both nurse and ill person to communicate effectively without ever establishing a meaningful relationship (i.e., a human-to-human relationship). Whether or not a meaningful relationship will be established between the nurse and the recipient of her care seems to be dependent on *what* is communicated in the interpersonal process, or the *content* of the communication. Such feelings as dislike, indifference, or unconcern are communicated as effectively as are the affective caring qualities of concern, interest and liking. *What* the nurse thinks and feels about the particular person with whom she is interacting is invariably communicated to the ill person, as are the nurse's basic intentions. By this is meant the ill person's perception of the extent to which the nurse "means well" or "tries to help." If a nurse lacks "good intentions" it is probably not possible to establish

N.B. Portions of the content on observation, interpretation, decision-making, nursing action and appraisal are adapted from "The Process of Psychiatric Nursing" in Travelbee, Joyce: Intervention in Psychiatric Nursing. Process in the One-to-One Relationship. Philadelphia: F. A. Davis Company, 1969, pp. 25–45.

relatedness with others. "Well-meaningness," or its lack, is inevitably communicated to others who will respond accordingly.

Thus it is that *what* is communicated in nursing situations will either enable a nurse to know the recipients of her care, or block the process of knowing; will either assist the nurse in establishing relatedness, or irrevocably destroy it. *What* the nurse communicates to the ill person will either assist him in coping with the long loneliness of illness and suffering, or will intensify and deepen his sense of isolation and alone-ness.

It is essential that the nurse understand the meaning of the ill person's communication in order to use this information in planning care. The ability to grasp or assess the content of communication in nursing situations is developed by systematically studying interactions. Nurses do not usually become aware, in any systematic way, of *what* is transpiring unless this process is studied. One approach to studying the interactive process is through the use of process records. The process record is written and analyzed; the interactive experience is then reconstructed in order to ascertain *what* transpired between nurse and ill person and evaluate the extent to which nursing intervention was successful.

What is discussed during the interactive process, i.e., the subjects of conversation, should be of such a nature as to be *meaningful* to the ill person. *A major assumption of this work is that the nurse should strive to engage in meaningful dialogue with each person with whom he (or she) interacts.*

Meaningful dialogue is characterized by purposeful reciprocal communication between both participants in the interaction. What is discussed is pertinent, relevant and appropriate. The content of the communications is directed toward the "here and now" problems of the ill person. One ill person stated:

> "I am worried . . . I want the doctor to come and take my sutures out so I can go home. I was going to ask the nurse this morning but she was busy telling me about the new disposable bed linens."

In this example, the nurse was too focused on self to pay attention to the ill person. There was no meaningful dialogue because there was no sharing and the conversation was not appropriate to the ill person's need at the time.

Necessary prerequisites to meaningful dialogue, on the part of the nurse, are knowledge and the ability to use it for the good of the ill human being, sensitivity, and an exquisite sense of timing in the interpersonal situation.

Certain skills and abilities are needed by the nurse in order to assess what is being transmitted in the interaction. It is also necessary that the nurse possess certain communication skills and abilities in order to use the communication process purposefully, i.e., to interact and communicate in such a way as to achieve the purpose of nursing. These skills and abilities are discussed in Part IV.

N.B. For a detailed discussion of process recording see Travelbee, Joyce: Intervention in Psychiatric Nursing. Process in the One-to-One Relationship. Philadelphia: F. A. Davis Company, 1969, pp. 117–137.

PART IV—THE COMMUNICATION SKILLS
OR ABILITIES

All nurses communicate but not all nurses are aware of the underlying reasons or rationale for communicating in nursing situations. Neither is every nurse aware of *what* she communicates in nursing situations.

Nurses vary in their ability to assess the effect of their behavior on others. Some nurses are highly sensitive and seem to have little or no difficulty in sensing the thoughts and feelings of others, while other nurses seem to lack this sensitivity. Some nurses intellectually understand the nature of the purposeful use of the communication process, yet are unable to translate this knowledge into action in nursing situations. There are still other nurses who operate intuitively and without knowledge. Such nurses, probably because of their self-insight and concomitant insight into the behavior of others, are usually able to establish relatedness. Other nurses lack both knowledge and sensitivity and tend to respond automatically and in a stereotyped manner in nursing situations.

Despite the nurse's present level of skills and abilities, there is much that each nurse can learn by systematically studying the interactive process, ascertaining the content of communication and deciding whether or not what is being communicated in the nursing situation is actually assisting the nurse to establish relatedness.

No nurse is without some degree of skill in being able to purposefully use the communication process; neither is any nurse a communication expert in the sense that she cannot develop further skill.

It is the responsibility of the professional school of nursing to help students with the skills they already possess, and to assist in further development. A student cannot develop the required skills and abilities unless faculty members themselves possess these abilities and strive to assist the student. The ability to communicate purposefully, i.e., to extract meaning out of interactions and to be able to use these meanings in nursing situations, cannot be learned in *one* course in the nursing school curriculum. Every course in the curriculum should assist students to develop these abilities. The clinical nursing courses provide an opportunity for students to *systematically* study the communication process. The communication skills and abilities are useful and valuable not only in nursing situations but in all areas of life.

DEFINITION OF TERMS

In this work, skill in nursing is defined as ". . . the ability to use one's knowledge effectively and readily . . ." [3] Ability is defined ". . . competence in doing . . . acquired proficiency . . ." [4]

Therefore an individual who is skillful possesses the underlying knowledge and is able to translate knowledge into action. It is believed that skill without knowledge is as useless as knowledge without the ability of using it.

---

[3] By permission. From Webster's Third New International Dictionary, copyright 1961 by G. & C. Merriam Co., Publishers of the Merriam-Webster Dictionaries.

[4] *Ibid.*

The skills of communication are learned as the student learns the disciplined intellectual approach to problems, and the therapeutic use of self. A nurse possessing these abilities is able to think logically, to reflect, reason and deliberate. She is able to analyze and synthesize, to draw upon and use concepts and principles from the natural, physical, biological, nursing and behavioral sciences in order to meet the nursing needs of others. A nurse possessing the therapeutic use of self consciously uses her personality and knowledge in order to establish relatedness, and to structure nursing intervention. Both of these abilities i.e., the disciplined intellectual approach and the therapeutic use of self, are learned slowly over a long period of time and it is usually a lifetime goal toward which we work for the synthesis of these abilities. The communication abilities are never completely learned—there is always more to be achieved in this area.

A nurse is considered to be skillful in using the process of communication to plan, direct, guide and evaluate nursing intervention when she demonstrates the behaviors implied in the communication abilities. Competency is also evaluated in terms of the extent to which the purpose of nursing is achieved and, more specifically, in the nurse's ability to interact and communicate in such a way as to (1) know ill persons, (2) ascertain and meet needs and (3) fulfill the purpose of nursing.

The communication skills are divided into two categories: abilities needed by all educated individuals, and specific abilities having implication in nursing situations.

GENERAL ABILITIES

1. Ability to read
    to comprehend what was read
    to interpret correctly what was read
    to apply knowledge gained through reading

2. Ability to express oneself in writing
    to use correct spelling
    to use correct grammer

3. Ability to express oneself in speaking
    to speak clearly, concisely and to the point
    to speak with (not at, or to) others
    to use appropriate vocabulary when conversing with others
    to speak with others at their level of understanding and to do this without con-
        descension

4. Ability to listen, hear and interpret
    to interpret accurately the verbal and non-verbal communication of others

SPECIFIC ABILITIES

5. Ability to observe and interpret observations
    to use observational data to generalize and infer
    to develop valid inferences
    to validate inferences with the ill person and others
    to use validated inferences in planning nursing intervention

6. Ability to direct or guide the interaction in order to accomplish goals
   to develop general and specific objectives prior to an interaction
   to be able to change objectives if necessary, in order to meet nursing needs

7. Ability to ascertain *if* communication is taking place and to understand what is being transmitted in the interpersonal process
   to assess what is being transmitted in the interpersonal process

8. Ability to recognize when to speak and when to be silent
   to develop a sense of timing

9. Ability to wait
   to proceed at the other individual's pace

10. Ability to evaluate one's participation in the interaction
    to evaluate the extent to which goals were achieved
    to plan further intervention on the basis of new data obtained

The extent to which these abilities will be developed is invariably a matter of degree. However, it is deemed essential that the nurse develop at least minimal competency in each of the abilities.

The communication abilities are interdependent and interlocking in that each is dependent on the other. The abilities may be viewed as a nursing hierarchy of steps, each step leading to the fulfillment of the purpose of nursing. If one step or phase is missing, if the nurse does not possess at least minimal competency in a particular ability, it is probable that the purpose of nursing will not be fulfilled. For example, if a nurse does not possess the ability to observe in a meaningful manner, then she will not be able to interpret any observation. Neither will she be able to develop inferences, validate them, or use validated inferences in planning nursing care.

There are certain prerequisites in developing the ability to communicate and interact in such a way as to achieve the goals of the interaction. One of these is that it is necessary for the individual to develop an understanding of his current communication pattern, or how he habitually interacts with others, in order to identify his weaknesses and strengths.

A primary prerequisite is the ability to focus on another individual. Without this ability no one can develop and/or improve skill in communication. It is possible to communicate without this ability, but it is not possible to become aware of *what* one is fully communicating without it.

The ability to focus on another person includes the ability to give undivided attention to the other person, to be "all there" psychologically as well as physically, "to be still' and receptive to the communication of another and eliminate, insofar as is possible, any distractions which tend to interfere with the communication process. It is basically a contemplative act. An individual possessing this ability not only listens, but is able to perceive all of the varying shades and nuances of meaning which are transmitted in the communication.

The ability to focus on another person is the ability to transcend self, yet to use all of one's faculties to understand what is occurring in the interaction, and thereby be enabled to guide and direct purposefully the interaction in order to fulfill the purpose of nursing. A nurse who lacks the ability to focus on another individual will not meet the nursing needs of the ill human being.

The ability to focus on another individual is a prerequisite to being able to use communication techniques in any meaningful way. Factors which tend to hinder the development of the communication abilities are discussed in Part VI, "Communication Breakdown."

PART V—THE COMMUNICATION TECHNIQUES

DEFINITION OF THE TERM "COMMUNICATION TECHNIQUES"

Communication techniques are methods used to accomplish the specific as well as the overall goals of nursing intervention. As such, the communication techniques include not only the use of verbal interchange with ill persons but also all non-verbal means used by the nurse to influence the recipient of her care. Techniques are valuable and useful in facilitating communication when used in a *judicious* manner.

Communication techniques are a means to an end, the end being the achievement of the purpose of nursing. More specifically, techniques are useful in getting to know ill persons, in establishing relatedness, and eliciting and meeting needs.

Communication techniques are not panaceas for ailing interactions. There are no magical phrases one can utter to establish relatedness. The skillful use of techniques will not assist a nurse in establishing relatedness, if the nurse's basic attitude towards ill persons is one of disinterest or unconcern. There is always the possibility that a nurse will become so interested in the *how* (i.e., the technique) that she will ignore the *why* (or reason for using the technique). However, techniques *are* useful when the nurse understands *why* she is using them and *what* she hopes to accomplish.

Because each nurse is unique she will be more comfortable in using certain techniques than others. No one should force himself to use a particular technique, if by its use, spontaneity and naturalness are sacrificed in the interpersonal process.

A guiding principle in selection and use of communication techniques is as follows: The nurse should use any communication technique whereby she is enabled to explore and understand the meaning of the ill person's communication.

Certain prerequisites are necessary before using communication techniques purposefully and effectively. These prerequisites are that the nurse possess and use a disciplined intellectual approach, combined with the therapeutic use of self. These prerequisites imply possession by the nurse of *the knowledge underlying the skills* and the ability to use this knowledge in order to achieve the purpose of nursing.

THE TECHNIQUES

The judicious use of the following techniques will facilitate communication:

Use of Open-Ended Comments or Questions

Examples: "And then you . . ."
"You were saying . . .?"
"And after that you . . .?"

These are bridge phrases or transition phrases. They do not block communication but encourage the individual to continue speaking. An exclamation that is sometimes quite effective is "Oh." "Oh" used with varying inflections, nodding of the head and other non-verbal communication will encourage individuals to continue speaking.

The nurse may also encourage the ill person to verbalize by using non-verbal means such as head or hand movements which convey the message "continue" or "keep talking." In some instances non-verbal methods may be more effective than verbal methods in assisting ill persons to continue speaking.

Use of The Reflecting Technique

The "reflecting technique" is probably the best known, least understood, and most popular communication technique. There are two general categories of reflecting techniques: one is to reflect (or repeat) certain words or phrases spoken by the other person in order to facilitate communication. This is known as *reflecting content*. When reflecting content the nurse repeats the individual's statement in the form of a question. An example of reflecting content is as follows:

Mr. Jones, "I want to go home."
Nurse,   "You want to go home?"
Mr. Jones, "Yes, I'm so worried about my children and my wife."

In this example the nurse demonstrates her willingness to explore with Mr. Jones his reasons for wanting to go home. The exploratory process would have been blocked had the nurse responded with such statements as, "What's the matter, don't you like it here?" or "What did your doctor tell you about going home?"

In the example given above, a short sentence was reflected. This example may give the impression that the technique of reflecting content is easy whereas in actuality it is one of the most difficult of all techniques. The nurse must decide which statement, out of a series of comments made by an ill person, is most likely to yield meaningful data when explored.

The second category of reflecting techniques is the reflection of feelings or impressions. An example of *reflecting feelings and impressions* is as follows:

Nurse,   "Good morning, Mr. Smith, how are you today?"
      Mr. Smith sighs but does not answer.
Nurse,   "Mr. Smith?"
Mr. Smith, "Oh, I'm pretty good, nurse."

The nurse gets the impression that Mr. Smith is depressed and somewhat angry about something. She reflects the feelings she has perceived by stating,

"You seem sad this morning, Mr. Smith . . ." or
"You look like you're angry about something . . . what's wrong?"

By reflecting feelings and impressions the nurse gives the individual an opportunity to talk about his feelings. Both nurse and ill person explore the probable underlying causes motivating the feeling. On the basis of the data obtained, the nurse plans whatever action is needed in order to alleviate the individual's distress. It may be that the only action the nurse *can* take is to be more supportive towards the individual in his time of crisis.

The reflecting technique can be valuable and useful but it can also be misused. The following example illustrates this point.

Mr. Adams, "I don't like this room."
Nurse,   "You don't like this room?"
Mr. Adams, "No, I don't like the bed."
Nurse,   "You don't like the bed?"
Mr. Adams, "No, I don't like anything about this room."
Nurse,   "You don't like anything about this room?"
Mr. Adams, (angrily) "Isn't that what I've been telling you?"

The above is an example of misusing a communication technique and thereby blocking communication. In this instance the nurse failed to heed the principle regarding the selection and use of communication techniques, namely, *the nurse should use any technique whereby she is enabled to explore and become clear as to the meaning of the ill person's communication.*

Use of The Technique of Sharing Perceptions

Orlando suggests that the nurse share her perceptions with the ill person in order to ascertain the meaning of the individual's behavior. According to Orlando, we perceive, have automatic thoughts about our perceptions, then feel a certain way about these perceptions and thoughts. An example follows:

The nurse perceives the ill person's hands are trembling.
She thinks the person is anxious, is cold, etc.
The nurse then feels a certain way about her automatic thoughts.

Orlando suggests that the nurse share perceptions with the ill person. In this instance the nurse would state, "Your hands are trembling can you tell me why?" This is an example of sharing perceptions. According to Orlando it takes less time to ascertain the meaning of behavior if the nurse explores only what she perceives.[5] If sharing perceptions fails, Orlando suggests that the nurse next share thoughts and then feelings.[6]

Deliberate Use of Cliches

A cliche is a trite, automatic question or response. Cliches are used automatically,—i.e., without reflection or thought. They are, in fact, excellent substitutes for thinking. Cliches include "pat-answers" and "stock replies" such as "Don't worry you have a good doctor," "You'll be all right," etc., and miscellaneous questions such as "How are you feeling?," "Did you eat your breakfast?," "Did you sleep well last night?," and so forth, especially when these questions are asked, not with

---

[5] Orlando, Ida Jean: The Dynamic Nurse-Patient Relationship. New York: G. P. Putnam's Sons, 1961, p. 44.

[6] *Ibid.,* p. 55.

the intention of eliciting meaningful information, but in order to have something to say to ill persons.

The professional nurse *may* deliberately choose to utilize cliches as bridge or transition remarks at the beginning of an interaction. If purposefully chosen, and used for a definite identifiable purpose, then their use may be countenanced.

The cliche "How are you feeling?" is probably used by more nurses than any other and has achieved the status of a "nurse-ism." This question can elicit information provided the ill person perceives that the nurse *is* interested, *really* wants to know *how* he is feeling, and will take the time to listen. If the ill person perceives that the nurse doesn't really want to know how he is, he will respond automatically to this question by such comments as "pretty good," "fine," "OK," "not too bad," "so-so."

A suggested alternate to asking "How are you feeling?" is to ask "How's *it* going?" The "*it*" in "how is *it* going" can be anything the individual chooses. Useful information may be elicited by using this particular question.

Summary

The communication techniques are devices or methods used purposefully in nurse-patient and other situations. These techniques are valuable and useful in facilitating communication when used in a judicious manner. The nurse should use any communication technique whereby she is enabled to explore and understand the meaning of the patient's communication. In the next section, the causes of communication breakdown and distortion are considered.

PART VI—COMMUNICATION BREAKDOWN

In order for communication to take place there must be a sender and a recipient, and the message must be understood by all concerned. Communication breakdown (or failure to communicate) occurs when a message is not received, or when a message is misinterpreted or misunderstood. Communication breakdown can also occur when one participant in the interaction receives and correctly interprets the message, but for some reason does not wish the other person to know that the message has been understood. Not wishing to communicate, or a "lack of good intention," can effectively block communication. In other instances, communication is blocked when one participant in an interaction responds automatically without deliberation, and thus hinders or blocks the other participant from expressing himself since this lack of deliberation gives the impression of lack of interest or of ignorance.

There are many causes of communication breakdown and distortion. Some of the major causes are discussed in the following paragraphs.

MAJOR CAUSES OF COMMUNICATION BREAKDOWN AND DISTORTION

1. Failure to Perceive the Ill Person as a Human Being

Meaningful communication cannot occur in interactions when a participant fails to perceive the other as a unique human being. Failure to perceive the ill person as a human being is usually due to the nurse's stereotypes and preconceptions about ill persons. A stereotype is defined as ". . . a standardized mental picture . . . representing an oversimplified opinion . . . or uncritical judgment . . ." [7] A preconception is ". . . a conception or opinion previously formed." [8] Stereotypes and preconceptions are usually developed when nurses develop inferences and opinions about the behavior of a small group of ill persons, then generalize these beliefs until *all* persons in particular groups are considered to be alike. Some preconceptions and stereotypes are as follows:

1. All males are cooperative when ill.
2. All females are demanding when ill.
3. All (Black, Italian, Jewish, Indian, Catholic, etc.) individuals behave in certain ways when ill.

Preconceptions and stereotypes interfere with a nurse's ability to communicate and establish relatedness; they are mind-sets which hinder the nurse from responding and appreciating the uniqueness of others. A nurse also fails to perceive the ill person as a human being if she treats him *as if* he were someone else (i.e., the nurse's relative or someone from the nurse's past).

2. Failure to Recognize Levels of Meaning in Communication

Communication breakdown may be caused by failure to recognize that messages transmitted during the communication process may have meanings other than the apparent "obvious" literal meaning. Communication is also blocked when nurses accept statements made by ill persons at "face value," with no reflection or thought; or when nurses answer questions too quickly without exploring the ill person's meaning and intention.

It is important to ascertain what ill persons really mean when they ask questions or make comments. For example, an ill person asks a nurse, "When am I going home?" This particular question could mean any or none of the following:

a. The individual might want to know the day and hour of his discharge from the hospital.
b. He might want to know if his doctor signed the discharge slip.
c. He might be inquiring if the nurse knows that he has been discharged by his doctor.
d. He might want to know how he is progressing in his illness. He may want assurance that he will recover—that he will not die—or he may want to know if he will die.
e. The need might be to make a phone call in order to attend to urgent business matters.

---

[7] By permission. From Webster's Third New International Dictionary, copyright 1961 by G. & C. Merriam Co., Publishers of the Merriam-Webster Dictionaries.

[8] *Ibid.*

f. The individual might want to know when he is going home because he is running out of money and is afraid that he will not be able to pay his hospital bill if he remains any longer in the hospital.

g. He might want to know because he needs to get back to work, is afraid he will lose his job, etc.

The nurse who responds to an ill person's inquiry by asking if he has asked his doctor this question is blocking communication. Communication is also blocked if the nurse answers that she does not know. The task of the nurse, in such a situation, is to elicit from the individual his reason for asking the question and to proceed from there.

Another example illustrates the need to explore the particular meaning that ill persons attach to commonly used words or phrases. A nurse asks an ill person, "How do you feel?" The individual replies, "Pretty good." If the nurse accepts this statement at face value she well may believe that "all is well" with the individual. However, it must be remembered that the nurse's interpretation of "pretty good" may not coincide with the ill person's interpretation of this phrase. It is the task of the professional nurse to explore with the ill person the meaning attached to phrases.

For one ill person, "pretty good" may mean that "the pain is not as excruciating today as it was yesterday." Another person may use this term to mean "I am feeling well today." The nurse does not know the meaning of this phrase according to the ill person; therefore she must validate with the ill person what is meant.

3. Failure to Listen

Communication is blocked when one participant in an interaction fails to receive (listen to, or hear) a transmitted message. Failure to listen is a major cause of communication breakdown. Listening is an active process requiring the expenditure of energy as well as the ability to focus one's entire attention on the other individual. The nurse may not be willing to expend the necessary energy; she may be tired, preoccupied, bored or disinterested. She may fail to listen because of the manner in which the ill person speaks, i.e., if he mumbles, speaks in a low monotonous voice, or displays other speech habits which tend to encourage not-listening.

Failure to listen to ill persons also may be caused by the nurse talking too much, and interrupting the individual when he is conversing. *A cardinal rule for nurses to follow in interacting with ill persons is as follows: Never assume that an ill person likes to talk as much, or as little, as you do. Instead, strive to adjust to the ill person's tempo and pace in conversation.*

The nurse's failure to listen is often interpreted by ill persons, and probably rightly so, as disinterest in them as individuals. In order to listen, the nurse gives undivided attention to the ill person and is "all there" psychologically as well as physically. She devotes her entire attention to the person. She does not gaze out of the window, fiddle with objects, drum her fingers, or look at her watch.

The professional nurse consciously strives to improve her ability to listen—to hear and interpret what is occuring in the nursing interaction. She strives to become increasingly perceptive in communicating with others, and is willing to expend the energy needed to listen and to communicate purposefully.

4. Using Value Statements without Reflection

A nurse uses value statements when she responds to an ill person's comments by using such statements as "isn't that fortunate" or "fine" or "wonderful," etc., before discovering how the ill person feels about the situation in question. For example, an individual tells the nurse that he is going home tomorrow, and the nurse responds by saying, "Isn't that wonderful!" Unless it is *obvious* that the individual is pleased, it is suggested that the nurse first elicit from the ill person how he feels about going home instead of operating on the assumption that "all ill persons feel wonderful about going home." If the individual does not feel "wonderful" about going home and wishes to explore his feelings with the nurse, he may not feel free to do so, especially in view of the nurse's response.

The statement "I'm going home tomorrow" may have been initiated by the ill person for any number of reasons, one of which may be that the ill person is worried about caring for himself at home. The nurse's response blocks further exploration, and, unless the individual is unusually persistent and explains his problems to the nurse, he will probably not allude to it again since he realizes that the nurse cannot or will not assist him in this matter.

5. Cliches and Automatic Responses

The use of cliches and automatic responses hinders and blocks communication. A cliche is a trite, tired, meaningless, hackneyed phrase or question. Cliches are used automatically without reflection or thought on the part of the nurse. Cliches include "pat answers" and "stock replies." Unless the nurse strives to become consciously aware of how she communicates she will probably revert to the use of cliches, which are employed to avoid thinking and also to maintain distance between the nurse and the ill human being. Some examples of typical cliches as used in nursing situations are:

A. An individual scheduled for surgery says to the nurse, "I am a little worried about my operation." Typical cliche-like responses on the part of the nurse may include any of the following answers:

1. "Don't worry, you have a good doctor."
2. "You'll be all right."
3. "I'm sure everything will be just fine."
4. "It's only minor surgery."
5. "You're worried about a little operation like that?"
6. "There's nothing to worry about."
7. "The man in the next room had the same surgery and he's doing fine."
8. "It'll be over with before you know it."
9. It's a simple operation. There is nothing to it."

All of the above responses will hinder or block the flow of communication. In this example, the nurse does not allow the ill person to explore the nature of his concern, and since she does not know what the problem is, not having discussed it, she is unable to assist the individual in resolving the difficulty. It is the task of the professional nurse practitioner to elicit from the ill person the nature of his concern and then to plan nursing intervention accordingly.

B. An individual is complaining of discomfort. The nurse says, "You shouldn't complain so much. Mr. Brown is much sicker than you are and he doesn't complain."

In this example, the nurse has completely ignored the fact that the ill individual and Mr. Brown are utterly different human beings, each responding to the experience of illness and suffering in his own unique manner. The nurse is in effect saying to the complaining person that he should not be like himself but instead be, and act like, Mr. Brown—an obvious impossibility. The nurse is also informing the ill person what type of behavior she (the nurse) finds acceptable.

In this example, communication is blocked and the establishment of a human-to-human relationship is not possible. The ill person's needs cannot be met, much less ascertained under such circumstances. The ill person, effectively blocked in expressing the nature of his discontent, has no recourse but to continue to complain or to give up seeking assistance from nurses. Although not a cliche per se, a similar device used by some nurses in the initiation of a bartering type of relationship wherein the nurse tells the ill person that if he cooperates with the nurses then the nurses will cooperate with him. An implied threat usually accompanies such a statement. That such manipulatory practices have no place in professional nursing practice cannot be overly emphasized.

C. A common cliche is telling ill persons, "I know just how you feel."

It is not possible to "know" just how another person feels; one can only imagine and one's imagination may well be inaccurate. In order to gain some degree of understanding of how another person feels it is necessary to elicit this information from the individual. This cliche-type remark effectively blocks the communication process.

D. Various questions nurses tend to ask ill persons are also considered as cliches, especially when nurses ask these questions without reflecting, or without the intention of eliciting any useful information to structure nursing intervention. Some examples are:

"How are you feeling?" (This is probably the most common cliche)
"Did you sleep well last night?"
"Did you eat your breakfast (or lunch or dinner)?"

All of the above questions *can* be purposefully used by the nurse in order to elicit meaningful data. The major difference between using these questions purposefully and using them as cliches lies in the purpose or intention of the nurse asking the question, her interest in the ill person, and her intention to elicit meaningful information which will assist her in planning nursing intervention.

Cliches are generally used, not so much to show interest in ill persons or to "reassure" and help them, but in order to make the nurse more comfortable. Of course, some nurses may use such cliches as "You'll be all right," honestly believing that they are reassuring individuals by telling them such things. Nurses who use cliches and automatic statements may "mean well," but they fail to reassure ill persons, fail to assist them, fail to meet their needs, and block the communication process. Ill persons arrive at the all too correct conclusion that there is no point in saying anything important to the nurse, because she is not going to understand anyway. Ill persons also may respond automatically because some nurses probably furnish such excellent examples for them to follow.

Cliches and automatic responses can be avoided by: first, becoming consciously aware that one is using them; second, by thinking before speaking; and third, by keeping in mind what it is one wishes to accomplish in nursing situations, namely, fulfillment of the purpose of nursing. Ill persons are not helped to cope with the stress of illness and suffering when they cannot communicate with the nurse, or if they do communicate to be blocked by the nurse.

The ability to think before speaking is a difficult discipline to learn, but it is the sine qua non of the communication process. The purposeful use of the communication process requires that the nurse has consciously thought out reasons for her comments and responses to ill persons. Communication process is hindered or blocked by using automatic responses, or tired cliche-like comments that are irrelevant and mean little or nothing to ill human beings.

6. Accusing, Blaming and Teasing

Another effective means of blocking communication is to accuse, blame or tease ill persons. Some nurses blame ill persons and verbally accuse them of causing their own illness or injury. The ill person may be accused, taunted, teased or in some way made to feel stupid, careless or inadequate. An individual who *knows* he caused his illness or injury is *not* helped by a nurse who accuses him of having brought his condition on himself. Some nurses give the impression that they are very busy and are not about to "waste time and sympathy" on anyone who deliberately causes his own hospitalization. The nurse behaves as if the individual's illness or injury is a personal affront to her. A case in point follows:

> While playing with friends a sixteen year old high school student fell beneath a tractor, crushing his right foot. Following emergency surgery he was admitted to a surgical nursing unit. The injured boy was well aware that his careless behavior led to his injury. He also realized that his ambition of a career in the military service was now an impossibility because of his injury. The evening nurse, while making rounds, greeted the boy with, "Oh, you're the kid who can't handle a tractor." The nurse acted annoyed when the injured boy asked for narcotics to ease his pain. Another nurse said to him, "You must have wanted a rest from school." She conveyed the impression that the boy had deliberately injured himself in order to evade school work! A nursing assistant, probably as a result of the example given by the "professional" nurses, never called the boy by name when conversing, but referred to him as "Crip."

By their behavior these nurses tried to induce guilt in the ill person, place him on the defensive and almost seemed to want the ill person to apologize for taking up their (the nurses') time. These kinds of behaviors are not only unprofessional, they are cruel, inhumane and punitive. Ill persons are dependent on the care given by health workers and hence are in a somewhat powerless situation. They are not likely to complain to health workers or to their supervisors about such treatment. Frequently ill persons and family members do not complain because they fear retaliation from nurses and other health workers. They do not complain while the ill person is hospitalized, but will bitterly relate these experiences to friends and others after the ill person has been discharged from the hospital.

Some nurses tease ill persons or attempt to induce shame in a misguided attempt to effect a change in the ill person's behavior. For example, they may tell an ill person who is crying to "stop acting like a baby." The nurse may also imply that the ill person is too big, too old, etc., to behave in such a childish manner. Behaviors such as accusing, blaming and teasing block the communication process. It is not possible for nurses to establish relatedness with ill persons when they use these kinds of tactics.

7. Failure to Interrupt

Another major cause of communication breakdown and distortion seems to stem from the nurse's belief that it is impolite to interrupt ill persons while they are speaking. For example, an ill person may talk for some period of time, may bring forth numerous and diverse ideas that require exploration. The nurse may not clearly understand *what* the individual means. Unless the nurse interrupts the individual's conversation, it is not likely that she will be able to remember, much less explore with the person, the meaning of his comments. It is therefore recommended that the nurse interrupt the ill person's conversation and clarify any unclear comments. *A guiding principle is that the nurse should explore with the ill individual any comment that she does not understand.*

Such are the major causes of communication breakdown and distortion. Failure to communicate cannot always be prevented; however, it can nearly always be recognized. In order to recognize communication breakdown and distortion the professional nurse practitioner continuously evaluates her ability to communicate and to extract and use meanings communicated to her in nursing situations. Improvement in nurse's ability to communicate is probably possible only if such an evaluation process is a continuous one.

Professional nurse practitioners do not consider themselves to be "communication experts," i.e., individuals who "know" so much and are so capable that they cannot improve. Professional nurses know they can improve their ability to use the communication process more purposefully and are continually seeking ways and means of doing so.

N.B. References used in this chapter are in the footnotes. These are not repeated.

SECTION *FIVE*

The purposes of this section are to identify and explore the nature of the helping process in nursing, namely the human-to-human relationship, and to consider specific ways in which nurses can assist ill persons to cope with the stress of illness and suffering.

In Chapter X the term "human-to-human relationship" is defined and differentiated from a "nurse-patient interaction." The characteristics of a human-to-human relationship are discussed as are the phases leading to the establishment of a relationship. A permeating belief is that the human-to-human relationship is the means through which the purpose of nursing is achieved.

In Chapter XI, "Nursing Intervention," the nurse's responsibility in assisting ill persons to find meaning in illness and suffering is explored. Specific ways and means of assisting ill individuals with various reactions to the stress of illness and suffering are discussed as are ways of assisting the ill person's family. A major belief is that it is the role of the professional nurse practitioner to assist ill persons to find meaning in the experience of illness, suffering and pain.

In Chapter XII, Surgery: A Human Experience is discussed. The preparation of the ill person for the surgical experience is explored.

Chapter X

THE HUMAN-TO-HUMAN RELATIONSHIP

A major assumption of this work is that it is the task of the professional nurse practitioner to establish a human-to-human relationship. A characteristic of the human-to-human relationship is that both nurse and ill person perceive and relate to each other as unique human beings, rather than as "nurse" to "patient." In order to establish human-to-human relatedness, the facades of "nurse" and "patient" must be penetrated in order to reach the humanity of each person.

The term "nurse-patient relationship" is not used in this text because it is believed that a "nurse" and a "patient" cannot establish a relationship. It is only when each individual in the interaction perceives the other as a human being that a relationship is possible.

The human-to-human relationship, in nursing situations is the means through which the purpose of nursing is accomplished, namely, to assist an individual (or family) to prevent, or cope with, the experience of illness and suffering, and to help him (or his family) to find meaning in these experiences.

Everything the nurse says and does for and with ill persons helps to fulfill the purpose of nursing. The final measure of nursing competency is always in terms of the extent to which individuals and families have been assisted with the problems of illness and suffering.

Each contact the nurse has with the recipient of ther care can be a step leading in the direction of a human-to-human relationship. This is especially true, if, in each contact, the nurse intentionally strives to know the recipients of her care and to ascertain and meet their needs.

The human-to-human relationship does not "just happen." It is built day by day as the nurse interacts with ill persons and others. It implies that the nurse knows what she is doing, thinking, feeling and experiencing. The nurse structures nursing intervention in full conscious awareness, making full use of available knowledge and understanding.

Another major assumption is that a human-to-human relationship is established after nurse and recipient of her care have progressed through four preceding interlocking phases. These phases are: (1) the original encounter, (2) emerging identities, (3) empathy and (4) sympathy. All of these phases culminate in rapport and the establishment of the human-to-human relationship.

The establishing of a relationship may proceed at any rate of speed—either slowly or rapidly. There may be a sequence of progression followed by retrogression to a previous phase. Some degree of progression and retrogression is inevitable as nurse and ill person work through the various phases together. Progress may cease or "level off" at any phase with the result of relatedness not being achieved. This cessation of progression may be temporary or permanent. However, it is the nurse's responsibility to identify reasons for failure to progress towards relatedness, and to intervene in such a manner to reactivate progression. In some instances, nurse colleagues may be useful in identifying factors that are hindering progression towards relatedness and rapport.

The term "human-to-human relationship" and the terms "relatedness" and "rapport" are considered as synonymous. The human-to-human relationship is characterized by rapport and includes all elements necessary for rapport.

Part I of this chapter contains a definition of terms and a discussion of "nurse-patient interactions," and further differentiates a nurse-patient interaction from a relationship. In Part II, the term "human-to-human relationship" and its characteristics are defined and discussed. In Part III, the phases leading to the establishment of a human-to-human relationship are considered.

PART I—DISCUSSION OF THE TERM "NURSE-PATIENT INTERACTION"

DEFINITIONS OF TERMS

The term "interaction" refers to any contact during which two individuals have reciprocal influence on each other and communicate verbally and/or nonverbally.

The term "nurse-patient interaction" refers to any contact between a nurse and an ill person and is characterized by the fact that both individuals perceive the other in a stereotyped manner. The nurse perceives the ill person as a category, i.e., as a "patient," not as a unique human being. The ill person perceives the human being who is the nurse as a stereotype of all nurses he has known or encountered.

DISCUSSION OF NURSE-PATIENT INTERACTIONS

There are all kinds of interactions—some helpful and useful to ill persons, some not useful. Some of the ill person's needs may be met during the interactive process, but in the interaction these needs are not met consistently and unconditionally. The human-to-human relationship, in nursing situations, is primarily differentiated from the nurse-patient interaction in that the nursing needs of the ill person are met consistently and unconditionally. Although one may speak of a "good nurse-patient interaction or relationship" or a "poor" one, the term "human-to-human relationship" is not qualified. A human-to-human relationship *is* good, *is* helpful, and the ill person's needs *are* met.

Interactions occur when the nurse communicates with the ill person, gives medications, performs nursing procedures, or gives prescribed treatments. Nurses interact with ill persons when giving direct physical care, engaging in health teaching, or when directing the ill person's activities.

KINDS OF NURSE-PATIENT INTERACTIONS

There are all kinds of nurse-patient interactions. Some interactions are characterized by superficiality, a lack of personal involvement or commitment on the part of the nurse, and by the fact that the ill person's nursing needs are not met. Some of the individual's needs may be met, but they are met inconsistently—some in a conditional manner, meeting certain needs and not others.

THE "AUTOMATIC INTERACTION"

There is a type of interaction having little or no significance to either individual involved. There is an automatic quality to this type of encounter; neither nurse nor ill person moves toward knowing each other; both communicate, but they do not relate and fail to proceed in the direction of a relationship. The nurse does not possess, and therefore cannot use, the disciplined intellectual approach or the therapeutic use of self.

THE HELPFUL NURSE-PATIENT INTERACTION

Some nurse-patient interactions are "helpful" and useful to ill persons even though the contact never proceeds to a relationship level. For example, a nurse may give excellent physical care to an ill person, not because she is interested in the individual, but because she wants to live up to the expectations of others such as her co-workers, colleagues, supervisors, and physicians, or she is trying to live up to her own expectations. Ill persons may be grateful to nurses who give such physical care even though they sense that the nurse is not interested in them personally. In such a case, this type of interaction may be helpful and useful to ill persons.

THE "INVOLUNTARY" NURSE-PATIENT INTERACTION

Some nurses never interact voluntarily, i.e., their only encounter with ill persons occurs when they *must* perform some required treatment. Such nurses generally carry out a function of nursing thoroughly, and that function is the "dependent" function of "carrying out the doctor's orders." There may be many reasons for this behavior, such as a lack of understanding of the nature of nursing, or the responsibility of the professional nurse. In some few nurses this behavior may be the result of the manner in which their position is perceived. Nursing may be "just a job" to these nurses and they are not willing to do any more than is absolutely necessary. They will perform all tasks for which they may be held accountable, such as performing treatments, giving medications, charting, sending in the proper requisition forms and so forth. But they will not voluntarily "just talk" with ill persons in order to anticipate or ascertain needs. As one nurse stated, "Let's just leave well enough alone. All you have to do is to go in their rooms and believe me they'll always want something. I have enough to do as it is without looking for more work."

With the possible exception of psychiatric nursing, nurses generally are not evaluated by their supervisors on the basis of their ability to relate with ill persons or support them in their time of crisis. Neither are nurses promoted because they are able to establish rapport with ill persons and their families. The nurse most likely to be promoted or considered a "good nurse" by the power hierarchy seems to be the nurse who "gets the work done," i.e., the nurse who carries out the doctor's orders, gives medications on time, sees to it that beds are made and baths are given before ten o'clock in the morning, sends in the proper requisition forms and doesn't complain too much. Such behaviors are given high priority and nurses are rewarded for engaging in these activities. It is quite possible for a nurse to be considered a "good nurse" by nursing supervisors even though the nurse never voluntarily interacts with ill persons.

Why is it that some nurses seldom interact voluntarily with ill persons? Many nurses are graduates of schools of nursing whose faculties overly stressed nursing techniques and methods. As students these nurses were never taught the importance of talking with ill persons in order to assist them in their time of crisis. Graduates of such programs are usually highly trained technicians; they are, however, unprepared to assist ill human beings to cope with illness and suffering. Because such nurses are unprepared, they tend to avoid interactions with ill persons whenever possible.

The nurse who *knows* she should spend time with ill persons to get to know them as human beings may not do so if she observes that her colleagues do not engage in such activities and do not consider them important. The young graduate who wishes to establish relationships with ill persons may not do so because of pressures from her peer group.

Nurses also may perform *only* those activities for which they may be held accountable as one way of "getting back" or "getting even" with their employers. This is especially true in those settings where the nurses feel underpaid and not appreciated by their employers.

THE "INCONSISTENT" NURSE-PATIENT INTERACTION

There is another kind of interaction characterized by conditional interest or conditional kindness on the part of the nurse. Some nurses will become interested in an ill person only under certain circumstances, such as critical illness. Some become interested in the ill person during a particular phase of illness, and not other times. Some nurses exhibit their "caring quality" most often when the person is utterly dependent, and not at other times. But even this type of interaction may be helpful and useful to the ill individual. A conditional interest or kindness may be perceived by the ill person as being better than none at all. And if it is perceived as such one would say that such interactions, though not approved because of lack of consistency, might be helpful and useful to ill persons, and better than no interest at all. It is that old question of "half a loaf being better than none." While this may be true in regard to bread, it is a maxim of dubious merit when used to explain (or excuse) poor and inconsistent nursing care.

Thus a nurse-patient interaction, whether helpful or not, may be the means through which some of an ill person's needs are met. However, each interaction affords an opportunity for the nurse to get to know ill persons, and to ascertain and meet their needs. It is the task of the professional nurse practitioner to plan, direct and guide purposefully the interaction in such a way as to develop a relationship.

Interactions will proceed in the direction of a relationship as the nurse and ill person move through the process of knowing, or of striving to know, each other. The nurse progressively uses intellectual operations and reasoning to structure nursing intervention which will alleviate the ill person's distress. There is progressive development of warmth in the interaction, a more consistent attitude and feeling of acceptance; interest and confidence grow as nurse and ill person move through the phases preceding rapport. There is a mutual perception of each other as a unique human being and a definite perception on the part of the ill person that he means something—he matters as a human being. Nursing actions become less automatic and more purposeful. Thinking, feeling and acting are not separated but merge together. Every nursing action is thus purposefully designed to assist the ill human being or individual in need of the services of the nurse can offer.

PART II—DEFINITION AND DISCUSSION OF THE TERM "HUMAN-TO-HUMAN RELATIONSHIP"

DEFINITION

A human-to-human relationship is primarily an experience or series of experiences between a nurse and the recipient(s) of her care. The major characteristic of these experiences is that the nursing needs of the individual (or family) are met. The human-to-human relationship is purposefully established and maintained by the professional nurse practitioner.

DISCUSSION

The human-to-human relationship is an experience or series of experiences between two human beings—a nurse and an individual (or family) in need of the service the nurse can render. However, it is a particular kind of experience, namely, a *mutually significant experience.*

The relationship is significant and meaningful in that *both* nurse and recipient have needs met as a result of this experience. Some may object to this statement, believing that nurses should *always* concentrate on meeting the needs of the other person, but never their own. This is unrealistic; the nurse is a human being and, as a human being, is needful. A nurse does not cease being human (or needful) during her eight-hour tour of duty. To expect otherwise is unrealistic. The exhortation "meet patients' needs but not your own" seems noble and altruistic, but if strictly adhered to results in dehumanization of the nurse. It is not possible for nurses to gain any degree of job satisfaction unless they are able to meet *some* of their needs in the work situation.

The nurse meets some needs through establishing relationships with ill persons and through meaningful contacts with co-workers and others. Certainly not all of a nurse's needs are met in the work situation; neither are the ill person's. But it seems that some needs *must* be met if the nurse is to experience job satisfaction. Nurses are not apt to be able to meet the needs of ill persons in any consistent way if their own needs are ignored.

The human-to-human relationship is a reciprocal process. A relationship is not established by the nurse alone; both nurse and ill person establish relatedness as they progress through the phases preceding rapport. However, the responsibility for establishing and maintaining the relationship rests with the professional nurse—not with the ill individual.

The human-to-human relationship is an experience characterized by a particular way of behaving, i.e., perceiving, thinking, feeling and acting. Each participant in the relationship perceives and responds to the human-ness of the other; that is, the "patient" is perceived and responded to as a unique human being—not as "an illness," "a room number," or as a "task to be performed." Neither is he stereotyped as the personification of "all patients" the nurse has encountered. In turn, the nurse is perceived and responded to as a unique human being—not as the personification of "all nurses." The way in which each participant views the other is rooted in reality and truth; each is perceived as he is, namely, as a unique utterly different human being. In order to perceive and respond to the human-ness of others the barriers of title, position and status must be transcended.

The relationship is reciprocal in that both nurse and ill person engage in similar activities as they move through the phases preceding rapport. It is the task of the professional nurse to observe the recipients of her care; however, in any face-to-face encounter, the observer (the nurse) is also the observed. Many other activities thought of as lying strictly within the province of nursing are also engaged in by ill persons. For example, the teacher (the nurse) is also a learner. In fact, every encounter provides an opportunity for professional nurses to learn.

Nursing Needs of the Individual or Family Are Met

The major characteristic of the human-to-human relationship is that the nursing needs of the individual (or family) are met. What do we mean by nursing needs? How is a nurse to ascertain the nursing needs of an individual, or family? Is there any systematic plan or method that a nurse may use which will guide her in more effectively meeting the nursing needs of ill persons as she progresses through the phases preceding the human-to-human relationship?

Definition of Nursing Need

A nursing need is any requirement of the ill person (or family) which can be met by the professional nurse practitioner, and which lies within the scope of the legal definition of nursing practice. A nursing need is also a requirement which, if met, assists the individual (or family) to prevent (or cope with) the experience of illness and suffering.

Steps in Meeting Nursing Needs

The following steps may be used as a guide in determining and planning to meet the nursing needs of ill persons and families:

1. *The nurse must be observant in order to ascertain if the person is in need.*

The ill person may inform the nurse of his need; however, as Orlando states, ill persons have difficulty many times in communicating their needs to nurses.[1] Nurses cannot always rely on ill persons to inform them of their needs. A nurse can, of course, infer the existence of a need through *systematic observation* of the ill person's behavior. Systematic observation implies that the nurse possess a fund of knowledge, skill and ability. She must know what to observe, how to observe, as well as be able to judge the relative importance of what has been observed. Florence Nightingale's thoughts about observation in nursing are as pertinent and meaningful today as they were when written more than a century ago. She states:

"The most important practical lesson that can be given to nurses is to teach them what to observe—how to observe—what symptoms indicate improvement—what the reverse—which are of importance—which are of none—which are the evidence of neglect—and what kind of neglect." [2]

"In dwelling upon the vital importance of sound observation, it must never be lost sight of what observation is for. It is not for the sake of piling up miscellaneous information or curious facts, but for the sake of saving life and increasing health and comfort." [3]

". . . it may be safely said, not that the habit of ready and correct observation will by itself make us useful nurses, but that without it we shall be useless with all our devotion." [4]

In this step the nurse, through observation and communication with the ill person, becomes aware that the individual is in need and develops inferences as to the nature of the need. The nurse may develop automatic interpretations or inferences as to the nature of the need to be met; hence the nurse should validate these inferences with the ill person.

---

[1] Orlando, Ida Jean: The Dynamic Nurse-Patient Relationship. New York: G. P. Putnam's Sons, 1961, p. 26.

[2] Nightingale, Florence. Notes on Nursing—What It Is and What It Is Not. Selected Writings from Florence Nightingale. (Compiled by Lucy R. Seymer.) New York: Macmillan Co., 1954, p. 194.

[3] *Ibid.*, p. 208.

[4] *Ibid.*, p. 199.

2. *The nurse validates the inference.*

In order to validate the inferences developed in step one, the nurse initiates an exploratory process, i.e., she explores with the person her inference that he is in need, and gives him an opportunity to discount or corroborate her inference. Orlando suggests that the nurse share perceptions, thoughts and feelings with the ill person in order to ascertain if the individual is in need, and as a means of determining the exact nature of the need.[5]

There are many situations in nursing, however, when nurses cannot explore with the ill person (or his family) his possible needs. In emergency situations the nurse must quickly assess the individual's condition, develop inferences on the basis of the available data, and make an on-the-spot judgment as to the probable needs of the ill person; then is initiated any action required to meet these needs. However, in most instances the nurse does have the opportunity to explore her inference regarding the need with the ill person. After validating the nature of the need, the nurse then moves into the area of decision-making.

3. *The nurse decides if she can (or should) meet the ill person's need, or if the individual should be referred to some other health worker.*

When the nurse identifies needs related to health care (other than nursing needs) it is her responsibility to refer the ill person to the health worker whose function it is to give required aid. However, it remains the nurse's responsibility to follow-up any referral made, and to work closely with members of other health disciplines. Referral is a means of assisting ill persons, and not a means of disposing of unwanted problems. There are instances in which it is difficult to ascertain if a need is indeed one which nurses can or should meet. Hospital or agency policies, as well as consultation with colleagues, may be needed to arrive at a decision. Unfortunately, some nurses completely relinquish all responsibility for any "follow-up" once they have referred an ill person to the appropriate agency or individual. This is especially true in regard to "meeting the spiritual needs of ill persons." The nurse may stop trying to meet these needs once she has notified the individual's rabbi, priest, or minister. Many articles have appeared in the literature stressing the importance of the nurse's function in meeting the spiritual needs of ill persons. Most of these articles stress the importance of the nurse having some knowledge of the major teachings of the various religious faiths; also stressed is the nurse's role in notifying the ill person's priest, rabbi or minister if the ill person requests such visitation or is in danger of dying. It cannot be denied that nurses, as educated individuals, should possess knowledge of the various religious faiths, and it is her function to notify spiritual counselors when necessary. However, it is often overlooked that the spiritual needs of ill persons are best met by the nurse who is spiritually oriented, and demonstrates the tenets of her faith in her behavior.

There will be some needs a nurse cannot meet. Obviously a nurse cannot practice outside the limits of the legal definition of nursing practice. Neither can she fulfill the ill person's needs if these needs conflict with the medical care plan.

---

[5] Orlando, *op. cit.*, pp. 44-45.

For example, an individual on a low sodium diet cannot be given a regular diet. The nurse can, however, inform the individual's physician of any complaints and contact the dietician to instruct and talk with the person. If the nurse is working in a setting where dietitians are not available, it is the nurse's responsibility to instruct the individual. It is important for nurses to become aware of the free (and readily accessible) teaching materials which are available through the various health associations. Instructing the ill person about his diet is necessary (whether this be done by dietitian or nurse); however, instruction alone will not necessarily assist the ill person in adjusting to, or coping with, the difficulties imposed on him by being on such a diet. It is the *nurse's* responsibility to assist the ill person in coping with the knowledge that his entire way of life may be affected by the fact of being required to remain on such a diet.

In step three, the nurse decides if she or another health worker is best prepared to meet the ill person's needs. If she decides that there is a nursing need she then begins to plan a course of nursing action. If the ill person should be referred to other health workers the nurse makes the referral *and works closely with the members of the other health discipline.*

4. *The nurse plans a course of nursing action (based on validated inferences).*

In this step the nurse (a) decides the method in which the individual's need should be met, (b) determines when the need should (or can) be met and (c) develops alternate means or ways of meeting the ill person's needs.

The method in which the ill person's need should be met depends on a multiplicity of factors. In order to make this decision the nurse must be able to draw upon and use concepts and principles from the natural, physical, biological, behavioral, medical and nursing sciences. The selection of methodology also requires that the nurse know the individual's medical history, physical status, diagnosis, etc., as well as have a thorough understanding of the ill person's medical care plan. All of this knowledge, however, may not assist the nurse unless she *knows* the individual with the need. It must be remembered that one may "know" all of the facts about an ill person, may thoroughly understand "his case," i.e., from the standpoint of etiology, symptomatology, course, prognosis and treatment, and still not *know* the ill person. *Knowledge about* an individual cannot be equated with *knowledge of* the individual. In nursing practice, knowledge *about* and knowledge *of* the individual are essential.

There is always a choice of methodology; the nurse invariably must decide *how* needs are met, even in those instances when it appears that there is no choice or decision to be made. A case in point is that of a postoperative person who cannot void. Assume that the nurse has tried all of the usual nursing measures and all have been unsuccessful and the physician directs that the individual be catherized. The nurse must decide *how* she can best perform this (or any) procedure taking into consideration her knowledge of, and about, this particular person. Judgment of the most discriminating type is needed in professional nursing. Nursing care will never become truly *individualized* until nurses are able to make discriminating judgments regarding the care of ill persons based on her knowledge of them—in all treatment given them.

Closely related to the question of methodology is the question of when the ill person's needs can (or should) be met. The determination of timing in meeting nursing needs is important. Some needs may be met immediately, others cannot. An anxious individual who is scheduled for surgery is not apt to have his need, "freedom from fear," met during one short brief encounter with the nurse. This is possible, depending on the skill of the nurse, but not probable. The nurse, using her judgment, her knowledge of and about the ill person, her understanding of the effects of anxiety on behavior, decides that she will interact with the individual for a number of short frequent intervals in order to assist the individual to cope with the experience of anxiety. Each encounter is planned and purposeful, i.e., the nurse understands what it is she wishes to accomplish (the desired behavioral changes in the ill person), how she proposes to proceed in order to accomplish the goal, and decides when intervention is most likely to assist the individual. These decisions are not "snap judgments" made on the spur of the moment. Much thought and reflection has preceded the development of these decisions, the nurse can explain the bases upon which the decisions were reached, and can identify the underlying theoretical concepts.

Nursing needs are not static; new needs and problems are always emerging. Although decisions are made to intervene in certain ways to assist an individual, the nurse frequently discovers that her method of relieving the ill person's distress is ineffective. The nurse must then be prepared to revise her approach and to develop and use alternate ways of meeting the ill person's needs. There is actually no *one* way of meeting ill persons' needs; there are a multiplicity of ways. Each ill person and nurse are unique and, although the nursing needs and problems of a large number of ill persons may be similar, the ways in which the needs can be met are not. The professional nurse of today needs to possess a large fund of knowledge and the ability to use it; but she must also be flexible and willing to change. The ability to recognize the need to change the approach to the care of ill persons is contingent on the nurse's ability to evaluate the care she has given.

5. *The nurse evaluates the extent to which the need has been met.*

The nurse must ascertain if the ill person's need has been met. She does this by observing changes in the individual's behavior, and by exploring with the individual whether or not the need has been met. The nurse, then, relies on observation and communication skills in order to ascertain whether or not the person's needs have, in fact, been met. Ill persons will, at times, state that their needs have been met when they have not. In such cases, if the nurse does not believe that the individual has indeed been assisted by her actions, she explores the matter with the ill person again, and gives him the opportunity to tell her whether or not her actions have indeed assisted him. It must not be forgotten that in the final analysis, the ill person is the final authority on his own needs. The evaluation or assessment process, although listed as step five, actually is continuous throughout the nurse's contact with the ill person.

The five steps, listed as a guide in determining needs of ill persons, are useful in ascertaining and meeting the nursing needs of individuals and families. It is *not* the only method or way of ascertaining and meeting nursing needs. Methods are useful *only* if they assist the nurse in meeting the nursing needs of individuals and families. Methods are only of use, however, if the nurse understands the theoretical basis underlying the particular approach or method used. Without such an understanding of methods and approaches these become meaningless, and the use of such approaches does not meet the nursing needs of ill persons.

If the nurse lacks essential knowledge she will not be able to ascertain needs, much less meet them, in any consistent manner. Good intentions and kindness are not substitutes for understanding and skill in the nursing process.

A disciplined intellectual approach is necessary since the professional nurse must know *how* to think, and possess the facts and principles with which to think. However, a relationship is not established solely through the use of reasoning and logical thinking; a nurse may identify an individual's problems, making a nursing diagnosis, decide on a course of action to solve the problem and still not establish relatedness. This is especially true if the nurse perceives the ill person as a problem and not as a human being. A blend of the disciplined intellectual approach and the therapeutic use of self is needed in order to establish relatedness.

The Social Relationship and the Human-to-Human Relationship

A human-to-human relationship is not a "friend-to-friend" relationship. There are, however, similarities and differences between the two. The usual criterion is as follows: in a social relationship the needs of both individuals are of concern; in a human-to-human relationship the focus is on meeting the nursing needs of the ill person or recipient of the nurse's care. This, however, is not a strict delineation since the needs of the nurse are also of concern. What, then, is the difference?

Being a friend has its own requirements as does being a professional nurse. Certain behavior is expected from friends, as contrasted from that of professional nurses. The friend is under no obligation to intentionally initiate a helping process in order to meet his friend's needs, whereas the nurse *is* obligated to meet the person's nursing needs. Neither is the friend obliged to study and constantly seek new ways to assist his friend.

Friends care about each other, like each other, and develop some degree of interpersonal closeness. How does this correspond with establishing relatedness? It is not absolutely necessary for a nurse to *like* the recipient of her care in order to establish relatedness; however, it is probably not possible to establish relatedness if the nurse intensely *dislikes* the ill person.

A professional nurse is not apt to experience intense dislike for any individual if she is able to perceive the ill person as a unique, irreplaceable human being.

What degree of interpersonal closeness is considered appropriate in the nursing situation? This question may be answered by assuming that there are varying levels of relatedness, the minimum standard being that the ill person's nursing needs are met. It would seem that the degree of interpersonal closeness experienced by nurse and ill person may vary from mutual respect of each other as unique human beings, to perception on the part of the ill person that he matters as a human being to the nurse, and, possibly, to the warmth of genuine fondness.

The human-to-human relationship in nursing and the social relationship are, therefore, quite unlike each other, the differences being inherent in the requirements and obligations of the participants to each other, as well as in tasks to be performed. There is also the matter of choice. Individuals choose their friends. With the possible exception of certain private-duty nurses, nurses are not able to select or choose the ill persons for whom they will care. Neither can ill individuals or their family members choose their nurses, again the possible exception being private-duty nurses.

The social and human-to-human relationships are not diametrically opposed; it is simply that each is different in qualifications, requirements and obligations.

PART III—PHASES LEADING TO THE ESTABLISHMENT OF A HUMAN-TO-HUMAN RELATIONSHIP

As stated previously, the human-to-human relationship is a goal which is achieved after nurse and ill person have progressed through several preceding phases. These phases are discussed in this section.

PHASE OF THE ORIGINAL ENCOUNTER

When a nurse encounters a person for the first time, she observes and develops inferences and value judgments about the individual, as the person usually does about the nurse. Feelings are aroused in the interaction as a result of the inferences developed.

Observation is the first and most important step in the nursing process. Observation and development of inferences which follow are important, since they serve as the basis for decisions made. These inferences are important because what one "sees" or perceives about another—the thoughts and feelings engendered—tends to determine how one will behave or react towards the other individual. Thus, observation and the development of inferences and value judgments form the basis for subsequent interaction pattern.

The initial judgment formed during the phase of the original encounter is termed "first impressions," "snap judgments," or a "feeling" about the other person. The judgments and inferences are triggered by the perception of interpersonal cues, and by verbal and non-verbal communication. Generally, if the first impression we have of another person is a "good" one it is probably because the individual reminds us of an individual from our past and is similar to, or resembles, an individual with whom we have established a certain degree of relatedness. Another reason why we develop "good" impressions of individuals is probably because they meet our need for recognition as unique human beings. First impressions tend to be determined by the background experiences of the individuals involved. The initial judgment we make of another person may be distorted. Distortion occurs in the interpersonal process when an individual attributes, to the person with whom he is interacting, character traits possessed by an individual from his past. The initial judgments may change or modify as the process of knowing continues, or they may remain unchanged. Some individuals boast that their first impressions of other persons are invariably accurate. The individual who believes his first impressions are always accurate usually engages in self-fulfilling prophetic behavior. That is, the individual reacts toward the other person in such a way as to elicit the behavior required to fulfill the prophecy. An individual who boasts that his first impressions are invariably accurate and that he "never changes his mind" is either a very rigid person or an individual who cannot admit an error in judgment.

Usually in the original encounter the individual views the nurse as "a nurse" and the nurse views the person as "a patient." There is little or no recognition of uniqueness; generally both nurse and other person are stereotyped and categorized during the original encounter, and it is only when each views the other as a particular unique human being that these stereotypes are shattered. Since neither individual knows the other, both will rely on stereotypes until these are changed and displaced by new insights into each other. To operate on the assumption that both nurse and recipient of care are strangers to each other is true to the extent that neither knows or appreciates the uniqueness of the other. The human being who is "the nurse" has not perceived the human being in "the patient." Although neither nurse nor "patient" knows each other in the sense that the uniqueness of each is perceived, both may have preconceived ideas obtained from some past interaction or some other source of information. The nurse draws upon her fund of experience with prior "patients," and the "patient" uses his knowledge concerning past experiences with nurses. Lacking prior experience with nurses, individuals may rely on hearsay, or on knowledge gained through reading, television, and radio; lacking these sources the individual will supply in fantasy what has not been actually experienced.

To assume we know nothing about the particular individual with whom we are interacting, except as revealed and validated in the nursing process, may be true on an intellectual level but it is not necessarily true on an emotional level, depending, of course, on the nurse's perceptive ability. This "emotional knowledge" may (or may not) be accurate, but valid or not it *does* affect the interaction.

Task of the Nurse

The nurse's failure to recognize the manner in which she is perceiving the other individual—that he has been stereotyped as "the patient"—will prevent the nurse from moving into the next phase. The task of the nurse is clear; it is to break the bond of categorization in order to perceive the *human being* in the "patient."

It is probably easier to perceive the individuality and human-ness of those ill persons who appeal to us or who meet our needs. However, it is the task of the professional nurse practitioner to respond to the human-ness of *all* of the recipients of her care. Whether or not the ill person is personally appealing to us in no way lessens this responsibility. Actually, it is often the "unappealing" individual who has the greatest need to be recognized and treated as a human being by nurses and other health workers.

The ability to perceive the human being in "the patient" is probably determined to a large extent by the nurse's ability to transcend herself, as well as her interest in others as separate human beings, instead of as categories or extensions of herself. Inability to progress to the phase of true human understanding is exemplified in the dehumanized, superficial, mechanical types of interaction wherein the "nurse" never perceives a human being in "the patient." As stated previously, it matters very much whether an individual is perceived as "a patient" or as a unique human being. *Only human beings establish relatedness, not categories or labels.*

Nurses who have habitually perceived ill persons as "patients" have to *want* to perceive ill persons differently and then make the effort required to perceive the human-ness of each ill person they encounter. It is by no means an easy task to accomplish. A habit of perceiving others must be broken and a new way of viewing ill persons substituted.

Once the nurse begins to experience the uniqueness of the ill person and the individual begins to respond, the next phase is reached, i.e., emerging identities.

PHASE OF EMERGING IDENTITIES

The phase of emerging identities is characterized by the ability to appreciate the uniqueness of another person, as well as the ability to establish a bond with the other individual. It is getting beyond and outside of self to some extent in order to perceive another, yet using self as the instrument to accomplish this purpose. It is to perceive another less as a category, and more as a separate identity, but to still interact with him on the basis of his effect on oneself personally.

It is an experience of thought and feeling toward the other person and a recognition of the impact of his personality. A bond is established between two individuals, and yet a separating process begins in the sense that individual identities are emerging and are perceived as unique. The ability to perceive the uniqueness of another may be an involuntary non-deliberative process, or a voluntary deliberate one.

During this phase, both nurse and ill person begin to establish a bond and to view the other less as a category and more as a unique human being. The nurse begins to perceive how the unique human being who is "the patient" feels, thinks and perceives his situation. The ill person, in turn, begins to perceive the nurse as a different unique human being, and not as the personification of "all nurses."

This phase is not characterized by the clarity of uniqueness as perceived in the phase of empathy, but a beginning is made. Similarities and dissimilarities are emerging and are being recognized. The phase of emerging identities is an intermediate one laying the foundation for empathy, and deepening the process of understanding each to the other. Understanding of each to the other, in this sense, is used to describe an experience, not a deliberate act of the will.

Inability to Perceive the Uniqueness of Others

Inability to perceive the uniqueness of the ill person is demonstrated whenever the nurse reacts to him as though he were a category or individual from her past. Anytime a nurse reacts to another individual as someone other than he is—unique, different, yet in some ways a similar human being—she is not perceiving him as he is. Neither is the nurse perceiving the individual's uniqueness when she thinks, "I know how I would feel if I were in his place." How the nurse would feel (or thinks she would feel) does not necessarily correlate with how the individual feels; the nurse is not focusing on the separateness of her experiences as opposed to the other person's, but is assuming that these experiences are identical, which is an unrealistic and invalid assumption.

The inability to perceive the ill person as a separate unique human being is the starting point of many difficulties in the nursing situation and serves as a barrier to relatedness. One such barrier, due to the nurse's inability to separate herself from the other person, is termed *"over-identification."* Over-identification is usually caused by the inability of the nurse to separate herself and her problems from those of the ill person's. In such a situation, the nurse does not perceive and respond to the uniqueness and separateness of the human being, instead the nurse responds to herself "in the patient." "Conscious awareness of how one is actually perceiving the patient, or if one is 'using the patient' is essential in order to avoid this problem. It may be necessary that someone outside the nursing situation help the nurse so involved, since many times nurses in such situations have little or no understanding of what is occurring." [6]

Having been through experiences or situations similar to those to which the ill person is subjected may either help or hinder a nurse from perceiving the uniqueness of the individual. For example, because a nurse has had a fractured leg does not imply that she is better able to perceive the uniqueness of an individual with a fracture. The nurse seeing the individual with this type of condition may ruminate in fantasy on her own experiences and discomfort, and therefore never "see" the other individual at all; instead she "sees" herself in the injured person. She may never establish the bond or contact necessary in order to perceive the uniqueness of the ill person because she may not be able to separate her experience from that of the other individual.

Separation of experiences and identities is essential as well as is the maintenance of a tie or bond each to the other. Similarities of experience are important in order to empathize or to understand another, but similarities may blind nurses to

---

[6] Travelbee, Joyce: What's wrong with sympathy? Amer. J. Nurs. 64:69, 1964.

the perception of the separateness which is so essential in the understanding process.

It is important that nurses go beyond "seeing themselves in others" and begin to "see the object of their attention." It is possible, unless a nurse develops a conscious awareness of this problem, to focus on herself to such an extent that she never contacts or establishes a bond with the ill person.

Individuals vary greatly in their ability to perceive and respond to the uniqueness of others. What hinders an individual from developing this ability? An individual may need to deny differences because he is threatened by the uniqueness of others. One simply does not see what he doesn't want to see. How can the uniqueness of others pose a threat? With some individuals it simply never really occurs to them that there are people with different personalities, values and beliefs. Some lip service may be paid to this concept as demonstrated in the "it's a good thing everyone isn't alike" attitude. Every individual is unique; however, when an individual whose differences are markedly pronounced is encountered, his differences may be discounted, ignored, belittled; or he may be considered uneducated and ignorant, i.e., considered a person who "doesn't know any better." The tacit assumption is that the individual's judge does know better.

Use of Oneself as a "Yardstick"

There is a strong human propensity to use "oneself" as a yardstick against which others are judged and measured.[7] When others do not "measure up" a "decision" is made either to ignore, negate, or belittle the differences—or the person with differences. The uniqueness of others can be threatening to some individuals because anxiety is aroused. When the uniqueness of others is perceived there is also a tendency to compare oneself or one's beliefs with those of the other person. This comparison can intensify anxiety because one may begin to suspect the validity of one's own belief system. Some individuals seem to feel that the uniqueness of others threatens their own uniqueness, or in some ways takes "something away" from them. In such instances it is probably not the differences (or uniqueness) per se which threatens them, as much as the tendency to envy the other person's talents, gifts or assets.

Envy

Interactions may engender envy in both nurse and ill person. Ill persons may envy nurses' skills and supposed "secret knowledge" and "know-how." Not infrequently women will inform nurses that they too had wanted to be a nurse. This statement may be simply a statement of fact, may represent a frustrated vocation, or may be indicative of envy toward one who was able to achieve a goal denied to

---

[7] Laughlin, Henry P.: The Neuroses in Clinical Practice. Philadelphia: W. B. Saunders Co., 1956, p. 112.

the patient. Ill persons may also envy the nurse's possession of good health and "independence." Certain nurses, on the other hand, probably due to strong dependency needs, may envy the secondary gains of illness which some ill persons "enjoy." What the envious nurse perceives, in such a situation, is not a unique human being, but a smug, comfortable individual whose needs are being met (whether this be true or not) while hers (the nurse's) are not. This behavior is usually demonstrated by the nurse's need to underestimate the effect of illness on the individual combined with the assumption that the person is "not as sick as he pretends to be." In some instances the illness itself is denied in that the nurse doesn't believe that the person is ill at all. If the nurse admits the individual is, in fact, ill, she may believe that his illness "isn't really too bad" or that other factors such as material possessions will compensate for the person's disability. One nurse, speaking of an individual disabled as a result of poliomyelitis, stated, "Well, I know he's disabled and all that—but after all he's pretty well fixed . . . He has a family to care for him. He owns his own home and I'll bet he's got a big fat bank account . . . after all he doesn't have any money problems . . ."

Transient feelings of envy towards another probably do not preclude the later development of relatedness, but they can be a barrier to its subsequent development. Envy prevents a nurse from perceiving and appreciating the uniqueness of the ill person.

More obvious reasons for an inability to perceive and appreciate the uniqueness of others may be due to a lack of interest in others, i.e., the individual is unable to transcend self and emotionally invest in another person. Some individuals are able to appreciate the uniqueness of certain individuals and not others. This will be discussed in the next section, "the phase of empathy."

The Task of the Nurse

The task of the nurse is to become aware of how she is perceiving the other individual, as well as the extent to which she is able to recognize the uniqueness of this human being whom we call "the patient." Another task is to assess similarities and differences between herself and the individual in order to assist in the development of empathy. Probably the critical requirement in this phase is that the nurse must be able to transcend herself to some extent. Inability to progress through this phase is exemplified in superficial types of interactions and by the "semi-helpful" interaction.

The phase of emerging identies continues to operate until relatedness is achieved, since this is the source of empathy and the means or vehicle whereby the individual can travel beyond the empathic boundary.

PHASE OF EMPATHY

Empathy is an experience which takes place between two or more individuals. It is basically the ability to enter into, or share in and comprehend the momentary psychological state of another individual.[8] It is a process wherein an individual is able to see beyond outward behavior, and sense accurately another's inner experience at a given point in time.

It is an almost instantaneous process characterized by the ability to comprehend the meaning and relevance of the thoughts and feelings of the individual concerned.

One shares in the psychological state of another but not to the extent of thinking and feeling *as* the other person. To empathize is to "share" in, but to stand apart from, the object of one's empathy. This "apart-ness" in empathy does not imply a cold objectivity; rather it implies a sense of sharing while being detached from the object of one's empathy. To empathize is to form a bond with another and experience closeness without being submerged by the involvement. During the empathic process the uniqueness and individuality of each person are more clearly perceived and appreciated.

It is a mutual understanding type of experience. Each person in the interaction realizes that something meaningful is transpiring; each knows that one is in touch with the other.

It is thus a conscious process; one knows when empathy is taking place. The end result of the empathic process is the ability to predict the behavior of the individual with whom one has empathized.

DIFFERENTIATION

Empathy is most often confused with such concepts as identification, projection and sympathy. Identification and projection will be defined, then differentiated from empathy. The concept "sympathy" will be defined and differentiated from empathy in the section in this chapter titled "The Phase of Sympathy."

Definitions

Identification is an unconscious process and a mental mechanism wherein an individual strives to be like another, or pattern himself after another. It is an unconscious imitation process. Conscious identification does occur as when an individual identifies with a character in a book or a play.

Projection is an unconscious process and a mental mechanism wherein an individual attributes to persons or objects in his environment his own unconscious undesirable tendencies or traits or his desirable tendencies or traits. The individual then treats the persons or objects as if these tendencies originated in them, and not in himself.

---

[8] Schafer, Ray: Generative empathy in the treatment situation. Psychoanal. Quart. 28:345, 1959.

Delineation

Empathy differs from identification and projection in that empathy is a conscious process. One knows if, and when, empathy is occuring. No such awareness occurs in projection or in identification. Both identification and projection are mental mechanisms, whereas empathy is not.

The end result of the empathic process is the ability to predict the behavior of the individual with whom one empathized; the end result of the identification process is to become like (or imitate) another. The end result of the process of projection is the ridding of oneself of undesirable tendencies by attributing these tendencies to others. It is a reality-distorting process in that the other individual is not perceived as he is. During the empathic process the uniqueness and individuality of each individual are more clearly perceived. Empathy is not reality-distorting; the thoughts and feelings of the other person are accurately perceived. These are the major differences between these concepts. For further differentiation the reader is referred to the bibliography at the end of this text.

Empathy in Nursing Situations

Empathy is not a continuous process, i.e., a nurse may interact many times with an ill person and only empathize once or several times. Once empathy has occurred (in an interaction) the pattern of the interaction is irrevocably changed; the relationship between the individuals involved can never be as it was before empathy occurred. Something has been acquired that cannot be easily effaced.

If the individuals involved later grow to dislike each other, the dislike is apt to have a more virulent quality than the dislike felt if empathy had not occurred. The sense of "hurt," of being "let-down" by someone with whom one felt some degree of closeness, seems to be more profound. It also seems to be more difficult to forgive someone with whom one empathized than someone with whom we had never developed empathy.

Either individual (nurse or ill-person) may regret the fact that empathy has occurred. The ill person may fear that too much has been revealed about himself to the nurse, and the nurse may not be able to cope with the knowledge gained through empathy and use it in a beneficial manner. Some degree of trust is needed in empathizing with another person. Therefore, trust may be destroyed depending on the nature of the knowledge gained and its wrong use. The gaining of an ill person's trust, and its use, canot be considered lightly.

The comprehension gained as a result of the empathic process is useful in predicting the behavior of the other individual. Prediction of behavior, then, is a goal in the empathic phase, whereas this is not the result in the phase of emerging identities.

Empathy does not "just happen." There are certain prerequisites and necessary conditions for developing empathy. These prerequisites will be considered in the next section.

Prerequisites to Empathy

Empathy is dependent upon similarities of experience between the two persons involved; therefore, ability to predict or comprehend the behavior of another is limited by one's personal background. *Research findings seem to indicate that a person's ability to empathize with others is determined by the degree or kind of similarity between two individuals.* According to Halpern and Lesser, "... a person's ability to empathize with similar people lies strictly with the boundaries of their similarity and disappears in personality areas in which they differ."[9]

People cannot readily comprehend or predict what has not been experienced on some level—it is like another attempting to describe a country he has never visited. While it is possible to appreciate and respond to the uniqueness of other persons, it is not possible to empathize unless one has a similar background or situation upon which to draw.

Since empathy can only operate on the basis of similarity, it is unrealistic to expect nurses to empathize with all ill persons. This, however, does not mean that nothing can be done about one's failure to empathize with another person. It is possible to expand one's empathic boundary and to grow in the ability to empathize with more and more individuals. (For specific suggestions regarding expansion of empathic boundaries see Appendix.)

This characteristic of similarity in empathy also may account for some of the difficulties the young student nurse has in trying to develop empathy. Young students may find it difficult to empathize because of a limited backlog of experiences upon which to draw. This characteristic of similarity also seems to account, to some extent, for the seeming innate ability of some older nurses' aides or nursing assistants to empathize with ill persons. Their rich personal background enables them to readily comprehend and understand because they have, in all probability, known or experienced many of the situations or conditions of the ill person. Young students tend to lack this rich experiential background.

Besides similarity, another prerequisite in developing empathy is the desire to comprehend or understand the other person. The desire or intent to understand another may be motivated by many factors: the desire to help (or exploit) the other person, or curiosity itself may be the motive. Whatever the motivation, there must at least be the desire to empathize combined with the intent to understand the other person.

Characteristics of Empathy

Empathy is characterized by the ability to predict the behavior of another. However, empathy, in and of itself, does not necessarily lead to closer relationships with others; that is, it does not imply that one do anything with the knowledge gained through the empathic process other than use it to predict behavior.

---

[9] Halpern, Howard M., and Lesser, Leona N.: Empathy in infants, adults and psychotherapists. Psychoanal. Rev. 47:38; No. 3, 1960.

Knowledge of another gained through the empathic process may be used constructively, i.e., this emotional and intellectual knowledge may be used to help the other person, or it may be used to manipulate and exploit the other person. (Confidence men are masters of the art of empathy.) This knowledge may also lie fallow and not be used at all.

Empathy is not characterized by an imperative need to do anything with the knowledge gained through the empathic process—other than to use it to predict behavior. Actually one might classify the act of empathy as indifferent—being neither good nor bad. How the knowledge gained through the process is used (or if it is used at all) leads one into the area of ethical and unethical interpersonal behavior.

It is possible to intellectually understand another's thinking and feeling and to predict his behavior, yet fail to do anything constructive with this ability— constructive in the sense that this knowledge will be used to help the other person. Like communication, empathy can be used to aid the helping process to draw others closer—or to hinder the later development of rapport and drive others away. One can empathize with another without necessarily establishing rapport, but if one achieves rapport it is because he has first been able to empathize and to use the knowledge gained through empathy to assist or help the other individual.

It is possible to empathize with others without liking them or having positive feelings towards them. A nurse may be able to predict the behavior of an individual accurately without liking the person; this is quite a common phenomenon. Liking someone seems to depend more on the extent to which that someone meets our needs; we generally tend to like those who meet our needs, and be indifferent toward those who do not. The degree of infantile omnipotence remaining in all of us seems to play a part in liking or disliking, the assumption being that if others realized how important we are they would like us.

The ability to intellectually comprehend another and to predict behavior does not seem to rest on liking (or disliking) the other person; but the degree and kind of similarities of experience between the persons involved are the important factors.

Value Judgments and Empathy

Probably during, or immediately after, one has gained empathic knowledge of another, value judgments are made. These judgments may be consistent with the original "snap judgments," or may change. In the phase of the original encounter, and to a certain extent in the phase of emerging identities, value judgments are made on the basis of inadequate information about the other person. The value judgments may be on an unrealistic basis, especially if the judgment is made, not in terms of the individual with whom one is interacting, but on the basis of an individual from our past.

Value judgments may also derive from the nurse projecting herself into the ill person. In empathy, value judgments are made more towards the human being with whom one has empathized. Using the knowledge gained through empathy, one "decides" whether or not to blame, accept, reject, or be "non-judgmental" towards the individual, or hold decision in abeyance and "wait and see." Even deciding to be non-judgmental is a judgment in the sense that something is believed about the other individual and a decision is made which will form a base for action.

The "Non-judgmental" Attitude

A review of the literature concerning the non-judgmental attitude reveals that most authors believe that an individual with this attitude possesses a particular way of perceiving other human beings, i.e., others are not blamed or judged. Many authors believe that the individual who is non-judgmental *has* value beliefs about the behavior of others but does not seek to impose these values or belief systems on others. Other characteristics include a lack of provincialism and humility (a much misunderstood trait, as is sympathy).

The author believes the term "non-judgmental attitude" is a misnomer since one judges or decides to be non-judgmental based on knowledge (whether rational, accurate, realistic or not) about the other person. *The non-judgmental attitude is a myth since all human beings tend to judge the behavior of others.* The criteria upon which most judgments are made usually are based on the extent to which an individual conforms to, or deviates from, the standards of conduct of the "judge," who invariably utilizes the personal yardstick. *Nurses should not strive to be non-judgmental.* The nurse should strive to become aware of the judgments she has formed about the ill person. It is only by being aware of the judgments that have been formed that the nurse can evaluate the effects of these judgments in the interpersonal encounter with the ill human being.

Nurses invariably form judgments about ill persons. Some ill persons are judged on the basis of their presenting behavior. For example, an ill person whose presenting behavior is "crankiness" may be judged and labelled as "a crank," "whiner" or "crock." Other ill persons are blamed for having caused their illness or disability. For example, an individual who contracts a venereal disease may be judged immoral, or an individual with a psychosomatic disorder may be judged and labelled as a "neurotic." Therefore it is essential that a nurse acknowledge the judgments she has formed about the ill human being and then decide what (if anything) she intends to do about it. Value judgments nurses form about ill human beings are invariably communicated to others who will respond accordingly.

In some instances, because of unconscious factors motivating the nurse's behavior, it is not possible to change the judgments the nurse has formed. The nurse can, however, strive to minimize the effects of these negative judgments when caring for the ill person. It is also recommended that the nurse introspect and strive to develop insight into her own behavior, i.e., strive to understand why the ill person's behavior threatens her to such an extent that she must censure and blame him.

A nurse develops positive judgments about others probably because she is able to accept the ill person. However, a nurse may empathize with an ill person and still not "accept" him.

Acceptance

Acceptance seems to be more akin to forgiveness in the sense that one weighs or judges the behavioral characteristics of another and, while acknowledging the "undesirable" or "negative" aspects of another, glosses over them, blurs them, while bringing into sharper focus those characteristics most pleasing and reassuring to one's self. Of such is friendship formed. Acceptance seems to be more of a selective forgiveness process; it is to display tolerance and possibly approval towards others, but not in the sense of "putting up with others." To excuse others because they differ from ourselves and those we have known is to accept others.

Acceptance either occurs automatically or remains a goal to be achieved. Certainly not all aspects of an ill person's behavior are automatically accepted; nor does the nurse "accept" an individual's illness. Illness and disability are *not* accepted because the nurse strives to effect changes in the ill person's condition and engages in purposeful activities in order to do so. Thus it is that the process of acceptance operates in circumscribed areas and is not all-encompassing and all-inclusive. *It is suggested that nurses not accept ill persons as they are, but purposefully and deliberately strive to change them.*

Some writers attempt to circumvent the difficulties inherent in the concept of acceptance by stating that one should accept the person, but not necessarily condone the behavior of the person. In actuality this is unrealistic since a person *is* his behavior. The forgiveness process must therefore encompass the person's behavior, as well as the person.

If the nurse is able to forgive the ill human being for being different from herself and strives to effect changes in the ill person's condition, she is then able to move into the next phase leading to relatedness, namely, sympathy. If the nurse is unable to achieve the above goals, progress ceases and the nurse is not able to move into the phase of sympathy.

Empathy is important but it is not enough; as has been shown, in and of itself it does not lead to relatedness but is an important step leading to relatedness. It is necessary to move beyond empathy into the realm of sympathy and compassion. To empathize is to intellectually understand another on the basis of similarity, to gain some understanding of the mental world of another; but it is not relatedness. Just to understand and predict behavior is not sufficient; the nurse must move into the area of action wherein she wants to assist the ill human being, not because it is expected of her by others—but because of the individual himself. To do this, sympathy is needed.

PHASE OF SYMPATHY*

The ability to sympathize emerges and results from the empathic process. It is a step beyond empathy in that in sympathy there is a basic urge or desire to

---

* N.B. Portions of the content in the section, "Phase of Sympathy," are excerpted and adapted from the article, What's wrong with sympathy? This article, written by the author, appeared in the Amer. J. Nurs. 64:68—71, 1964.

alleviate distress. *This desire to alleviate distress, absent in empathy, is a distinguishing characteristic of sympathy.*

Definition

Sympathy is an experience which takes place between two or more individuals. According to Webster's Third New International Dictionary, sympathy is the capacity to "... enter into or share the feelings or interests of another ... the character or fact of being sensitive to or affected by another's emotions, experiences or esp. sorrows ..." [10]

It is a process wherein an individual is able to comprehend the distress of another, be moved or touched by another's distress, and desires to alleviate the cause. One "shares" in the feelings of another and experiences compassion; therefore, it is not possible to both sympathize and stand apart from the object of one's sympathy. Sympathy cannot operate in an atmosphere of objective detachment and alienation. When one sympathizes one is involved but *not* incapacitated by the involvement.

Sympathy in Nursing Situations

Sympathy implies genuine concern about the misfortune or distress of another, combined with a desire to aid the afflicted individual. But though the urge to relieve distress is present, it does not always follow that the sympathetic person will constructively know how to aid, or be able to give needed assistance. It does, however, indicate that there is in sympathy an urge to allieviate distress that is lacking in empathy.

Sympathy is not a phase in the process of knowing, although it will probably aid and deepen one's relationship with another; it is, rather, a predisposition, an attitude, a type of thinking and feeling which is communicated to the other person. This thinking and feeling are characterized by deep personal concern and interest. When a nurse sympathizes with an ill person she communicates to the individual that he matters to her; she wants to assist him, is concerned about him, and wants to help him, not because he is bed 19 and she is expected to give him nursing care, but because he is himself and no one else.

The warmth of the caring quality that is sympathy is frequently communicated to the other individual verbally, but often it is non-verbal. The tenderness and compassion that are sympathy may be expressed by a look, glance, gesture, or manner in which the nurse performs her ministrations. It is most often the nurse's manner or behavior that conveys sympathy (or its lack) in nursing situations.

What does expressing and receiving sympathy mean? It means that the nurse enters into and shares the distress of the ill person, thereby relieving him of the burden of carrying it alone. It means that the distress of the other individual is of concern to the nurse and she institutes action to relieve this distress.

---

[10] By permission. From Webster's Third New International Dictionary, copyright 1961 by G. & C. Merriam Co., Publishers of the Merriam-Webster Dictionaries.

The presence or absence of sympathy in the nursing process affects the ill person not only on a psychological level, but on a physiological level, and may have some bearing on the manner in which the ill person is able to muster resistance to his illness; it may make the difference between the will to live or die. Sympathy may produce a needed act of will when its emotional support is correctly used by the nurse.

Sympathy is not the same as being courteous to ill persons—it is more than that. Neither is it just being kind to people. Nurses can be both courteous and kind in a frightening dehumanized manner, conveying neither warmth nor understanding. Sympathy is warmth, kindness, a transient type of compassion, a *caring* quality experienced on a feeling level and communicated to another. It cannot be feigned or pretended, despite the most elaborate communication techniques. Like rapport, one possesses it or not.

It means that this human being we call the nurse is concerned about the human being who is the "patient," and seeks to alleviate his distress. It means that the nurse is not afraid to show interest, or to feel concern, but not, however, to be engulfed by care or concern to the point of inactivity. It means that the nurse cares, but in caring gives emotional support and sustains another human being in time of crisis.

It means that the nurse is an authentic human being who is sympathetic and can demonstrate sympathy; or that, lacking this quality, she is a dehumanized individual communicating with other dehumanized individuals. Without sympathy the nurse offers, at best, a superficial interaction—lacking warmth and personal caring qualities. Sympathy, as we have seen, is a step beyond empathy; it adds to empathy the personal caring quality, and the urge to relieve the distress of another person.

Comparison Between Empathy and Sympathy

Empathy is a process wherein an individual is able to comprehend the psychological state of another. Because this comprehension occurs, the individual is then able to predict the behavior of the other person. However, empathy is a neutral process since it does not imply that the individual take action on the basis of the comprehension which has been gained.

Sympathy, on the other hand, implies a desire to aid the other individual in order to relieve his distress. As Koestler states, "empathy becomes sympathy when to this mental resonance is added the desire to collaborate or help." [11] There is a warmth or urge to act in sympathy not present in empathy. The empathic person can perceive another's distress, identify its source, and anticipate the behavior which will result from it. But the sympathetic person feels another's distress. He is touched by it and wants to do something actively to assist or alleviate the condition.

---

[11] Koestler, Arthur: Insight and Outlook. New York: Macmillan Co., 1949, p. 360.

The aim of sympathy seems to be the transmission of concern, with desire of alleviating the cause of the concern. One would be sympathetic only as long as the cause of concern existed. Therefore, unlike compassion, sympathy is not a permanent attitude—one constantly in operation; it is transient, changing in focus and object. However, empathy continues as long as one individual deliberately and consciously strives to perceive and comprehend the inner experience of another person.

Both empathy and sympathy require a perceptual openness to experience, and the mental freedom to make use of one's personal background of experience, in order to understand and appreciate the experiences of others. Both require an active and alert mind without a feeling of defensive barriers against involvement.

When one empathizes one is not moved or touched by that which concerns another—one simply understands what another is experiencing without desiring to do anything to aid the distress. Sympathetic persons assist others, not because it is their assigned job, but because they are motivated by compassion, which underlies, and is a fundamental element of, sympathy.

Empathy is important since it is the forerunner of sympathy, and a stage in the process of achieving sympathy. But sympathy extends beyond empathy since a sympathetic person takes action to relieve the distress of another. Certainly taking action to meet an ill person's need is an essential nursing function; it would therefore seem essential that empathy be transformed into sympathy if this basic goal is to be achieved.

Objections to Sympathy

A review of periodical literature and current nursing textbooks representing various clinical areas reveals, though it is considered important for nurses to empathize with "patients," that there has been little or no attention given to the importance and need of sympathy in the nursing process. It may be that the lack of nursing literature dealing with the concept of sympathy is due to confusion of the term "sympathy" with the popular connotation of "feeling sorry for someone," or "pity," and all that is implied in these terms. Weigert says, "just as the word love has beome a coin debased by usage, and misunderstood in more than one sense, the word sympathy also has no longer the ring of a spontaneous emotion. It is suspected of hypocrisy, sentimentality, blind partiality and sado-masochistic exploitation." [12] Sympathy has become a suspect emotion.

Over-identification

Countless nursing students have been warned about the dangers involved in being sympathetic with "patients." "To be sympathetic" with ill persons has been construed, by some, to mean that the nurse "over-identifies" with the individual to

---

[12] Weigert, Edith: Role of sympathy in the psychotherapeutic process, Amer. J. Psychoanal. XXII:9, No. 1, 1962.

the point of immobility and inaction, or that the nurse becomes so emotionally involved and enmeshed in the ill person's problems that she cannot meet the individual's needs, because she is too busy meeting her own needs. The typical picture of the "too sympathetic nurse" is one who joins the ill person in his emotional binges, cries when the individual cries, and becomes depressed when the ill person becomes depressed. This is not sympathy; it is rather failure to proceed beyond the phase of the original encounter. The nurse has actually related to "herself" in the ill person, in order to relieve the tension of her own unmet needs.

Such nurses generally describe themselves as "too soft-hearted" or too "tender-hearted." In actuality, they are not concerned about others and tend to view them only as extensions of themselves. Conscious awareness of how one is actually relating, or if one is using the ill person, is essential in order to avoid this pattern. Someone outside of the immediate situation may be needed to help the nurse so involved, since many nurses in such situations have little or no realization of what is occuring.

Emotional Involvement

Involvement is the ability to care *for* and *about* other human beings and to translate this *caring* into helpful behavior. The human being is known by his behavior, not by kind thoughts he may have about others—thoughts which may never be translated into action. Involvement, then, is a commitment to a way of life; it is an ongoing process. It is not an attribute a person *has*, it is a sensitivity to something he *is*. It is something he has become through the use of his will.

There are all kinds of involvement and all kinds of people who become involved. Hitler and Stalin were dedicated individuals; they were consistently involved. However, one must look at the object of one's involvement: the end result as well as the means used to accomplish one's goals. One of the major goals of involvement, as has been stated, is to develop the ability to care for and about other human beings. Another goal is to develop an awareness of actions which dehumanize and make non-persons out of human beings. The involved nurse engages in a determined fight against this type of activity or behavior. It means to struggle against, to protest anything (or anyone) that would maim, wound, or kill the human spirit. Any thing or condition which prevents human beings from utilizing their humanity or which destroys beauty, or serenity of the heart, mind or spirit is a legitimate target of protest. These goals may be accomplished by group or individual action. It is interesting to speculate how much improvement in nursing care would result if nurses en masse refused to give consent to, or condone by omission or commission, any act which dehumanizes the ill person or permits ineffective and unsafe care.

If a nurse is to establish a helping relationship she must become emotionally involved. The nurse must seek to feel and experience along with the ill individual. But it is essential that the nurse be fully aware of what she is feeling and experiencing. It is obvious that a nurse must not become so blinded by her feelings that she cannot discern what is happening in her relationship with the ill person. Relationships must be structured in full conscious awareness of what one is doing and thinking, as well as in terms of the goals to be accomplished in each interaction.[13]

There is, of course, the possibility that sympathy may be distorted and misused in the interpersonal process. The fault does not rest in the emotion, but in its use! Nor is it a remedy to condemn the emotion because it may be twisted and used to meet one's own needs; any human feeling may be distorted until it is but a caricature of the feeling it originally represented. One may as well denounce the use of automobiles because they cause damage when not properly controlled.

Sympathy cannot operate in an atmosphere of alienation. It is probably an act of courage to permit oneself to feel sympathy for another, because with the experience of sympathy may come pain. This is especially true when one is powerless to aid the object of one's sympathy or, when despite one's best efforts, the distress of the afflicted person is not even diminished, much less relieved. When one succeeds in assisting others, one is enriched and fulfilled; but when one fails (and all will fail at one time or another), frustration will be experienced, followed by a tendency to blame the other person. The hurts of failure may cause a nurse to protect herself by denying her feelings and by crushing them lest they arise and catch her unprepared. One may not be willing to pay the price of failure, and so begins detachment and protection of self. One is then not hurt by others, but neither is one's experience enriched by contact with others.

To sympathize is to give part of oneself to others, and in the giving and sharing to become vulnerable. This, however, is the vulnerability of the strong who neither fear life, nor fear to be authentic human beings. Loving humanity in the abstract does not affect one in this manner; but the act of entering into, sharing, and giving of oneself in a deep personal way exposes one to the shocks of commitment and all that this entails.

Involvement is not a problem. The professional nurse is involved, but she is not in any way incapacitated by the involvement. Knowing what one is thinking and feeling in relation to the ill person but also understanding the goals to be achieved in nursing situations are the best safeguards against immature types of emotional involvement. Being involved *helps* the professional nurse to assist the ill human being. Involvement does not hinder nursing action; it facilitates it as long as the emotional involvement is on a mature level. It is only by becoming involved that the nurse can relate as human being to human being, can communicate meaningfully and sustain the individual in his time of crisis.

Without involvement the nurse will not experience concern for ill persons, much less express sympathy to them. It is not possible to know ill human beings, much less assist them in any consistently constructive manner, without involvement. Nurses who do not become involved maintain "nurse-patient distance" and behave in a depersonalized mechanical manner. Neither nurse nor ill person benefits

---

[13] Travelbee, Joyce: What do we mean by rapport? Amer. J. Nurs. 63:71, 1963.

by non-involvement. The nurse is deprived of satisfying and meaningful contacts with ill persons; indeed, is deprived of job satisfaction itself. Ill persons are deprived of the support they may require in order to cope with the stress of illness. Involvement, however, is not nearly as great a problem in nursing situations as is its lack.

Objectifying Pity

Besides "emotional involvement," another objection to sympathy probably arises from confusing the quality of sympathy with objectifying pity—a distortion or twisting of the emotion of pity. Pity is defined as "sympathetic heart felt sorrow for one that is suffering physically or mentally or that is otherwise distressed or unhappy." [14] Pity, a warm human feeling, when distorted results in objectifying pity. Objectifying pity is a dehumanizing way of viewing others, and communicating and relating with them as if they were objects and not human beings. It is best exemplified in the "oh, you poor *thing*" attitude. The individual becomes an object, is viewed and related to as if he were a *thing*, or as something less than human.

Objectifying pity is not sympathy; neither is it empathy. The aim of this type of pity is not intellectual understanding of another, nor is it the ability to predict behavior; neither is it characterized by a sincere desire to help alleviate the distress of another, although lip service may be paid to doing so. This type of pity seems to be characterized by a smothering, condescending, superior attitude.

The great majority of individuals do not want to be pitied, and are indeed made angry by being pitied by nurses or anyone else. A small minority of ill persons act as if they are seeking pity or sympathy from nurses. This is exemplified in the "poor defenseless me" attitude, or the "I feel sorry for myself" attitude; this behavior seems to indicate an active desire that others "feel sorry" for them. Nurses tend to have difficulty in handling and working through their feelings about such persons. Usually these individuals are judged as those who "feel too sorry for themselves." The assumption seems to be that anyone who feels sorry for himself doesn't need anyone to feel sorry for him. These people engender anger and guilt feelings in nursing personnel, who, unless they are aware of the underlying dynamics of this phenomenon, may tend to act in a punitive way.

Ill persons who "feel sorry for themselves" may be attempting to relate with others in the only way they are able to relate. Such individuals need understanding, not condemnation. Recognition of the dynamics, and understanding why the individual must seek objectifying pity, will assist nurses in caring for them. These persons require a judicious reality-oriented, sympathetic attitude, not pity, which he will not receive from the nurse anyway. A judicious reality-oriented sympathetic attitude implies that the nurse is able to meet, to some extent, the press of the unmet need for attention and sympathy—to admit to the individual and calmly

---

[14] By permission. From Webster's Third New International Dictionary, copyright 1961 by G. & C. Merriam Co., Publishers of the Merriam-Webster Dictionaries.

agree with him that "yes, it was a rough experience; yes, it is difficult being hospitalized; it is not easy etc." instead of lecturing the person how fortunate he is that he isn't worse off! One agrees with the ill person whenever his complaints are reality based, supports him whenever possible, attempts to feed his starved need for attention, to lower his anxiety level, and to anticipate his demands.

The problem is not that these individuals have been given too much sympathy—they have received too little. If the nurse can recognize the desperate fright and utter loneliness of such persons, empathy followed by sympathy may develop.

"Harmful Effects of Sympathy"

Probably due to a basic confusion regarding sympathy and the concept of objectifying pity, nurses have almost a mental block against the concept of sympathy; there seems to be great hesitation in expressing sympathy to ill persons lest it "harm them" in some way. It is not clear what this harm constitutes. This attitude may represent a vestige of Anglo-Saxon stoicism, or a reaction to a lack of sympathy given ourselves as individuals or as professional people, and therefore we are unable to give to others what we ourselves have not received. It may be that in being denied sympathy we cannot conceive of anyone else getting what we were denied in our needs. Who has not desired, but not received, some measure of sympathy when tired, distressed and misunderstood, harassed, or suffering mentally and physically? That we did not seek sympathy says something about our character structure, but the fact that we did not seek what we needed at that time does not mean that we did not desire it.

Another objection to sympathy is that the ill person will enjoy the attention so much that he will not strive to get better; if his hospital stay is too relaxing and without anxiety the individual will regress and never want to get better. Thus the humanizing qualities of the nursing process are viewed as dangerous and harmful. The basic assumption underlying this belief seems to be that most individuals are so poorly integrated and weak that sympathy will in some way "ruin" them. It is difficult to comprehend how the transmission of concern, personal interest, and the desire to alleviate distress, which is sympathy, can make ill persons regress. No one was ever ruined as a result of kindness and sympathy, but many have suffered needlessly from the lack of these qualities in nursing process. It is difficult to comprehend by what manner nurses have moved away from the expression of sympathy in nursing situations except to account for it by fear of expressing objectifying pity to ill persons or the additional fear of "becoming involved."

Sympathy is a necessary and essential element that is required in order to achieve relatedness.

Result of Sympathy

What is the end result of the sympathetic process? The relationship of nurse to ill persons, although still somewhat tenuous, is strengthened and enhanced. The ill person perceives the nurse as a unique human being in her own right, as well as perceiving her as a helping human being eminently qualified and capable of assisting him. The nurse has been able to translate the experience of sympathy into nursing action and has relieved, or diminished, the ill person's distress. The ill individual perceives that the nurse has assisted him, not because he is a "patient" and she is a nurse whose duty is to assist him, but because she is interested in him as a unique human being.

As a result of the experience of sympathy, the ill person begins to trust the nurse; however, complete confidence in the nurse is lacking during this phase. Sympathy is a transient experience—one which strengthens the bond of each individual to the other. Because it is transient, its effects may be short lasting. It is also still possible that rapport may not be achieved. This is especially true in those instances when the ill person tests the nurse in order to ascertain her reliability, and the nurse does not meet the patient's expectation.

However, generally speaking, trust is an outcome of the process of sympathy. According to Webster's Third New International Dictionary, trust implies "an assured attitude towards another which may rest on blended evidence of experience and more subjective grounds such as knowledge, ... admiration, ... respect.[15]

Trust must be earned. Very few individuals are naive enough to trust nurses automatically. The nurse must prove by her behavior that she is reliable and dependable. Some ill persons require much evidence of the nurse's dependability before they will begin to trust her, while other persons require little evidence. Trust is probably developed most rapidly when scrupulous attention is paid to every request made by an ill person, no matter how trivial or unimportant such a request may appear to nursing personnel. There will, of course, be instances when the nurse cannot grant the request, or cannot immediately fulfill the request, but an explanation as to why the request cannot be granted or fulfilled immediately and some indication as to when the request can be fulfilled are essential if trust is to be developed. When such requests are "forgotten" by the nurse, the ill person may well question whether or not he will be able to depend on nursing personnel when he is "really" in need.

Complete confidence of the ill human being in the nurse is experienced when the individual learns that he can depend on the nurse and that she will not fail him. Confidence is experienced by the ill person and the relationship proceeds into the phase of rapport.

Task of the Professional Nurse

The task of the professional nurse, in the phase of sympathy, is to translate this phase into helpful nursing action. This helpful nursing action requires a combination of the disciplined intellectual approach combined with the therapeutic use of self.

---

[15] By permission. From Webster's Third New International Dictionary, copyright 1961 by G. & C. Merriam Co., Publishers of the Merriam-Webster Dictionaries.

Sympathy alone will not meet the nursing needs of people. Sympathy must be translated into intelligent, helpful nursing action. The sympathetic nurse must not only wish to help, but must know how to assist, and possess the knowledge and skills so necessary to helping the process.

The phase of sympathy is a precursor of the phase of rapport. Sympathy merges into, and becomes an important ingredient in, rapport. Sympathy is an experience which precedes rapport and continues on into the process of rapport, which is the epitome of the human-to-human relationship.

PHASE OF RAPPORT*

The establishment of a human-to-human relationship, and the experience that is rapport, is the terminus of all nursing endeavor. Rapport is that which is experienced when nurse and ill person have progressed through the four interlocking phases preceding rapport, and the establishment of a human-to-human relationship, namely, (1) the original encounter, (2) emerging identities, (3) empathy, and finally (4) sympathy. All of these phases culminate in rapport and the establishment of a human-to-human relationship.

Terminology

The terms "relationship," "relatedness" and "rapport" are used interchangeably. All are experiences perceived and undergone by both nurse and ill person. One distinction can be made, however; the human-to-human relationship encompasses the experiences of rapport and relatedness. Rapport is the experiential aspect of the human-to-human relationship. The term "relatedness" is used as a synonym for rapport.

Definition

Rapport is a process, a happening, an experience, or series of experiences, undergone simultaneously by nurse and the recipient of her care. It is composed of a cluster of interrelated thoughts and feelings, these thoughts, feelings and attitudes being transmitted, or communicated, by one human being to another. Rapport is basically the manner in which two individuals perceive, and behave towards, each other. These thoughts and feelings vary somewhat according to the uniqueness inherent in every nursing situation. However, some common aspects exist and are identifiable in the nursing situation characterized by rapport.

The experience of rapport is necessarily undergone by both nurse and ill person; however, due to the relative position of the two, each with different backgrounds, each being separate and unique human beings, it is evident that the nurse

* N.B. Portions of the content in the section, "Phase of Rapport," are quoted or adapted from What do we mean by rapport? This article, written by the author, appeared in the Amer. J. Nurs. 63:70-72, 1963.

will experience rapport somewhat differently than will the ill person. The ill person's experience will also usually be different even though encountered by nurse and ill person simultaneously. The nurse and ill individual remain separate and distinct human beings who share a series of experiences together. The experiences nurse and ill human being have shared are *mutually significant,* meaningful ones, for both. Each has been involved—each to the extent of his capacity for commitment.

Prerequisites to Rapport

Rapport is experienced when nurse and ill human being have progressed through the four phases preceding the establishment of a human-to-human relationship. Rapport is a phase beyond sympathy. During the phase of sympathy the nurse experiences the urge, or desire, to assist ill persons, and institutes nursing actions to achieve this end. This, however, does not mean that the sympathetic nurse will help (or know how) to alleviate the individual's distress. Unless the nurse has structured nursing intervention in full conscious awareness, making full use of the knowledge available to her, and has sought evidence that she can indeed alleviate the ill person's distress, there is no guarantee of actual help; nor has the nurse any real way of knowing that her intervention can be of assistance to that individual.

In order to achieve rapport it is necessary that the actions initiated by the nurse are consistent in their alleviation of the ill person's distress, an implied assumption being that the nurse has not *added* to the distress.

According to Webster's Third New International Dictionary, alleviate means to: "LIGHTEN, LESSEN: RELIEVE, MODERATE: as to make easier to be endured . . ." [16] The nurse therefore strives to alleviate distress, to lighten or lessen it or to make it easier to be endured; she cannot always assist in removing the cause of the distress, and it is unrealistic to assume otherwise. An individual with a fatal illness will not be cured, nor will the course of his illness necessarily be altered because of the nurse's ministrations (although this may occur). She can, however, assist the ill person to cope with the experience and minimize the impact of the distress of illness.

The prerequisite that the actions initiated by the nurse have consistently alleviated the ill person's distress is contingent on many factors: the nurse's knowledge and ability to translate that which is known into actions beneficial to the particular individual for whom she is rendering care. It includes all of those elements inherent in the disciplined intellectual approach, and more besides. Rapport is contingent on the manner in which the ill person has been helped by the nurse. The manner in which the nurse assists the ill person is, of course, dependent to some extent on what the nurse knows, and is able or willing to do. But it is also dependent on the nurse's perception of human beings, i.e., what she truly believes about others as opposed to what she professes to believe. What is truly believed will be reflected in behavior towards ill persons and others.

---

[16] By permission. From Webster's Third New International Dictionary, copyright 1961 by G. & C. Merriam Co., Publishers of the Merriam-Webster Dictionaries.

A nurse may be able to ascertain and meet some of an individual's nursing needs, and may be able to some extent to alleviate the ill person's distress; but rapport is still not experienced. Rapport is achieved by the nurse who possesses and uses the disciplined intellectual approach combined with the therapeutic use of self. Rapport is a part or expression of the nurse's personality. It is bound and enmeshed into her philosophy of life; it is a *part* of her value system. Rapport is not only something a nurse *has*, it is something she *is*.

Characteristics of Rapport

Both nurse and ill person perceive and relate as human being to human being, instead of as nurse to "patient." The "patient" and "nurse" stereotypes are forever shattered in nursing situations characterized by rapport. This does not, in any way, imply an "unprofessional relationship." It simply means that two human beings can interact without the need to use distancing tactics. It is the ability to be still and experience the other as a human being—to appreciate the unfolding of each personality one to the other. Some may object to these statements on the grounds that the nurse is not hired to "appreciate" an ill person's personality; neither are ill persons admitted to hospitals for the purpose of getting to know nurses as human beings. A relationship is not a mutual admiration society, although mutual admiration may exist in a relationship. These criticisms are valid if viewed in a restricted limited context. The basic reality of the nursing situation, however, is that both nurse and ill person are thinking, feeling, experiencing human beings and to view them as otherwise is to negate reality. To experience the unfolding of another's personality is simply another way of saying that one is able to appreciate another human being. The fact that the human being happens to be ill is not a justifiable barrier precluding such appreciation.

This is not to suggest that the ability to appreciate the human-ness of the ill person is all that is required to render nursing care. A nurse does not simply stand by and "appreciate" an ill person who is going into shock; she acts quickly and takes the steps necessary to reverse this process.

Those who have stressed the humanistic aspects of nursing care have been criticized (sometimes validly) for neglecting to give adequate emphasis to the physiological needs of ill people. Nurses are also criticized for seeming to regard the human being as "pure psyche," totally and completely removed from a human body. This view is probably an over-reaction to the view that the ill person is *only* an ailing biological organism, or a mass of physiological needs. Both extremes are fallacious and unrealistic. Man is an entity and his psychological and physiological needs are inseparably intertwined. Giving a thirsty individual a glass of water meets a physiological need, and, depending on the relationship of the nurse to the individual, and how this assistance is rendered, may also meet a psychological need. It is probable that reassurance and emotional support affect the physiology of the human being, and meet some physiological needs. How can these needs be, in fact, separated?

These extreme views are not as prevalent today as they have been in the past; they do, however, still exist. Nonetheless, it is hopeful that this type of dichotomized thinking about the human being is changing. These extremes unfortunately are being surplanted by another view, i.e., the growing tendency to regard the ill person as a "nursing problem." This tendency *can* result in dehumanization of the ill person in the same manner as regarding the person as an illness, or a room number. At the risk of belaboring the point it must be remembered that *ill persons are not problems—they are human beings with problems.* To view an ill human being as "a problem to be solved" negates the humanity of the person and reduces him to an "interesting problem" which is probably a variant of the old "interesting case" viewpoint. Rapport is not readily established by nurses who hold such perceptions of people, since such are unable to appreciate the human-ness of the recipients of their care.

The ability to appreciate the human-ness of the ill person is characterized by the capacity to *be*, as opposed to *doing*. It is not problem-solving; neither is it necessarily characterized by intellectual activity. Rather, it is more of an openness to experience, not an emptiness. Such moments, and they are but moments, are permeated by a type of ambient, enveloping, all pervasive quietness and understanding of each to the other. There is no need or desire to verbalize this experience—it *is*, in and of itself. Rapport is characterized by such moments of relatedness.

Another result of the ability of nurse and ill person to perceive and relate as human being to human being is the freeing of energy once needed to maintain the facades of "nurse" and "patient." The effort and energy previously used for this purpose can now be used more constructively by both nurse and ill person. The ill person can use the energy to combat his illness. The nurse is now free to use this energy, once converted into efforts to maintain "nurse-patient distance," into helpful nursing actions.

In the phase of rapport, the ill person progresses beyond the stage where he must test the nurse to discover how reliable she is. Trust, an outcome of the phase of sympathy, is supplanted by confidence. According to Webster's Third New International Dictionary, confidence "indicates a feeling of sureness about another that is based on experience and evidence without strong effect of the subjective . . ." [17] Confidence thus is a step beyond trust. It is obvious that a great deal of energy is expended by ill persons who do not trust or have confidence in nursing personnel. This is especially true if ill people believe they must continually check on nurses, or question everything being done to and for them, because they lack trust or confidence in those who care for them. Every encounter offers an opportunity to increase the confidence of ill persons in those who care for them.

Communication problems may still develop in situations characterized by rapport, but their occurrence is minimal because when problems emerge they are readily recognized and are fairly easily resolved. In the milieu that is rapport, the ill human being can be more authentically spontaneous in conversing with the nurse.

[17] By permission. From Webster's Third New International Dictionary, copyright 1961 by G. & C. Merriam Co., Publishers of the Merriam-Webster Dictionaries.

There is less of a need, on the part of the ill person, to "weigh his words" in order to judge the effects of his comments on the nurse. The effects of the ability to feel free to communicate with another is described by Craik who wrote:

> "... the comfort, the inexpressible comfort of feeling safe with a person, having neither to weigh thoughts, nor measure words, but pouring them all right out, just as they are, chaff and grain together; certain that a faithful hand will take and sift them, keep what is worth keeping, and then with the breath of kindness blow the rest away." [18]

This does not mean that the relationship between nurse and ill person is now characterized by social chit-chat, or that the nurse simply "enjoys" the ill person's conversation (although the prohibitions against both seem somewhat arbitrary). During every phase of the nursing process the professional nurse practitioner *intentionally* strives to interact, and to communicate in such a way that the goal of knowing ill persons is achieved, thus ascertaining and meeting the nursing needs of these individuals. Everything the professional nurse does in nursing situations is directed toward fulfilling these goals.

Another outcome of rapport is that both nurse and ill person grow as human beings as a result of this experience, probably because each participant has experienced the vivid aliveness of a meaningful, human-to-human encounter. There are some individuals who have seldom (if ever) had the opportunity to experience even transient moments of relatedness. The ability to relate in such a way is the core of the experience that is rapport.

Rapport is not static—it is a dynamic process, an experience of many facets. There are probably varying degrees, as well as varying levels, of rapport. Some nurses, probably because of their past life experiences combined with educational preparation, are able to move rapidly through the phases preceding rapport and maintain a higher level of rapport with ill persons than are other nurses. It may be that such nurses possess an unusually highly developed degree of creativity which they are able to canalize and use in the service of others. An imaginative, creative, knowledgeable nurse is more likely to envisage the various alternatives, solutions or semi-solutions possible in a nursing situation, and is less likely to be restricted to a dichotomized type of either/or thinking. The ability to think creatively and imaginatively, in and of itself, does not guarantee that the nurse will be able to assist others. The creative nurse is more prone (because she can envisage alternatives) to a restricting form of over-intellectualization wherein the ability to act becomes paralyzed. Such a nurse thinks and imagines, and has such an active rich mental life that this inner life may become an end within itself, and result in not being used in the service of others. In the experience that is rapport, action springs from thought and is related to it. It is, of course, easier to act without thinking, or to think without acting, than do both together. In the experience that is rapport there is a perfect blend of thought and action.

Thus are the characteristics of rapport—an ever-changing multi-faceted experience. Rapport is an experience which does not "just happen"; it is established and

---

[18] Craik, Dinah Maria Mulock, as quoted in The Shorter Bartlett's Familiar Quotations. (Christopher Morley and Louella D. Everett, eds.) New York: Permabook (Pocket Books Inc.), 1962, p. 89.

built day by day in the nurse's contacts and interactions with the ill person so that, as both nurse and ill person progress through the phases preceding relatedness, a relationship is eventually established.

Rapport—What It Is Not

Rapport is not just another way of loving humanity. It is quite possible to love humanity and yet be unable (or unwilling) to assist others. Loving humanity places no strain on the nervous system. It is far easier to love an abstraction than to translate this abstraction into helpful nursing actions. Neither is rapport just another synonym for love—although a characteristic of rapport is the capacity to care for and about others. It is not just warm, kindly feelings between two individuals who like each other, although these feelings may exist. It is quite possible to establish rapport without ever experiencing emotion. Actually the experience that is rapport is more dependent on the will than on the emotions, although the emotions cannot be excluded.

Rapport is not just a high-level ivory tower abstraction; it is an actual experience. It is more than a sentimental attitude. It cannot be seen, although one may infer its existence by systematically observing the behavior of both participants in an interactive process. It can, to some extent, be validated by interview and planned inquiry.

A nurse is able to establish rapport because she possesses the necessary knowledge and skills required to assist ill persons, and because she is able to perceive, respond to, and appreciate the uniqueness of the ill human being. She cares for and about those for whom she renders nursing care. The ability to truly care for and about others—to translate the quality of caring into action in nursing situations—is the core of rapport.

N.B. References used in this chapter are in the footnotes. These are not repeated.

Chapter XI

NURSING INTERVENTION
Fulfilling the Functions of Nursing

Nursing intervention is directed towards achieving the purpose of nursing. The purpose of nursing is to assist an individual, family or community to prevent or cope with the experience of illness and suffering, and, if necessary, to assist individuals and families to find meaning in these experiences.

The functions of the professional nurse practitioner have been discussed previously in Chapter I, "The Nature of Nursing." In this present chapter, particular attention will be given to the function: assisting individuals and families to find meaning in illness and suffering; ways and means will be stressed regarding fulfillment of this particular function.

A major belief of this work is that the human being is motivated by a search for meaning in life experiences, and that meaning *can* be found in the experiences of illness, suffering, and pain. When such meaning is found the individual is able to use the experience of illness as an enabling life experience, i.e., enabling in the sense that it is possible for the individual to achieve self-actualization and that which lies beyond—self-transcendence.

Viktor E. Frankl, the originator of Logotherapy, states that . . .

"... man is ... ready to suffer, on the condition ... that his suffering has meaning ... suffering would not have a meaning unless it were absolutely necessary, e.g., a cancer that can be cured by surgery must not be shouldered by the patient as though it were his cross. This would be masochism rather than heroism." [1] "Whenever one is confronted with an inescapable, unavoidable situation, whenever one has to face a fate that cannot be changed, e.g., an incurable disease ... just then is one given a last chance to actualize the highest value, to fulfill the deepest meaning—the meaning of suffering. For what matters above all is the attitude we take towards suffering, the attitude in which we take our suffering upon ourselves." [2]

---

[1] Frankl, Viktor E.: Man's Search for Meaning: An Introduction to Logotherapy. New York: Washington Square Press, 1963, pp. 179-180.

[2] *Ibid.*, p. 178.

Jaspers states,

"As soon as the individual wakes he does not merely want to live out the day but wants to live for something. He wants to experience some meaning in his life." [3]

The assumptions which underlie this work are based on Frankl's concepts of Logotherapy. These assumptions are as follows:

1. Individuals can be assisted to find meaning in the experience of illness and suffering. The meanings can enable the individual to cope with the problems engendered by these experiences.
2. The spiritual and ethical values of the nurse, or her philosophical beliefs about illness and suffering, will determine the extent to which she will be able to assist individuals and families to find meaning (or no meaning) in these difficult experiences.
3. It is the responsibility of the professional nurse practitioner to assist individuals and families to find meaning in illness and suffering (if this be necessary).

In Part I of this chapter the nurse's responsibility in assisting ill persons to find meaning in illness and suffering is explored and the prerequisites needed by the nurse to assist the individual are discussed. The nature and scope of the problems faced by nurses in assisting ill human beings are considered, as are the barriers which tend to hinder the nurse in helping ill persons.

In Part II, terms are defined and the meaning of major concepts is explored. In Part III, specific ways and means of assisting ill persons with various reactions to the stress of illness and suffering are discussed. Ways of assisting the ill person's family are discussed in Part IV.

PART I—THE NURSE'S RESPONSIBILITY

What can nursing offer the ill person who, although not fatally ill, nevertheless finds his life robbed of all meaning by the onset of a life-long illness? What has nursing to offer the individual whose life has been irrevocably changed by the onset of a long-term incurable illness? One may well question whether finding meaning in illness is, in fact, a nursing responsibility; or if the responsibility of the professional nurse practitioner is to assist the ill person in maintaining the highest optimal level of health. One cannot argue with this statement, but does it not depend on one's definition of the term "optimal level of health"? In many nursing situations, ill persons require more than good physical care, health teaching, or encouragement, although these activities are important and should not be minimized. *The professional nurse has a more difficult responsibility in that she must be able to assist ill persons to find meaning in the experience of illness, suffering and pain.* Nurses have not always recognized, much less assumed, their professional responsibility in this most difficult area.

---

[3] Jaspers, Karl: General Psychopathology (translated by J. Hoenig and Marian W. Hamilton). Chicago: The University of Chicago Press, 1963, p. 696.

One might question if assisting individuals to find meaning in illness and suffering is a *nursing* responsibility or the responsibility of some other member of the health team. It is certainly the physician's responsibility to assist the individual in accepting his illness and learning to live within the limitations illness imposes. But it is not wholly the physician's responsibility. It is also a function assumed, to some extent, by social workers, ministers, priests, and rabbis. However this responsibility is shared with other health workers, it is nevertheless *primarily* a nursing responsibility. The nurse is "on the scene"—she is there more than any of the other health workers. The nurse must be able to cope with *any* problem which seriously affects the ill person's well-being. There is little evidence at this time (but it is probable) that the genesis of many "nursing problems" is the ill person's inability to accept illness, much less find any meaning in this experience.

Can a nurse assume that she is giving "total nursing care" if she ignores this most difficult area? This does not mean that the nurse can personally assist the ill person to always find a solution to his problem (it may be necessary to refer the individual to another health worker); however, the nurse is ultimately responsible for the individual receiving needed assistance. *The nurse is accountable and responsible.* It is not sufficient to refer the ill person to someone else, and in the act of referral assume that one's responsibility is ended. Follow up of the extent to which the ill person is being assisted is a nursing responsibility. It is unfortunate but true that the function for whom everyone is responsible, and accountable, is the one for whom no one feels responsible. A function assumed by *all* health workers becomes a function performed by *none*.

A nurse does not strive only to alleviate physical pain or render physical care—she ministers to the person. The nurse cares for the individual, not a body part. The existence of suffering, whether physical, mental or spiritual *is* the proper concern of the nurse. It is her responsibility to see to it that the ill person receives the assistance he requires. No nurse would fail to assist an individual in physical pain; neither can she absolve herself of the responsibility to assist a human being suffering from the anguish of meaninglessness.

It must be stressed that ill persons who are not able to find meaning in their life, who perceive illness and suffering as inexplicable and meaningless, are not necessarily neurotic or psychotic. Nor is psychiatric intervention necessarily required. A knowledgeable nurse who understands and believes that illness and suffering can contain profound meaning and who is able to establish relatedness, will be able to assist most ill persons who suffer from their inability to cope with these most difficult human problems.

PREREQUISITES

In order to assist ill persons to find meaning in illness the nurse herself must believe that illness can contain profound meaning—meaning which can enable the individual to cope with his difficult experiences. *This belief also presupposes that the nurse has a vastly different concept of illness than is generally held, i.e., the only possible perception of illness is that it is undesirable and intrinsically evil.* This is not to suggest that the nurse must believe that illness is, in and of itself, a positive good, or that illness is to be preferred to health. It does imply that the nurse is able to comprehend that illness and suffering can be profoundly meaningful life experiences *provided* the ill individual also comprehends, or is assisted by the nurse to find, *meaning* and *purpose* in these experiences.

The orientation of health workers is a major barrier to accepting the concept that illness is an experience that can be self-actualizing rather than meaningless. Nurses and other health workers are creatures of the culture in which they live, and tend to hold to the general beliefs of that culture—that illness and suffering are to be avoided, if at all possible, and that an ill individual who is "unproductive," bedridden, in pain, or completely dependent on others would be better off dead. Health workers generally learn about illness by studying such subjects as anatomy, physiology, pathology, and other similarly related courses. The meanings illness can have for the individual are not given the same amount of emphasis.

Most health workers are "cure-oriented" and derive great satisfaction from assisting ill persons to recover. However, many individuals suffer from illnesses which cannot be cured and many ill persons do not get well, i.e., in the sense of being completely freed of their disease process. What is the attitude of health workers towards individuals who do not recover? When "little can be done" in terms of cure, how does this affect the attitude of health workers? Do physicians and nurses tend to view the ill person's lack of improvement as a reflection on their professional competence? There is growing evidence in the literature to support the claim that health workers, once they perceive that ill persons will not recover, begin to withdraw psychologically and physically, especially from the individual with a long-term illness. A general aura of helplessness and hopelessness soon prevades their attitude and is usually communicated to the ill person by the health worker. The "there is nothing we can do" or the "he would be better off dead" types of attitudes are not only corrosive in terms of establishing relatedness, but may drive a sick person to despair. How many problems have been engendered by health workers who hold such beliefs?

SCOPE OF THE PROBLEM

With the growing number of individuals whose life span has been lengthened by advances in the medical sciences there has also been an upsurge in the number of individuals suffering from long-term illnesses. At the present time, these illnesses cannot be cured. Assisting these individuals to find meaning in suffering and illness is a complex task. It is not only the individual suffering from an acute or fatal illness who needs assistance. One must also include large numbers of individuals whose life experiences have been drastically curtailed, or modified, as a result of the onset of an illness, which, though not fatal, is nevertheless long-term and incurable. Consider the somewhat "simple problem" of an individual with a cardiac condition who has been placed on a 500 mg low sodium diet. On the surface this problem may not seem important, particularly complicated, or may not indicate that the ill person needs help to find meaning in illness. Superficially it may appear that the individual requires only health teaching relative to his diet. Health teaching is important; however, it is but one aspect of the problem and teaching alone may not be sufficient to assist an individual to modify the eating habits of a lifetime. The individual is being asked to modify or change his way of life, *not* just his diet; this fact may not be immediately apparent even to the ill person. It is an old true-ism that one "begins where the patient is" in terms of health teaching, but it is also the task of the professional nurse practitioner to foresee some of the problems the ill person will probably encounter, and to prepare him to cope with them, since the problems are many. If the individual is successful in adhering to his diet at home, he is faced with the many nagging problems that dining out may entail. An invitation to dinner at the home of a friend can, instead of being an enjoyable visit, become an annoying arithmetical problem of calculating the amount of sodium in every portion of food eaten. Thus, such a "minor" problem can soon become an intolerable burden, especially if the individual perceives his life robbed of enjoyment and meaning by the very measures he must take to control the symptoms of his illness. Because of the many vexing problems the individual encounters he may believe that "it is not worth it" and will abandon any attempt to adhere to such a regimen. In the same manner, an individual suffering from diabetes may not adhere to his diet, or take the prescribed dose of insulin, because he perceives his life robbed of all meaning by the measures he must take to conserve health. Such individuals are not necessarily neurotic or "stubborn." It is highly probable that recalcitrant "diabetics" believe the measures they must take to conserve health are simply "not worth it." It is especially when such persons are undergoing stress caused by personal problems that they are likely to "give up" and abandon all attempts to maintain health. Individuals do not always engage in rational, realistic thinking. Unfortunately, the emotions are not as "well educated" as the intellect.

How often nurses and physicians are perplexed and annoyed by an ill person's refusal to follow a "simple diet" and thereby conserve health. Health teaching, lectures on the importance of adhering strictly to his diet, and fears of what will occur if he does not follow diet instructions, soon lose their force if the individual perceives that his life is robbed of enjoyment, satisfaction and meaning by the very measures he must take to control his illness. *The human being must be assisted not only to perceive meaning in illness but also in the very measures he must take to conserve his health and control his illness.* Health workers might well ponder the degree of self-denial (if not actual sacrifice) they so glibly request of others. Habits formed over a period of years are embedded in the personality and not so easily broken, neither are individuals always capable of immediate or prolonged self-denial.

The problems encountered by the individual on a low sodium diet have been discussed at some length as an example of a type of problem frequently overlooked by health workers. It is not a particularly dramatic problem, and may seem somewhat commonplace when compared to difficulties that other individuals encounter. But it is, nevertheless, a very real problem to the individual who is encountering it.

The major task of health workers in regard to such individuals is to assist them to find some meaning in the acts of self-denial and sacrifice they are asked to make. Without the perception of meaning in these acts, it is not probable that an individual will be motivated to persevere over any extended period of time in practicing such a high level of self-denial.

Before considering the nurse's specific responsibility in assisting ill persons in finding meaning in illness, or ways in which she may approach this most difficult task, it is necessary to consider what is meant by the term "to find meaning" in illness and suffering.

PART II—DEFINITION OF THE TERM "TO FIND MEANING IN ILLNESS AND SUFFERING"

Meaning is the reason given to particular life experience by the individual undergoing the experience. It is the "why" of Nietsche's often quoted comment, "He who has a *why* to live for, can bear almost any *how*." [4] It is probable that most individuals, at one time or another in their life, ask themselves these questions; however, it is in the experience of illness and suffering (our own and the experiences of those we love) that the need to answer these questions seems so compelling. In no other situation in life does it seem as necessary to find answers to these most difficult questions as in the experience of illness and suffering.

By this term is also meant a conscious awareness of the reasons why one is undergoing these experiences. These reasons are characterized by clarity and by the fact that they are understandable, i.e., they satisfy the individual, make sense to him, and are relevant to the experience that the individual is undergoing.

The term "meaning" is used in a restricted sense and refers only to those meanings which enable the ill individual not only to submit to illness, but to use it as an enabling life experience, i.e., enabling in the sense that it is still possible for the individual to achieve self-actualization and that which lies beyond actualization: the ability to transcend self as a result of these experiences.

The experiences of illness and suffering, per se, have no meaning in and of themselves. Only the ill person experiencing the impact of these conditions can attribute or discover value or meaning in these experiences. Meanings originate in the human being, not in the situation in which the person finds himself. Meaning is not inherent in life experiences; only the human being, immersed in and living through a particular life experience, arrives at meaning.

Since every human being is unique it follows that meaning discovered in the experience of illness and suffering will be unique to the individual undergoing the experience. Because meaning can be detected only by the ill individual it follows that health workers, family, or friends of the ill individual cannot "give meaning" to the ill person although they can help the person to arrive at meaning.

---

[4] Frankl, *op. cit.,* p. 164.

What is the genesis of meaning? If one accepts the premise that the human being is utterly unique and irreplaceable it follows that every person has particular tasks in life which can be performed or fulfilled only by himself. The individual is responsible for performing his particular life's tasks since no one else can perform them. Individuals who do not accept their unique responsibility are quite apt to succumb to the anguish of meaninglessness. It is believed that meaning can be found to the extent that the ill individual realizes he is *still* useful in regard to the tasks which can only be undertaken by himself alone. To be useful is to feel necessary. When one feels necessary (to or for someone, or something) he feels as though his life has significance. When an individual is able to perceive this truth he is also apt to be able to perceive the profound meaning illness can contain. However, most ill individuals and their families need *continuous* assistance from health workers and others in order to cope with these experiences, and eventually to find meaning in them.

Unfortunately, when the individual or family member has a great need to discuss these problems he finds few who will even listen to him, much less finds anyone who will give him an opportunity to explore some possible meanings to these perennial life problems. Thus it may be that when assistance from others is most needed the individual discovers he is most alone. Too often the ill individual is deserted psychologically; those who should be able to assist him (health workers) either cannot or do not know how to do so. The individual has no recourse but to struggle with the problem alone. Some individuals are able to cope with this problem, others are not; so they arrive at the conclusion that what has happened to them is utterly senseless and inexplicable. And what can be more demoralizing to an ill individual than to believe that his illness and suffering are meaningless? What is the individual left with but his loneliness and sense of futility which may border on despair? The tragedy is not that these situations occur, or that health workers are not always wise enough to help. The tragedy is that the problems are not even recognized by those whose responsibility it is to help and comfort. (Specific ways in which the professional nurse practitioner can assist the individual will be discussed in Part III of this chapter.)

PART III

How does one assist an ill human being to find meaning in illness and suffering? Specifically, the nurse assists the human being (1) to find meaning in the measures he must take to conserve health to control the symptoms of his illness, i.e., in acts of self-denial and sacrifice he will be required to make; (2) to accept illness and to live a full life despite the limitations which illness imposes. If the nurse can accomplish this she will have done much for the ill human being.

Some individuals perceive illness as inexplicable and meaningless, i.e., individuals who react to the stress of illness by developing the "why me?" reaction. There are also individuals who, although able to accept illness to some extent, nevertheless need support and help in order to continue coping with stress. These persons are also in need of the nurse's assistance. One may wonder if the nurse can possibly help individuals with such difficult problems. But the fact remains that nurses—prepared or not, willing or not, whether or not they recognize a cry for help—are constantly being called on to assist ill persons with such problems. It cannot be denied that these problems are complex or that our knowledge is limited; however, such reasons are invalid if used to justify refusal to try to aid ill persons with such problems.

No one is an expert in assisting individuals to cope with illness and suffering, i.e., an expert in the sense of knowing all there is to know about such human problems, or expert enough to be able to assist all ill individuals. It is not an easy task to assist individuals to find meaning in that which seems meaningless. It is a most difficult complex task requiring understanding, judgment, tact, skill and courage, on the part of the nurse. There is no one method best suited to aid such individuals. There is no one golden phrase that the nurse can utter which will magically assist these individuals. There are no short cuts, easy methods, or ready-made techniques; it is at best a slow painstaking process, but a rewarding one.

At the risk of being redundant, it is necessary to re-emphasize a basic belief or prerequisite needed by the nurse in order to assist ill persons to arrive at meaning. This belief is: *any nursing action designed to assist ill persons to arrive at meaning will be effective only to the extent that the nurse truly believes that meaning can be found.* If the nurse does not truly believe this, any nursing measures used to help ill persons find meaning will be to no avail.

What is required of the nurse is a particular type of orientation, or belief, about people—a belief which must permeate her every contact with others. This belief is that every human being has dignity and merit by virtue of his humanity. No matter how "useless" (in the "worldly" sense) or apparently unproductive an individual may seem—he is not divested of his humanity by virtue of his apparent "uselessness."

The nurse is the intercessor, mediatrix, advocator and protector of the weak, the helpless, the disabled, the disfigured, the unborn, those maimed in body and mind, and for all of the so-called "useless" and "non-productive" people. Since the first edition of this book appeared, a number of states have passed laws which legalize the performance of abortions or liberalize existing laws. In the author's opinion, this change is an ominous one reflecting a declining commitment to reverence for life. Permitting the destruction of an unborn child may be but the first step towards permitting another kind of legally sanctioned destruction, i.e., euthanasia. Some health workers are being infected by the prevalent cultural belief that the non-productive, "useless" person is better off dead. It is but a short step to advocating the "release" of the hopelessly ill, the old, the mentally ill and the mentally retarded—all in the name of "humanity." It is the author's conviction that the nurse *must be* an advocate of life—not death. These words will seem severe to some and unnecessary to others. It is only because the matter is so important and so seldom discussed that it has been given so much consideration.

The nurse who believes that an ill person would be better off dead obviously does not believe that life experiences, i.e., illness, suffering and pain, can contain profound meanings. One wonders if it is "love of humanity" which motivates a nurse to believe that an ill person would be better off dead, or if the nurse desires to escape from the feelings of vulnerability engendered in herself when she cares for such individuals. Is it really pity for the sufferings of a hopelessly ill individual that causes the nurse to believe that this person would be better off dead and beyond all suffering? Or is it that the nurse dreads any encounter with the ill person (or his family) because she feels helpless and does not really know how to assist the individual? Is the nurse not motivated by the pain of her own helplessness? When the ill person dies so dies the pain of the nurse's inadequacy (for the time being) until she confronts another such ill person and then the process begins again.

Values determine behavior, and individuals act on the basis of their belief systems. However, no one—nurse, ill person, or family member—is assisted when the nurse believes that an ill person is a burden. It is only when the nurse begins to comprehend the profound meanings that illness can contain that her beliefs will change. Until such a time, this type of nurse will consider finding meaning in illness as a waste—useless and futile. Therefore, these are the basic beliefs, or prerequisites, required by the nurse if the ill person is to arrive at meaning.

OVER-VIEW

In Part III, both general and specific ways of helping ill persons to find meaning in illness are discussed. The typical behavior patterns of individuals who are unable to accept illness are described. A discussion of the problem of self-pity is included, followed by a description of the extreme phases of the "why me?" (or non-acceptance) reaction. Effective ways of assisting the individual in pain are explored. Part III concludes with a brief discussion regarding ways of assisting ill persons in finding meaning in the measures which they must take to control illness and conserve health.

HELPING INDIVIDUALS TO FIND MEANING IN ILLNESS

The nurse's task is to assist the ill person to arrive at a meaning for illness *without* imposing her own meaning on the ill person or family. The nurse is able to assist the ill person to find meaning *only* if she is able to establish and maintain a human-to-human relationship. Establishing a relationship, in and of itself, does not provide an ill person with meaning, it only affords a context or gives the ill person an opportunity whereby he can be helped to arrive at meaning.

Not all ill persons will require this assistance; the nurse must first ascertain whether or not assistance is required. In order to do this, the nurse initiates the same helping process in assisting ill persons to cope with meaninglessness as she does in ascertaining any other nursing need. She observes the individual's behavior, explores with the individual her interpretation of this behavior (in order to validate or discount the interpretation), plans a course of nursing action (based on validated inferences), then evaluates the extent to which the need has been met. The helping process remains constant despite the type of problem the ill person may have.

When does the nurse assist the ill person with the problem of meaninglessness? During each interaction the nurse strives to assist the individual with this problem. She assists in a quiet, thoughtful manner. She must rely on her judgment since there are few guideposts or principles to assist her. In one sense, assisting individuals with meaninglessness is like a tenant moving into an unfurnished house—all the tenant has is what he brings to the house. The same situation prevails in approaching ill persons and helping them cope with meaninglessness. All the nurse has to offer is what she brings to the nursing situation.

GENERAL CONSIDERATIONS

In order to assist ill persons to cope with meaninglessness, the nurse must first examine the extent to which ill persons and family members accept illness. Does the nurse presume that acceptance follows knowledge? How often nurses assume that because an individual has been informed about his condition, told what to do to preserve his health, he will automatically be able to accept illness with all its limitations! "Knowing" is often confused with accepting. It is not, however, synonymous with acceptance. We know little about the process of acceptance or ways of helping ill persons to accept life experiences. Wolff believes that acceptance is an endless process, not a "one shot affair." [5] There is much truth to this belief since no one accepts a difficult situation on a once-and-for-all basis. A case in point is that of a twenty-six-year-old man who had suffered a traumatic amputation of the right arm. He stated:

> "They (the nurses) tell me I have to adjust—to get used to being left-handed. What do they know about adjustment? It's easy for them to say that . . . they have two good arms. I have to adjust every time I try to dress myself . . . when I eat or try to pick up something or carry something. Every time I watch a ball game on television I have to adjust. I don't need all of that hog-wash about adjustment . . ."

Some of the irritation expressed by this man was undoubtedly multi-determined, but some of it was quite realistically directed towards nurses who do not understand that adjustment and acceptance are continuous processes.

SUGGESTIONS

The following suggestions may prove helpful provided the nurse understands that it is *only* within the context of a human-to-human relationship that such methods may assist ill persons to arrive at meaning.

The nurse is urged to pay strict attention to the ill person's requests no matter how trivial these requests may appear to nursing personnel. Providing

---

[5] Wolff, Isle: Nursing Role in Counseling Parents of Mentally Retarded Children. United States Department of Health, Education and Welfare, Children's Bureau, Welfare Administration, 1964, pp. 4-5.

physical comfort also is a means of alleviating psychological distress. An ill person is not apt to express his deep concern to, or to trust, a nurse who does not meet his immediate nursing needs, whatever they may be.

It is also suggested that the nurse avoid *needless* probing into the reasons why the individual believes that his illness is inexplicable and meaningless. Once the nurse has validated (with the ill person) the fact that the individual perceives his illness as meaningless and has explained the reasons why he believes he is being afflicted, it serves no useful purpose to continue to discuss these reasons as this elicits little new or useful data; in fact, it may intensify or exacerbate the individual's emotional response. Prolonged probing in this area with the intention of helping the ill person "to ventilate" and "express his fears" may create more problems than it solves; ill persons may experience a resurgence of anxiety, depression and anger at a time when their ability to control or handle these feelings is weakened. This is not to deny that individuals frequently experience great relief in being able to discuss their problems with a knowledgeable, understanding nurse. What *is* deplored is the growing tendency to carelessly and needlessly probe into the psyche of others. The result is that the nurse may inflict more pain in her desire to be helpful and may break down the only controls or defenses which the individual has available to combat his difficulties.

How can the nurse approach the problem of meaninglessness? She first recognizes *the ill person's major problem area to be inability in accepting his human-ness and the tendency to exempt himself from the frailties of his human nature.* The first task of the nurse is then to assist the individual in accepting his human condition. Once the ill person has accomplished this he is enabled to arrive at some meaning or reason for illness which will be relevant for him. *The first task of the nurse then is to help ill persons accept their humanity.*

It must be remembered, however, that it is only within the context of a human-to-human relationship that the suggested methods and approaches will help individuals arrive at meaning. The suggested approaches should *not* be used indiscriminately or without much reflection on the part of the nurse. The professional nurse does not use *any* of the suggested approaches until she ascertains and validates with the ill person the nature of his distress. If it has been validated with the ill person that he believes illness is inexplicable and senseless, the nurse may then plan to use one or any of the suggested approaches. The nurse continually assesses the extent to which the individual is helped by the nursing measures being used; evaluation is a continuous process in every nursing situation.

Methods and approaches used to assist ill persons to accept their human-ness, and eventually to arrive at meaning, follow.

SPECIFIC METHODS AND APPROACHES

The methods of assisting ill individuals to accept their human-ness are divided into two major categories. Circuitous (or indirect) methods include (1) the parable method, (2) the veiled problem approach, and (3) the personal experience approach. Direct methods include: (1) questioning in jest but with intent and purpose, (2) the *purposeful* relating of opinions and (3) discussing the beliefs about the nature of man held by the great religious teachers and leaders.

Circuitious Methods (Indirect Methods)

Instead of confronting the ill person with the fact that he seems to believe that he should be exempt from misfortune the nurse chooses an indirect approach, hoping thereby to assist the individual to realize his wrong conclusion. The nurse does not supply the ill person with meaning but assists the patient to arrive at meaning.

Parable Method. The parable method seems particularly suited for some ill persons. In using this particular method the nurse, during her interaction with the ill person, relates a parable or tells a story which illustrates the point that no human being is exempt from illness. One particularly useful parable or story is "The Parable of the Mustard Seed."

> Gotami was born in India. She married and went to the house of her husband's people to live. She bore a son but the boy died. She began to grieve. She took her son with her from place to place asking for medicine for him. People scoffed and laughed at her. One man took pity on her and told her to seek the assistance of the foremost individual in the world. Taking her son with her she asked the great Teacher for medicine for her son. The Teacher told her thst she had done well in coming to him for medicine. He told her to go throughout the city and in whatever house no one had suffered or died from that house to bring a grain of mustard seed. She went from house to house and never succeeded in finding a house where no one had suffered. She realized that her son was not the only child who suffered and that suffering was a law common to mankind. [6]

This parable may need to be adapted, for some ill persons, because of the reference to death in the original parable. It may also be modified, depending on the point the nurse is striving to make. The particular usefulness of parables is that they are not easily forgotten and tend to be remembered by the ill person over a fairly long period of time. After reflecting on the meaning of the parable, the ill person may begin to understand its relevance to the situation which he faces. A sense of timing, of knowing *when* and *how* to use the parable method, is invaluable. If the nurse does not feel comfortable in using this particular approach other methods are suggested. The nurse is cautioned *not* to overuse this method by regaling the ill person with various parables in an attempt to "rush him along." This method seems most effective when only one or two parables are used, and when related at a time when the ill person is most ready for them.

Veiled Problem Approach. Another method which may be used in conjunction with (or instead of) the parable method is the use of indefinite pronouns, or the first-person plural pronouns such as "we," "us" or "our" in alluding to the ill person's problem area. The purpose of this method is to deflect the emotional impact of the problem by thinly disguising or veiling that which is being discussed.

---

[6] Burtt, E. A. (ed.): The Teachings of the Compassionate Buddha. New York: The New American Library of World Literature Inc. (A Mentor Book), 1955, pp. 43-46.

However, *both* nurse and ill person are aware that it is the ill person's problem which is being discussed.

This method is somewhat limited in its usefulness; however, it does allow the ill individual an opportunity to react more impersonally (to some extent), and to become more objective about the problem under discussion.

Personal Experience Approach. There seems to be a generally accepted belief that nurses are *never,* under any circumstances, to relate their personal experiences to ill persons, the reason for this prohibition being that the ill person may believe the nurse is more interested in herself than in him. This prohibition has much merit; however, it is believed that there are times and occasions when nurses *should* share personal experiences with ill persons. If the nurse believes that an ill person may benefit as a result of hearing of a personal experience of the nurse she does not hesitate to relate it. The relating of the experience is intentional and purposeful, being designed to assist the ill person to accept his human-ness.

What type of experience may the nurse relate? The nurse relates the type of experience which she believes will assist the individual and is relevant to the person's condition. For example, while relating with an ill person who believed that he should be exempt from illness, the nurse told the individual of her reaction, when, as a child, she first learned that "even doctors and nurses could become ill." She told him how upset she became when she first learned this. The ill man replied that he always "knew" doctors and nurses became ill but it had never really occurred to him until the nurse mentioned it! It was the relating, by the nurse, of this seemingly insignificant personal experience which caused this man to accept his human-ness and to discount his exemption from illness.

Nurses can think of innumerable personal experiences which may be used to illustrate an idea, give suggestions, or focus on a particular problem area. For example, any personal experience in which the nurse first realized that "good people" could become ill, and other such personal experiences, may be used. The personal experience method is used *only* to assist ill persons, as is any other nursing action or measure. It is not used to provide a social hour for the nurse.

Circuitous or indirect methods seem to be more effective in assisting individuals to arrive at meaning than do more direct methods of explanation or exhortation.

Direct Methods

Direct methods include the purposeful use of such techniques as (1) questioning seemingly in jest but with full intent and purpose and (2) the *purposeful* relating of opinions and (3) discussing the beliefs about the nature of man held by the great religious teachers and leaders. Direct methods are used in conjunction with the indirect or circuitious method, or may be used alone.

Questioning in Jest. Depending on the degree of relatedness between nurse and ill persons, the nurse may purposefully use the technique of questioning (seemingly in jest) but with full intent and purpose. Only the most experienced nurse should undertake the use of such a method. If misused, this technique comes perilously close to the "shaming" technique so frequently used by lay people and some non-professional (and professional) personnel. The nurse uses this technique as a means of assisting individuals to acknowledge their human condition. A case in point follows. A sixty-year-old male, recovering from a cerebrovascular accident, described his reaction to the use of such a method by a staff nurse:

> "I had a hard time of it after I had my stroke . . . Oh, the nurses took good care of me but I kept worrying whether my legs would be all right again. Dr. M. said I'd be able to walk . . . he said it just took time. Well, I'm sure he knows what he's talking about . . . but I just kept on brooding and one day I felt so bad I cried . . . a grown man and I haven't cried in years . . . Do you know Miss A. (staff nurse)? Well, she's been caring for me all along . . . she came in and saw me crying. She looked at me and said, "What makes you think you're Superman?" It sounded like she was kidding but I knew she wasn't. It sounds awful the way I'm telling you but she said it in such a way that I knew she was saying, "It's all right to cry—you're human." Well, I was finally able to stop crying and you know, Nurse, something healed inside of me that day. Oh, I still get disgusted and down in the mouth . . . but it wasn't like it was before. . ."

In this situation the nurse was able to assist the ill man because of her previous interaction pattern with him in which she had ascertained his difficulty, had validated his problem, and had initiated a course of nursing action which was of assistance to him. The question the nurse asked was specific and purposefully designed to assist the individual in accepting his human-ness. A proper sense of timing, of knowing when to use such a technique, seems essential for its successful use. Nurses are cautioned not to use such a device unless deliberation, consideration and reflection have preceded its use; unless the nurse has established this degree of relatedness the use of such a technique could destroy the relationship.

Explaining. Explaining, or telling the person that he is subject to all of the frailties of the human condition, is not an effective technique. Explaining ignores the obvious fact that the distressed individual is motivated more by emotions than by logical reasoning. Explaining or "telling ill persons" should be avoided unless the nurse's opinion is asked for by the ill person.

Discussing Religious Beliefs. Every human being has some basic beliefs about the nature of man, i.e., his origin, ultimate destiny, purpose for existing, and his assets and liabilities. Many individuals first learn these beliefs by attending services at churches, synagogues, temples or other places. Many individuals maintain their beliefs about the nature of man as taught by the religious leaders of their particular faith. The nurse who has an understanding of the major religious beliefs held by adherents to a particular faith or creed can utilize this knowledge in assisting ill persons to accept their human-ness by discussing these beliefs with the ill person.

One ill woman was helped to accept her humanity and change her belief that illness is a punishment from God by discussing with the nurse a major teaching of her (the ill person's) faith, namely, that Christ, in his humanity, suffered although he was blameless. This discussion was initiated by the nurse following a comment by the ill person that she did not know why God was "picking on her."

The nurse, then, can assist some ill persons to accept their humanity by discussing with them their religious convictions regarding the nature of man and the reasons why "good people" suffer. These reasons are based on the tenets of the particular person's religious belief system.

This method does not assist all ill persons, but it can be effective in helping some ill persons to accept their humanity and develop a clearer understanding of why human beings suffer and become ill. It is also believed that few nurses utilize this method due to cultural prohibitions about discussing "religious" matters with ill persons.

THE NURSE'S OPINION

If the nurse is asked for an opinion she carefully explores *why* the person is asking the question. She then determines *how* to respond to the question in such a way as to assist the person. For example, the individual may ask, "Nurse, why do you think this [the illness] happened to me?" Many individuals do not ask such questions because it never occurs to them that nurses can be of any assistance. Some ill persons, however, will ask the question if they respect and trust the nurse.

Assuming that during the nurse's previous interactions with the ill person the individual has stated that he doesn't know why he is ill since he's always been a "hard worker," etc., assuming also that the individual honestly wishes to know the nurse's opinion regarding his illness, then there is no reason why the nurse cannot state an opinion *provided*, of course, the opinion is such that it will help the individual, not harm him, as, for example, by discouraging the person. Naturally, unless the nurse has thought through the meanings which illness has for her she will not be able to give an opinion, much less discuss the problem with the ill person in any beneficial way.

How can the nurse answer such a question? No individual is ever really prepared to answer this question since no one possesses that much wisdom. If a nurse waits, however, until she is fully prepared to answer the question she will never respond. The nurse, therefore, weighs the question carefully, reflects on it and makes a decision as to whether or not her answer will aid the ill person. Some nurses circumvent the question altogether. There are no general guidelines or rules in this area. However, one veteran nurse answered the question, "Nurse why did this happen to me?" in the following manner:

> "Why does anyone become ill? I could answer you by talking about germs and infections, but this is not what you asked. I believe we become ill because we are human beings. I don't believe it has anything to do with how good a person we are, or how old or young we happen to be. We don't always understand it but it is the price we pay for being human. I've been a nurse for over thirty years and I've seen a lot. I'm not surprised when people become ill. But do you know what really amazes me? It's the courage people have that they don't know they have . . ."

The ill person reported that he was assisted by the nurse's reply. However, this is but one example; too many factors must be considered before advocating the use of such a method. Only the nurse's clinical judgment and her deep understanding of the individual ill human being can assist her in reaching such a decision.

Such are some approaches and methods a nurse may use to assist ill persons to arrive at meanings for illness.

In discussing the problem of meaninglessness it is suggested that the nurse strive neither to overly emphasize or underestimate the very real difficulties and problems which ill persons encounter as a result of illness. Negating and belittling the very real problems which ill persons face in a well-intended attempt to "cheer" them are usually interpreted (by ill individuals) as an indication that the nurse has little understanding. On the other hand, overemphasis on problems may overwhelm the ill person, thereby increasing feelings of helplessness and hopelessness.

It may not be necessary to assist ill persons to cope with meaninglessness; the individual may receive sufficient support and assistance through the human-to-human relationship with the nurse, and may be able to arrive at meaning with no further assistance. The very fact that the nurse is concerned—that she cares for and about the ill person—may suffice and enable the individual to cope with his distress. However, ill persons who react to illness by developing a non-acceptance (or why me?) reaction will require the assistance of the professional nurse practitioner.

Helping ill persons with specific reactions to illness, such as the "why me?" or non-acceptance reaction, will be considered next.

HELPING THE NON-ACCEPTING ILL PERSON

Non-accepting ill persons are those who respond to illness by developing a "why me?" reaction. These individuals may be grouped into two major categories, depending on the predominant behavioral response displayed by the individual. These two groups include the "unjustly afflicted" and the "punished individual." Self-pity is a problem for individuals in both groups. Feelings of self-pity may be so intense and persistent that the individual is almost overwhelmed by them. Or the individual may undergo transitory, less intense bouts of "feeling sorry for himself." Self-pity is discussed separately since it is so prevalent and is a major problem to the non-accepting patient.

Non-acceptance of illness can have serious consequences. Such individuals may disregard medical advice, or fail to take the necessary measures to control illness and conserve health. The inability to find meaning in illness may result in death. If unassisted, it is believed that some non-accepting individuals may enter into an extreme phase of suffering, i.e., the malignant phase of despairful not-caring. The process is reversible in this phase; it is seldom reversible in the next phase—the terminal phase of apathetic indifference. In this phase the individual loses the will to live and may die.

It is important for the nurse to remember that the behavior exhibited by ill persons may have many causes. The nurse does not *know* the reasons underlying behavior until she explores her inference with the ill person and validates them. Such behaviors as fear, anxiety, depression and self-pity *may* be caused by the individual being unable to perceive meaning in illness. The nurse does not know that such is the case until she explores her inferences with the ill person and validates these inferences.

Helping The "Unjustly Afflicted" Individual

The unjustly afflicted individual makes comments to the effect that he believes that illness is an unfair, unjust affliction. The nurse may realize that the individual finds it difficult to understand why he was afflicted and usually states that he has always been a "good person," "a good husband," "a good father," etc. The individual behaves as if he should be exempt from misfortune because of his "good" qualities.

The underlying premise seems to be that good persons are not supposed to suffer; he is good, therefore there is no reason why he should be made to suffer. Such an individual fails to realize that he is a human being with a human nature and thus is subject to all of the frailties of his human-ness. His goodness (or badness) cannot negate the fact that he belongs to the family of man and is therefore prone to illness, suffering and pain. Many such individuals have considered illness or accidents as events that happen to others—never to themselves. They have assumed that somehow they would be exempt from misfortune.

Such an individual dwells in a magical world where misfortune happens to others—not to him. When he becomes ill, the illusion of invulnerability shatters. In some respects the "unjustly" afflicted person acts on the premise that he is super-human—not human. In illness the individual can no longer ignore his humanity. He may not wish to accept his human-ness, but he can no longer ignore it. In order to transcend one's humanity it is first necessary to accept the fact that one is human and therefore not exempt from all of the frailties of human nature. The individual must also accept the difficult truth that being a "good person" or a "hard worker" does not exempt one from misfortune. The task of the nurse is to assist the ill human being to truly accept these facts.

Behavioral Range. The unjustly afflicted individual displays such emotional responses as anger (which may range from annoyance to bitter rebellion), some degree of self-pity, depression and anguish. Some degree of fear and anxiety is usually blended into the emotional response. The unjustly afflicted person is a very angry individual and this anger is evident in comments previously mentioned which such patients tend to make, such as "illness is an unfair, unjust affliction." The individual finds it difficult to understand why he became ill. The nurse may realize that the ill person needs assistance in finding meaning because of the types of comments made by the individual or by the questions he tends to ask. The nurse heeds any comment made by an ill person to the effect that he believes his illness is an unfair affliction—an affliction which somehow he doesn't deserve. Such an individual finds it difficult to understand why he has been afflicted and usually states that he has been "a good person," etc.

The individual seems to believe that "good persons" are not supposed to become ill; he is good, therefore there is no reason why he should have to suffer.

The ill person seems baffled and somewhat bewildered; he cannot seem to comprehend *why* he became ill.

Specific Helping Measures. It is the task of the professional nurse practitioner to assist the ill human being to accept his human-ness. It is suggested that the nurse use the circuitous methods in assisting the unjustly afflicted individual.

The "Punished" Individual

The punished individual displays such emotional responses as depression, anxiety, and some degree of self-pity. Depression seems to be his predominant feeling tone. In some individuals the reaction may resemble a retarded depression. Another outstanding characteristic of the "punished" individual is the tendency to focus on his "badness" and his belief that illness is the punishment meted to him for his "bad behavior."

The punished individual makes comments to the effect that he hasn't been a "good person." He may relate the number of times he missed going to church or explain that he hasn't been a "good father," "a good husband," etc. Many ill persons who perceive illness as a punishment once believed in the tenets of their faith, then "fell away" from their religion or began to disregard the tenets of their faith. Usually such individuals experience varying amounts of guilt for having departed from practicing their religious beliefs; when such persons become ill they may experience an upsurge of guilt feelings. In attempting to explain the illness, they may believe that it was sent to punish them for their past misdeeds.

This is a tenuous type of reaction in that if the person recovers he is apt to forget his belief that he is being punished. On the other hand, if the person's illness progresses he is quite apt to shift the "blame" from himself to God. The ill person's reasoning is as follows: if God exists then He is a kind and merciful God; a merciful God would not be so unkind as to punish him. Since he believes that he is being punished, the ill person then concludes that there is no God. If there is no God then there is no meaning (if even a negative one of being punished) in what the ill person must bear and suffer.

As in the case of the unjustly afflicted person, the punished person tends to deny his human-ness. These individuals do, however, strive to find meaning in illness (even though the meaning found is a negative one).

Helping Measures. Like the unjustly afflicted individual, the punished person has a tendency to deny his human-ness. The circuitous methods and approaches are used to aid the punished individual. The more effective methods seem to be the "parable method" and the "veiled problem approach." The indirect methods seem to be more useful in assisting such individuals than the direct ones.

Ill persons who believe that God is punishing them for their past misdeeds may be assisted by spiritual direction or counseling by the clergymen of their respective faiths. The nurse is urged to collaborate and work with the minister, priest or rabbi. If the nurse is not familiar with the ill person's religious beliefs she can readily obtain this information. A collaborative working relationship with the individual's minister, priest or rabbi is helpful to nurse and ill person alike and may widen the nurse's understanding of the religious beliefs of others.

A major barrier in assisting the punished person seems to be the nurse's reluctance to speak with ill persons about their religious beliefs and convictions. This reluctance probably stems from the belief that one should "never discuss politics or religion with others" lest an argument ensue. Illness, however, is not just a physical or emotional problem; it is also a spiritual encounter. If an ill human being wishes to talk about his religious beliefs there is no reason why the nurse should not listen to him, make carefully thought out comments to him, or ask pertinent questions. *To fail to do is tantamount to neglecting the spiritual needs of ill persons.*

PROBLEM OF SELF-PITY

Both the "unjustly afflicted" and the "punished" individual suffer from feelings of self-pity. Being "sorry for oneself" includes feelings which accompany the idea that one is being "picked on" or "put upon"—that one is being unjustly treated. Little is definitely known about the dynamics underlying self-pity, but it is probable that self-pity is a blend of anger (turned inward towards the self resulting in depression) and anxiety. In some individuals the reaction may be so severe as to resemble an agitated depression.

Most individuals, at one time or another, have experienced transitory periods of self-pity. These bouts of self-pity are usually engendered by an incident, or series of incidents, which undermine one's security and self-esteem. A person who has been subjected to a series of traumatic experiences is likely to experience self-pity. Disappointments and losses of all kinds, such as the loss of a loved one or loss of personal possessions or of one's integrity, may induce self-pity. Individuals who lead dull and boring lives devoid of pleasure are likely to experience bouts of self-pity. The self-pitying individual usually experiences feelings of sadness and anger. There is a strong tendency to affix blame on the person(s) deemed responsible for one's condition. In most persons, bouts of self-pity are transitory and self-limiting and the individual does not require assistance in coping with this problem.

However, non-accepting persons—those who respond to illness by developing the "why me?" reaction—may require special help in dealing with their feelings of self-pity. Those to whom illness has been a shattering experience, i.e., in terms of bringing them face to face with their own vulnerability, are apt to experience intense feelings of self-pity over a fairly long period of time.

The behavior of self-pitying individuals seems to have a provocative, almost goading effect on others. There are few individuals who can listen to "poor-me" type comments without experiencing some degree of irritation and anger. There are probably many reasons for the effect that self-pitying individuals have on others. Anxiety and depression are "contagious" emotions. Individuals working with the self-pitying person can become "infected" (to some extent) by the individual's mood. Self-pitying individuals are not "good patients" (i.e., in terms of the stereotype of a good "patient": namely an individual who seldom complains, requires little assistance, cooperates, is grateful for any attention he receives, and who gets well). Another possible reason for health workers' attitudes towards such individuals stems from the erroneous belief that the self-pitying individual is a weak-willed person who is "deliberately" feeling sorry for himself. The person is viewed as an individual who could "snap out of it" if he really wanted to do so.

If, however, the nurse reflects upon and begins to comprehend the utter emptiness, the fear, the horror of meaninglessness that the individual is experiencing, her feelings towards the ill person will change. She may still become momentarily annoyed, but such feelings will be transitory and will not result in ineffective or punitive measures.

Actually there is no other group of individuals more maligned and misunderstood or given so little sympathy and understanding. There is probably no other group so neglected or so in need of the services which a professional nurse can render. And there is no more effective way to measure a nurse's true love for humanity than to observe her interactions with ill persons who exhibit self-pitying behavior.

An individual who suffered from intense feelings of self-pity described her experience as follows:

"It's like standing at the bottom of a deep valley—it's dark there and you're alone . . . you can't get out and you're afraid. You try to climb out but you can't. I hated myself and the way I was acting but I couldn't stop myself. Dr. J. told me to quit acting like a baby, but that just made me feel worse. Miss A. (staff nurse) bawled me out because I didn't want to get out of bed and walk. I was so weak and it hurt so much all I could do was cry. One day Miss A. didn't even try to get me up . . . But with Miss B. (staff nurse) it was different . . . she never fussed at me but somehow she always managed to get me up . . . Oh, I'd cry a little and act like a baby sometimes but I never felt that Miss B. was disgusted with me . . . it was like she had faith in me . . ."

This particular individual's experience illustrates, to some extent, how an individual feels when immersed in self-pity and illustrates both effective and ineffective means of assisting such persons.

It is probable that most health workers or family members will tolerate a certain degree of expressed self-pity provided such expressions do not continue over any extended period of time, the limit usually being exceeded when health workers and others become annoyed, distressed, or alarmed by the individual's behavior. As self-pity increases there is usually a concomitant increase in "uncooperative" behavior. The individual may refuse to "cooperate" by refusing consent to treatments, and may fail to follow medical advice or to adhere to hospital rules and regulations.

Somewhere along the continuum of reactions, health workers or family members begin to exert pressure to change the ill person's behavior. A fairly common maneuver is to attempt to "shame" the individual and thereby change his behavior. It is extremely doubtful that an individual experiencing intense self-pity will be helped by being regaled with stories about non-complaining individuals who are much "worse off" than the ill person. When shaming fails, the individual is usually given "a good talking to" and is exhorted to "snap out of it" or is told to "pull himself together" (an interestingly graphic phrase used to describe an impossible feat).

Another maneuver, one used by some health workers, is to tell the ill person that he will not get well unless he "cooperates." A variant is the bartering type of approach, i.e., the ill person is informed, "if you are nice to us—we will be nice to you." This type of comment usually contains a hint or implies a threat of what may occur if the patient isn't nice and doesn't meet the health worker's expectations of a nice person.

Some well-intended individuals strive to help the ill person by telling him what they believe to be the meaning or cause of his illness and suffering. Some of these well-meaning individuals impose meanings which are irrelevant to the situation as the ill person perceives it. These meanings may also be untrue. (For detailed account of the use of this method, see the book of Job. Note comments made by Job's "comforters," Eliphaz, Baldad, Sophor and Eliu.)

None of these maneuvers is effective in terms of helping the ill person cope with the feelings of self-pity arising from inability to accept illness, and the manifold problems illness and suffering impose. Family members who use such ineffective methods mean well, and such relatives and friends are deeply distressed by the ill person's behavior, truly having the individual's interests at heart. However, if the ill person does not cease complaining and becomes increasingly angry and rebellious, family members and health workers may withdraw psychologically and/or physically from him. There is a tendency to withdraw from an individual who makes one feel uncomfortable or helpless.

When family members and health workers withdraw or avoid him, the ill person is deprived of human contact at a time when he most needs it. The withdrawal of human contact tends to increase the individual's feelings of self-pity— providing him with one more reason or justification for "feeling sorry for himself."

As a result of the various tactics used, the ill person's behavior may change (temporarily) in that he may try not to reveal his true feelings. However, the attempt to suppress these feelings is rarely successful, nor can the ill person control the expression of these feelings over any long period of time. A seemingly trivial frustration may precipitate an outpouring of angry rebellious feelings.

When shaming, being talked at, and withdrawal fail to elicit the expected behavior—some family members react by displaying objectifying pity which is exemplified in the "oh, you poor thing" attitude. Being subjected to objectifying pity usually always weakens the ill person's controls and increases his feelings of anger and resentment.

Without assistance the ill person's suffering becomes more intense, his angry feelings intensify, and he may progress into the malignant phase of despairful not-caring. This is the phase of the dark night of intense psychological turmoil and suffering.

Such ill persons, if these medications are prescribed, may frequently request narcotics (or sedatives), not to ease physical pain or induce sleep, but as a with-drawal tactic to deaden or kill their inner suffering. If not assisted, these ill persons may enter into the malignant or terminal phase of suffering. The individual may cease to strive to cope with the problems that he is encountering. Sometimes, *it is not so much that the person wants to die, but that he finds nothing to live for.* Death, then, is the repudiation of an existence which offers only meaningless suffer-ing.

The individual who finds no meaning in illness, who is harassed, humiliated and misunderstood by his family and friends, is indeed burdened. If, in addition, he is also misunderstood by those whose function it is to help and comfort, he is indeed bereft. Nurses who would exert every conceivable effort to aid an injured person who is hemorrhaging, or the individual in shock, sometimes do not compre-hend that an ill person who finds no meaning in illness is *as* needful as the person who is hemorrhaging. Both the individual who is hemorrhaging as well as the person who finds no meaning in illness are seriously ill. Both may die unless the nurse assists them.

When assisting the self-pitying individual it is essential that nurses avoid such ineffective tactics as attempting to "shame" the person by lecturing or giving him "a good talking to." The threatening "bartering" type of approach cannot be countenanced under any circumstance. Neither can the use of avoidance or with-drawal tactics be countenanced.

It is essential that nurses examine their thoughts and feelings about individ-uals who exhibit self-pitying behavior in order to avoid the approaches used by Miss A. (staff nurse) in the preceding example. Nurses are not superhuman. They are quite apt to react automatically towards ill persons who whine, complain, and seemingly do not appreciate the very real efforts which nurses make to assist them. However, gratitude is *not* the price a nurse exacts in exchange for nursing care. It is, of course, human to like ill persons who appreciate the services one is privileged to render; and there is nothing wrong with such feelings. What the nurse must guard against is expecting gratitude and cooperative behavior in return for the care she gives. While such conditional acceptance may be typical of a lay person's behavior, it is not typical or to be expected from the professional nurse practitioner.

Because such ill persons are overwhelmed with angry feelings it is not easy to care for them. It is a most difficult emotionally exhausting task. If a nurse does not have the insight and patience required in caring for such persons, it is best that another nurse be assigned to care for them since suffering can be inflicted on the ill individual by unskilled, insensitive nurses.

Specific Helping Measures

In communicating with the self-pitying individual it is helpful to agree with the person whenever his complaints are reality based. For example, the nurse calmly agrees with the ill person, "yes, it was a rough experience—yes, it was not easy for you." The nurse expresses such comments in a matter-of-fact tone of voice.

She neither overstates nor understates the ill person's problem. If an ill person says that an experience has been unpleasant or is difficult the nurse accepts the individual's perception as being true and valid for the person. On this basis it is possible to agree with the ill person's perception of an experience even though the nurse, from her vantage point, may view the situation quite differently.

> For example, an individual may complain bitterly about the number of injections he receives, how painful these injections are and how much he dreads them. The nurse may have a tendency to discount the person's complaints, especially if, in her experience, most ill persons who receive such injections do not complain. There is also the possibility that a nurse who prides herself on her ability to give a "painless" injection may interpret such complaints as a reflection on her technical competence.

Whatever the nurse's perception may be, the fact remains that the ill person's perception is true and valid for *him*. The nurse uses the ill person's perception of his experience to assist him, and does not impose on the ill person her expectation as to how he (the ill person) should behave or respond. Besides, the nurse is not the ill person, she is not ill, and neither does she feel the injections.

The effects of agreeing with the ill person's perception is that it provides a means of support. The individual realizes that he has been understood by the nurse who does not negate, deride, or overly emphasize his complaints or comments. Such an approach allows the ill person an opportunity to examine his perception. When the nurse verbally agrees with the person it has the effect of permitting the ill person an opportunity to reflect upon the validity of his complaint. A common end-result of such a process is that eventually the ill person may begin to comment that "well, it isn't really as bad as all that" or similar remarks.

Needless to say, this approach is quite different from that used by lay persons who tend to negate or overly emphasize the ill person's perception of his problem. The ill human being who is approached in this manner does not have to keep convincing others that his complaint is valid. Nurses should be alert to the fact that the self-pitying individual is particularly sensitive to any comments or implications that he may be exaggerating the degree of his suffering. Anyone who experiences self-pity is suffering. The nurse does not *really* know if the individual is exaggerating or not. *If* the individual is exaggerating he is doing so for a reason. It well may be that the ill person believes that no one will believe him or pay him any attention unless he does embellish his complaints or exaggerate. There is nothing wrong, per se, with wanting attention. Every human being wants attention. It demonstrates a lack of understanding when nurses make such comments as "all he wants is attention." Such a comment is usually made in a disdainful tone of voice— the nurse expressing or implying her disapproval of such a person. Who does not wish attention when ill? Who does not want to be noticed, respected, or understood? Who does not want nurses to care for and about him when he is ill? If an ill person seems to be constantly seeking attention of health workers, then the nurse tries to ascertain *why* the individual is behaving as he is, and attempts to assist him. Only if the meaning of the behavior is understood can the nurse plan a course of nursing action. Blaming helps neither the nurse nor the ill person to arrive at reasons for behavior. Blaming blocks relatedness. It alienates and inflicts additional suffering on the ill individual. A nurse who blames an ill person for his behavior cannot help but communicate her blaming attitude to the individual, who will invariably respond to this attitude. The individual must begin again to strive to convince the nurse that he needs assistance; his demands increase and the vicious cycle is operant again. If a person needs attention—attention should be given—not, however, in a grudgingly condescending manner, or in such a way as to convey to the individual that he is being given attention only to "shut him up." Such "attention" is unworthy of a professional nurse practitioner and cannot be countenanced under any circumstance.

The problem of the self-pitying individual has been discussed at some length because self-pity is a common behavioral response to illness. All that has been suggested regarding the self-pitying person applies generally to all individuals who experience illness as meaningless. If the individual is not assisted to find meaning in illness he may enter into the advanced phases of suffering. These phases are the malignant phase of "despairful not-caring" and the terminal phase of "apathetic indifference."

THE "DESPAIRFUL NOT-CARING" AND THE "INDIFFERENT" INDIVIDUAL

It is the task of the professional nurse practitioner to prevent individuals from advancing to the malignant and terminal phase of suffering. However, little research has been conducted in regard to finding effective ways of helping ill persons in the advanced phases of suffering. It is believed that if a nurse is able to establish relatedness with such individuals, and uses the supporting and comforting measures already described in this chapter, most individuals will be prevented from advancing to the extreme phases of suffering. However, nurses need to be cognizant of ways to help such individuals in the event that they enter into one of these phases.

An individual in the malignant and terminal phases of suffering may not necessarily be suffering from a "serious" illness, i.e., from the standpoint of prognosis. The individual may have a so-called "minor" illness; his reaction to illness, however, is far from minor.

The "Despairful Not-Caring" Individual

Despairful not-caring is experienced when the individual has suffered mentally, physically and spiritually over too long a period of time without assistance and without surcease of suffering. These persons are dominated by angry feelings of hopelessness which are bitterly expressed. If not assisted, these individuals may progress to the terminal phase of suffering. *Despairful not-caring is an interpersonal emergency and requires immediate concerted action.*

The despairing person protests that he "doesn't care what happens to him," but the vehemence of his protesting is an indication of how deeply he truly cares.

A case in point is that of Mrs. O., seventy years old, who was hospitalized for reduction of an old healed fracture of the right hip. The woman was given an extensive medical work-up and hence was hospitalized eight days prior to surgery. Surgery was deemed successful and Mrs. O. was considered to be in "good condition." However, the staff nurses began to complain about the patient's behavior. The Head Nurse described the woman's behavior as follows:

"Her personality has changed. She used to be so pleasant . . . now she complains all of the time. Dr. X. (physician) says she's doing fine . . . but she won't cooperate. Today, for example, she refused a.m. care. She said she just wanted to be left alone but if you leave her alone she still complains. She talks like she's mad at the world. Her family comes to see her regularly, but she tells them that they needn't bother to put themselves out for her . . . she gets furious with them if they're a minute late coming to see her. She told me that she is going to fire her her doctor . . . she said she had no use for him . . . we don't know what to do with her . . ."

Helping Measures. If possible, individuals in both the malignant and terminal phases should be cared for by clinical specialists in psychiatric nursing. If this is not possible, staff nurses working with such individuals should have the assistance of psychiatric nursing consultation. Staff nurses assigned to care for these individuals must be given sufficient time to work with them. The plan of nursing care should be carefully developed. Whenever possible the same nursing personnel should be assigned to care for these individuals.

Extraordinary consideration should be shown such ill persons. The individual's immediate needs are met as soon as possible. If at all possible the nurse should attempt to anticipate the individual's needs. If the ill person trusts the nurse, progress ensues. However, trust is established *only* after the individual learns that he can rely on the nurse. Nurses should pay attention to every request and defer to the ill person's wishes whenever possible. All ill persons need kind, non-punitive supporting care, but the despairful person is doubly in need of such care.

Left unaided it is probable that the despairful not-caring person will enter into the terminal phase of suffering. Despairful not-caring is a phase of extreme suffering and such individuals require immediate skillful assistance.

The "Apathetic Indifferent" Individual

Individuals in the terminal phase of suffering usually do not complain or bitterly express angry feelings of hopelessness. These individuals seem imperturable. The cry for help is stilled, probably because they believe that no one can or will help them. Nurses describe such individuals as having "lost their will to live." They seem to be "beyond caring." As in the case of despairful not-caring persons, individuals in this phase may not necessarily be suffering from a "serious" illness, i.e., from the standpoint of prognosis, to suffer intensely. These ill persons may have so-called "minor illnesses" and indications are that they "should get well," but they don't because they have lost the will to live.

As difficult as it may be to assist the despairful individual, it is still far easier to assist the individual in this phase than when he enters into the terminal phase. The condition is almost always reversible in the malignant phase of despair, but may be irreversible in the terminal phase of apathetic indifference.

Little is known about the "will to live"—what it is and what it is not. We do not know what complex of percipitating factors may motivate an individual to give up and, in a sense, almost "will" his death.

Helping Measures. What measures can be taken to assist such persons? Certainly the nurse can try some or all of the suggestions previously mentioned in this chapter, and any other ways that the nurse can think of to reach the individual and establish an emotional bond. These measures, however, may not assist the ill person unless he is somehow motivated to continue living.

What questions must one ask in such a situation? *What is required is not an answer to the question why the ill person wants to die, but rather what is he willing to live for?* In other words, what is required to regenerate the glimmer of life within the person? The nurse does not know, nor can she have any idea of, what may motivate the individual until she has more detailed information about the person than is commonly written on the individual's admission sheet.

The help of social service should be enlisted in order to gain this needed information. The nurse needs detailed information about the ill person—his background, interests and values—before she can truly plan nursing care. What kinds of information may be most valuable? The nurse needs to know if there is any human being whom the ill person cares for and may be willing to live for—any family member, friend, neighbor or acquaintance. She needs to know if there is any pet or inanimate object valued by the individual. Is there any idea or cause the person is willing to live for? Any unfulfilled dreams, unfinished work which may motivate the person? What was the individual interested in? Is there any fragment of beauty that once moved the person? What kind of music does he like? Does he have a favorite song? If so, what is it? What is his favorite food? How does he like it prepared or seasoned? What are his reading preferences? If the nurse is able to elicit such information from family or friends she can then use this information in planning an approach. The ill person can be brought into contact with individuals who are significant to him. Objects or things that have meaning to him can be brought to him. He can be given his favorite foods, and so forth.

If, however, little or no information is available about the person's background, the nurse must strive in every way possible to motivate the individual to continue living. She has no recourse but trial and error, hoping that somehow she will find a way to assist the person. All nursing personnel are enlisted to make a concerted effort to establish an emotional bond with the person.

Some nurses are able to literally assist such patients to re-enter life. However, there has been little research on this subject, and nurses who have successfully aided such persons often do not know what they did or said that produced a change in the ill person's behavior. How to aid such individuals is fertile research area, and unfortunately, a most neglected one.

HELPING INDIVIDUALS WHO "ACCEPT" ILLNESS

The acceptance reaction is the least common of all responses to illness and suffering. Although this reaction is uncommon, nurses will encounter such persons. Individuals who exhibit acceptance as a reaction to illness are able to receive illness without protest (i.e., in the sense that an injustice is being done). These persons have never exempted themselves from misfortune nor have they negated their human-ness. What explains their ability to accept illness? Probably a major reason is their ability to realize what it means to be a human being. Some ill persons are able to accept illness because of their religious convictions. Such acceptance is based on a realization of the human condition combined with a profound belief in the tenets of their creed.

Accepting persons do not behave as does the stereotyped, "good patient." The person who can accept illness is not a silent, martyr-ish sufferer; he does complain, will make his needs known, and will make requests of health workers.

These individuals are pleasant without being effusive and are usually quiet instead of chatty and gregarious. They give others an impression of "whole-ness" and completeness. There is an aura about them of quiet dignified strength. Somehow the accepting person gives others the somewhat disconcerting feeling that he (the ill person)—not the health workers—is in control of the situation. However, such individuals are not condescending to others; quite the opposite—they are usually extraordinarily considerate and gentle individuals.

Helping Measures

What possible problems could such individuals have? Being able to accept illness does not exempt the person from anxiety, fear, or even doubt (on occasions) as to the validity of his beliefs. The person may rebel, at times, against his illness and may display fear or anxiety, but usually these feelings are short-lived. The helping measures such individuals require are encouragement and reassurance; the concern and there-ness of the nurse will be needed especially when the individual begins to waver or doubt. *The task of the nurse is to assist such individuals to maintain their integrity.*

Such individuals are very rare and a nurse will probably encounter only a few of them in her entire career. One might ask: If there are so few of these individuals, why even mention them? It is believed that if the nurse has the privilege of caring for such an individual but *once* in a lifetime she is indeed fortunate. The nurse can learn more from such persons than she can ever teach them; she will be given more than she can ever possibly give. The nurse is urged to make use of the opportunity of caring for such individuals; the nurse cannot help but grow as a human being because of this contact.

Helping the Person in Pain

Assisting individuals who suffer severe pain over a prolonged period of time is a most complex, difficult assignment. It is a formidable task to assist individuals to find meaning in illness; however, helping individuals to find meaning in pain is almost a Herculean task.

It is difficult to communicate the experience of pain to another in such a way that the other person has some understanding of what is being experienced. Probably the experience of pain can never really be communicated in such a way that another can truly comprehend it and can grasp exactly what the individual is undergoing.

Helping Measures

What specific measures can the nurse take which will be of benefit to the individual who must endure pain over a prolonged period of time? How can the nurse best help the person who realizes that he must cope with pain for as long as he lives?

LeShan recommends a "loving-demanding" approach. High demands should be made of the person; he should be helped to remove the focus of concentration from himself and his pain to outside events. LeShan further recommends occupational therapy, work, and relating to others as being helpful measures.[7] Pity of the objectifying type makes the individual less able to cope with pain and may reinforce regression.[8] LeShan further believes that the "loving-demanding" approach gives the "greatest support and help to the patient." Further, the goal which health workers should strive towards is that of assisting the patient to gain composure, dignity and mastery.[9]

What other supportive measures can be used? Certainly such individuals need encouragement and, at times, almost an infusion of courage. The ill person gains strength to continue if his struggle is appreciated by others. Depending on the individual, there is no reason why the nurse cannot verbalize this appreciation. The nurse can, by words or attitude, communicate to the ill person her understanding that the individual has endured much. She communicates to him that she and the other nurses will help him—he is not alone.

These individuals tend to cry quite readily. There is no one method or way of helping the individual who cries. The ability to weep—to release emotional tension by crying—is, of course, helpful to many persons. There are, however, no set rules for assisting the ill person who cries. A nurse who stands quietly by may assist some ill persons but *not* others. There are times when it is *better* for the individual if the nurse pretends not to notice the ill person's tears. Commenting on the fact that the ill person is crying or probing into reasons as to why he is crying may shatter the individual's controls. A case in point follows.

> Mrs. D. is a forty-six-year-old woman who is dying of cancer. She has been in severe pain for a period of five months. She cries quite readily when the pain becomes intense. Assume that the nurse has *validated,* with Mrs. D., the reason for her crying, then what is to be gained by probing into the reasons as to why Mrs. D. cries when in pain?

---

[7] LeShan, Lawrence: The world of the patient in severe pain of long duration. J. Chronic Dis. 17:125, No. 2, 1964.

[8] *Ibid.,* p. 121.

[9] *Ibid.,* p. 125.

Such tactics frequently lessen the individual's controls. The result is not an individual who feels better because he has cried, but a depleted emotionally and physically exhausted individual. Clinical judgment is required in order to assess the situation and choose one set of nursing measures over another.

Individuals in pain frequently express such comments as, "I would be better off dead" or "What use am I like this?" If the nurse believes the individual *would* be better off dead then her usefulness in caring for the person is ended. What the individual needs is not confirmation that he would be "out of his misery" if dead; rather he needs *reasons to continue living* when suffering intense pain. What might some of these reasons be? Each individual has a particular task in life. Each person is unique and irreplaceable as a loved one or one who loves and, according to LeShan, this knowledge gives support to the individual and enhances his ability to cope with illness.[10]

Individuals who have relatives and friends who visit them are often strengthened by the knowledge that they are still needed and useful, still loved and wanted. Some ill persons strive to be an example to others; some wish to be remembered in a particular way. As one woman dying from cancer stated,

> "I know I don't have much longer to go . . . the only time I really feel bad about it is when my husband brings my little girl to see me (smiles). My daughter keeps asking me when I'll come home. She's only seven years old and such a beautiful child . . . That used to hurt me when she asked me when I was coming home and it still hurts some. I know I won't get well—the pain is much worse. Do you know what I really want? I want my little girl to remember me because I love her so much. I want her to remember me smiling—that's why I always ask for a shot for pain about an hour before visiting hours . . . I want to hide my pain when she comes to see me . . ."

This particular individual gained strength and courage and was able to endure intense pain. She was motivated to leave her daughter the only gift she could—the legacy of a smile.

Frankl tells of a general practitioner suffering from severe depression as a result of the death of his wife. Frankl confronted the physician by asking what would have happened if he (the physician) had died first? The man replied that it would have been terrible for his wife,—she would have suffered much. Frankl then replied, "You see doctor, such a suffering has been spared her and it is you who has spared her this . . . but now you have to pay for it by mourning her." According to Frankl the effect of this conversation was that he succeeded in changing the individual's attitude towards his fate and enabled the man to perceive some meaning in his suffering.[11]

Might not such measures be helpful to individuals who suffer severe physical pain? It is human for the ill individual to lament his suffering, but it is also helpful if he can find meaning in it by realizing that his burden is not senseless. He has taken onto himself (although not willingly) suffering, and has spared others by his acceptance of it.

---

[10] *Ibid.,* p. 123.

[11] Frankl, *op. cit.,* pp. 178-179.

HELPING ILL PERSONS TO FIND MEANING IN HEALTH MEASURES

Ill persons need assistance in finding meaning in the very measures they must take to conserve health and control illness. Many nurses recognize that ill human beings need help in finding meaning in illness; however, helping ill persons to find meaning in health measures has not been given as much emphasis.

In our society when an individual becomes ill he is expected to cooperate and follow medical advice. The individual with diabetes is expected to remain on his diet or take his insulin regularly; the individual with epilepsy is expected to take the prescribed anticonvulsive drug, and so on. Health workers expect ill persons to cooperate and "be reasonable." Ill human beings are asked to break the habits of a lifetime and to develop new habits. They may be expected to modify or change their entire life pattern, or requested to perform acts of denial and self-sacrifice in order to conserve health. How much assistance is given these individuals?

Certainly, most nurses are cognizant of the need ill persons have for health teaching and conscientiously strive to fulfill their responsibilities. In most instances, however, one finds that emphasis is placed on techniques or methods. The ill person is instructed "how-to," i.e., how to give himself injections, to calculate his diet, is told what signs or symptoms to look for, is given "health teaching" materials, and is sent on his way. The expectation of health workers is that since he "knows what to do," the individual will automatically be able to care for himself. Ill persons need information; there is no doubting it. However, more is needed by the human being than a knowledge of techniques.

What frequently occurs is that the ill person, for a time, may adhere to the prescribed regimen, but, as he encounters problem after problem, he may begin to perceive his life robbed of meaning and enjoyment by the very measures he must take to conserve his health. He may then abandon any attempt to adhere to such a regimen. Such behavior may seem "unreasonable" to health workers. Nevertheless, it is quite prevalent, and very human.

Helping Measures

How may nurses assist ill persons to find meaning in the measures they must take to control illness and conserve health? The nurse first strives to establish relatedness with the individual. It is within the context of a human-to-human relationship that the nurse institutes helping measures.

It is suggested that the nurse foresee some of the problems the ill person will encounter and prepare him (and his family) to cope with these problems. A consideration of so-called "minor problems" which the ill person is apt to encounter, as well as some ways to handle these problems, should be incorporated into the teaching plan. Nurses are urged to teach and discuss health measures with the individual when his family is present. The ill person's closest relative—the person who will be responsible for caring for him when he leaves the hospital—should be included in these conferences. The ill person's closest relative many times is the individual who must motivate the ill person to continue to take the measures needed to conserve his health. Family members not only have a right to know the health measures the ill person must take, they must also have this information in order to properly care for the ill person, and in order to encourage and motivate him.

It may be that, at some future time, greater use will be made of group meetings to assist ill persons with long-term illnesses. Individuals with common health problems (and their families) could attend such meetings and discuss problems caused by the illness. These meetings would be primarily for the purpose of motivating and encouraging the ill individual (and his family) to cope with, and solve, the many problems which he encounters. Information could be disseminated and common problems, and ways in which to solve them, could be discussed. These groups could be inaugurated by national health organizations, hospitals and clinics. Leadership tasks could be performed by members from the group with consultation, as needed, from nurses, physicians, psychologists, social workers, and others. Some groups are already in existence (although on a very small scale); many more are needed.

At some future time also, greater use will probably be made of video tapes and programmed instruction in health teaching. Nurses, however, must be prepared to use the newest technological innovations in the service of the ill human being.

PART IV—HELPING THE ILL PERSON'S FAMILY

It is not only the ill human being who needs assistance in finding meaning in illness, the sick person's family also may require the help of the professional nurse practitioner. The ill person *is* a member of a family and what affects one member of a family will inevitably have its effects on the other family members. The way in which family members react towards the ill person's illness is invariably communicated to him.

Nurses view ill persons' relatives and visitors in many different ways. Some nurses unfortunately perceive ill person's relatives as necessary evils who must be tolerated, or as nuisances who plague her with questions. Some nurses "blame" family members for "stirring up trouble." As one nurse complained. "He (the ill person) never complains until his wife comes to visit him, then he wants everything under the sun." All of these negative perceptions have one element in common, i.e., the ill person's relative is viewed as a problem, not as a human being with problems. How little understanding and consideration is given the ill person's family when nurses hold such views. The nurse who ignores the ill person's relatives because she is "not there to care for the visitors but to care for ill persons" deludes herself. Whatever affects the ill person's relatives affects the ill human being, and the reverse is also true.

Helping Measures

Indirectly the nurse assists the ill person's relatives by rendering expert nursing care to the ill family member. More directly the nurse makes an effort to know the ill person's family. If at all possible, she makes rounds during visiting hours and shows an interest in the ill person's visitors. She talks with them and listens to them. She is available in the event a family member wishes to discuss any aspect of the ill person's nursing care. The nurse is aware of community agencies, and, if necessary, interprets the services that these agencies provide to the family members.

Depending on hospital policy, relatives may be allowed to remain with the ill person, especially if the individual is seriously ill. These family members frequently remain with the ill person for hours at a time; some remain twenty-four hours a day. Their vigil may continue for weeks or even months. These persons are frequently physically exhausted and emotionally depleted. The emotional strain and utter monotony of sitting and waiting exacts its toll. Nurses have more of an opportunity to know these family members than she does the relatives who come only at visiting hours. Some recognition by the nurse that she appreciates the ordeal the family is undergoing is very meaningful to them. Besides showing interest in the relatives as well as in the ill person, the nurse might concentrate on performing those small acts of kindness which take so little time but which mean so much to the recipient. If she knows that the ill person's relatives drink coffee, she can bring them hot coffee. This small act of kindness is greatly appreciated, especially in the early morning hours before the hospital restaurant opens. She might bring the relatives something to read, give them pillows for the chairs, and perform numerous other thoughtful acts. None of these small acts of kindness require much time, but they are seldom forgotten by the ill person's relatives. When a nurse assists a family member she also assists the ill person. The more encouragement and support she gives relatives, the more will the relatives be able to encourage and assist the ill person.

Family member may also find it difficult to understand why their relative became ill, and may express the belief that the illness is "unjust" and "unfair" because the ill person has always been "a good person." The suggested methods and approaches designed to assist ill persons to arrive at meaning may also be used to help the relatives of ill persons.

If a nurse could remember that whenever she assists a family member, whenever she encourages or supports him, talks with him, is considerate of him and performs small acts of kindness she *is* assisting the ill person. If she could remember this, then perhaps relatives would be accorded the consideration which is due them.

N.B. References used in this chapter are in the footnotes. These are not repeated.

Chapter XII

SURGERY—A HUMAN EXPERIENCE

Surgery is more than a procedure; it is an experience undergone by a human being—a human being who will respond to this experience in his own unique way. There are, however, certain commonalities of experience shared by most individuals who undergo surgery. Generally, most individuals facing surgery encounter problems centering around their attempts to meet two basic needs: the need for *cognitive clarity* and the *need for security.*

The need for cognitive clarity refers to the individual's need to comprehend what is going to happen to him. An individual who *knows* what to expect is less likely to resort to fantasy in an attempt to understand his experiences. An individual who does not understand what is going to happen to him will supply in fantasy that which is not known in reality. The individual's behavior will then be motivated by what he fantasizes will happen to him. These fantasies may be incorrect and can be a source of great anxiety and fear to the person facing the stress of surgery.

The second need of the individual facing surgery and one closely related to the need for cognitive clarity is the *need for security.* The need for security is synonymous with the need for safety. In this situation *the need for security refers to the individual's need to believe he will survive the surgical experience* and that he will be given expert care and not abandoned in his time of crisis. The need for emotional support and reassurance is acutely felt by persons facing the stress of surgery.

It should be remembered, however, that there is nothing magical about knowledge. Knowledge, per se, does not necessarily dispel *all* fear and anxiety. An individual who "knows" his leg will be amputated or "knows" he is scheduled for open-heart surgery is not necessarily made "non-anxious" by such knowledge. Knowing, however, is the first necessary step towards accepting reality. There is simply no way to accept reality unless one knows what that reality may be.

The role of the nurse is clear. She renders expert physical care and strives to meet the individual's need for cognitive clarity and security throughout the surgical experience. It is believed that many "nursing problems" are created by failure, on the part of nurses and other health workers, to recognize and meet these particular needs.

It is generally assumed that individuals facing surgery experience varying degrees of anxiety, this is considered normal. *It is further hypothesized that there is a direct relationship between the extent to which the individual's need for cognitive clarity and security are met and the individual's anxiety level.* What is *not* generally recognized by most health workers is that with the possible exception of persons admitted for emergency surgery (as in the case of victims of accidents) the individual admitted to a hospital for surgery has already undergone a series of anxiety provoking experiences. The sequence is as follows. The individual experiences symptoms or notes signs of illness and seeks medical assistance. The nature or kind of symptoms experienced may provoke much anxiety. For example, chest pain, in an individual whose father died of cancer of the lung, may arouse much fear. Some individuals do not experience symptoms of illness. Their condition and subsequent need for surgery may be detected by a physician during a routine physical examination. The individual is usually subjected to various laboratory tests and procedures in order to confirm the diagnosis. Waiting for the results of these tests usually induces more anxiety in the individual. When the individual is told surgery is definitely indicated he then must decide whether or not to undergo this experience. Whether the person decides to submit to surgery or not depends on many factors. Two important determinants are the physician's relationship with the ill person and the amount and kind of information given the individual by the physician. Usually physicians give ill persons some information about the nature of their problem: the reasons underlying the proposed surgical intervention, the kind of surgery to be performed, the risks involved and the probable outcome of the operative procedure.

The decision to submit to surgery is by no means an easy one for many individuals to make. The ability to decide is invariably affected by the individual's anxiety level. It is never an easy matter to willingly submit one's body to surgery without experiencing anxiety and fear. Thus it is by the time an individual is admitted to the hospital for surgery he has already encountered many anxiety-provoking situations. The very act of separating from one's familiar environment and loved ones and entering a hospital can intensify one's anxiety. Facing surgery is an intensely lonely experience and cannot really be shared with others. Under the best of circumstances, and even when surrounded by, and helped by, many people, the individual who faces surgery encounters this experience *alone* since no one can substitute for him or take his place.

Since each human being is unique it follows that the factors causing anxiety may vary greatly from one individual to another. The nurse cannot hope to be helpful to the individual facing surgery unless she comprehends the effect of anxiety and fear on the human being and is able to recognize the behavioral manifestations of anxiety.

PART I—DEFINITION AND CHARACTERISTICS OF ANXIETY

Anxiety is broadly defined as *a subjective experience characterized by tension, restlessness and apprehension prompted by real or imagined threats to need gratification.* Anxiety and fear are considered synonymous in this work. Anxiety is not pleasurable and the individual develops various ways to reduce or cope with it. The energy generated by anxiety is discharged into overt or covert behavior. The behavioral manifestations are dependent upon the degree of anxiety experienced by the individual as well as upon the efficacy of the coping (or mental) mechanisms used to circumvent its effects. A certain amount of anxiety may be useful. However, as an individual's anxiety level increases, and if he is unable to counteract its effect, his personality may become disorganized by progressively mounting anxiety resulting in a psychotic state.

The overt and covert manifestations of anxiety are legionary and may include tachycardia, dilated pupils, diaphoresis, shallow respiration, tremors, anorexia, nausea, insomnia, vertigo, fatigue, headache, narrowed perception (or "tunnel vision"), increased motor activity, exaggerated responses to petty annoyances, inability to concentrate and irritability to list only a few manifestations.

Anxiety affects perception in that as anxiety mounts perception becomes increasingly fragmented. Anxiety also affects an individual's ability to learn. A small degree of anxiety is helpful in its alerting effect and may be necessary as a motivating factor in learning. However, too much anxiety affects the individual's ability to "take in" information, and to correctly evaluate reality. Too high an anxiety level can impede the learning process.

Anxiety thus affects the individual's ability to perceive, to think, to judge, to decide and to learn. It affects the total individual in body, mind and spirit.

CAUSES OF ANXIETY

Anxiety is prompted by real or imagined threats to need gratification. In the case of an individual facing surgery, the major threats to need gratification may include the threat of non-being, or death, the threat of loss of bodily integrity through surgery and the threat of loss of love or abandonment by others. Some individuals fear loss of control over their own bodies and having to submit passively to others. Thus it is that some individuals fear the anesthesia more than the surgery per se.

An individual's fear of surgery may be partly determined by the meaning of the body organ or part to the individual. If a woman believes a hysterectomy will make her "less of a woman" because she can no longer bear children, her emotional response to surgery will differ greatly from a woman who does not equate loss of a uterus with the loss of femininity. The anticipated results of surgery may increase or lessen an individual's anxiety level. An individual who believes his health or condition will be improved following surgery will react quite differently than an individual who was asymptomatic prior to surgery.

The kind of surgery to be performed may evoke specific fears and anxieties. Individuals who are scheduled to undergo throat surgery may fear suffocation. Heart surgery may evoke fears of sudden death. Individuals who must undergo brain surgery may fear becoming psychotic, paralyzed or "retarded."

The nature or extent of surgery to be performed and the degree to which the effects of surgery are visible to others may create anxiety. The difficulty is compounded by the irrevocable nature of certain kinds of surgical procedures. As for example, an individual who must have an arm or leg amputated *knows* his way of life will be irrevocably changed by the surgical procedures. Even though the individual may be able to walk again by wearing a prosthesis, he is, nevertheless, irrevocably changed. These individuals frequently undergo grief reactions and mourn the loss of the body part. Such reactions are considered normal.

Any disfiguring surgery which is visible to others can cause mental suffering and distress. The fact that others can see one's disfiguration, the fear that other human beings may turn away in disgust, or that they may pity one, can create much mental turmoil. Not only must the individual adjust to the way in which he believes others perceive him, he also must adjust personally to the changes in his body. The individual's idea or perception of his body must be changed. *The body image is the individual's concept or picture of the way in which he perceives his body and believes others perceive him.* When a person is disfigured he must change his body image and incorporate a new concept of how his body is perceived by himself and others. Even though the effects of surgery may not be blatantly visible to others, they may, nevertheless, be perceived by the individual as mutilating. This is especially true in those instances where surgical intervention effects a change is bodily functioning, for example, in individuals with a colostomy. The individual, in this instance, sustains the loss of a body function and must learn to adjust to a new and strange mode of functioning. The individual must, in effect, be toilet trained again. Even the most well-adjusted adult may respond with anxiety, shame, dismay or disgust at having to cope with controlling his feces and regulating his bowels.

Another cause of anxiety in individuals facing surgery is fear of pain and discomfort. Individuals do not readily discuss their fears of pain and discomfort lest they be labelled "cowards" by others. Fear of pain may, in a sense, be a manifestation related to another group of problems, i.e., fear of depending on others, mistrust of others, or fear of loss of control over one's destiny. The individual may, because of his past life experiences, believe others are not dependable. An individual who has relied primarily on himself may find it very difficult to adjust to a situation where he *must* depend on others. The individual may believe that if he wants something done he must do it himself. To give others power over him then creates anxiety. An individual who believes that he will experience great pain following surgery because he is not sure that others will help him is indeed burdened.

Lack of information or cognitive clarity about the impending surgical procedure creates anxiety. An individual who does not understand exactly why surgery is to be performed or does not know the probable outcome of the surgery, or his chances of surviving surgery, may experience much anxiety. Generally, the less an individual knows about an experience he must undergo, the more he will supply in fantasy the knowledge he lacks in reality.

Personal problems may induce anxiety in the individual anticipating surgery.

The costs of hospitalization and surgery may be a source of very real concern and anxiety to the individual. Hospitalization insurance usually pays only a portion of one's hospital and doctor bills. Many persons must take out a second mortgage on their homes or borrow money in order to have surgery performed. Some individuals fear their hospitalization insurance will be cancelled by the insurance company if their bill is too high. The individual also must have the financial resources to pay his rent or mortgage, and take care of other bills. Some individuals have "sick pay allowance" or go on sick leave during their period of hospitalization; others, however, unless they receive disability payments from an insurance company, have no income when they are unable to work. Some individuals carefully plan their budgets so that a family member can have needed surgery. However, if complications develop or the individual must be hospitalized longer than was anticipated, the family savings (if any) may be completely spent.

Concern about the care of dependents during hospitalization may generate anxiety. For example, a widow who has young children and must undergo surgery may become very anxious about her children. Not every person has a family or friends to turn to in times of need. A middle-aged unmarried woman who cares for a totally disabled mother also faces an anxiety-provoking problem if she must undergo surgery. In such cases the children may have to be placed temporarily in foster homes and the disabled mother may have to go to a nursing home, provided such facilities are available. The individual who lives alone encounters unique problems. Such an individual might be concerned about the very real problem of caring for himself following discharge from the hospital.

Thus far we have discussed causes or sources of anxiety in the individual anticipating surgery. There are many other highly idiosyncratic causes of anxiety. Sources of concern vary. Anxiety, however, is invariably a problem for the individual facing surgery. It cannot be assumed that an individual facing major surgery will be more anxious than an individual facing "minor" surgery. *There is probably no such thing as "minor" surgery, especially to the individual undergoing the surgery.*

WAYS OF COPING WITH ANXIETY

Anxiety is manifested in overt and covert behavior. Each person has ways of coping with, or circumventing, anxiety. The methods or mental mechanism used tends to vary with each individual. Generally, individuals cope with the anxiety generated by impending surgery in the same manner that they have coped with other crises in their life.

An individual may control anxiety by denying the seriousness of his condition or his need for surgery. He may deliberately strive to "forget" his need for surgery by plunging into outside activities. Some persons minimize the probable impact of the surgical experience by insisting that theirs is "after all, only a little operation." Others relieve anxiety by their almost magical belief in the powers of the surgeon. "If *he* operates on me I *know* I'll be all right," is an expression of magical belief. Some individuals somaticize their anxiety and develop bodily aches and pains or other symptoms. Others utilize anxiety in such a way as to assist them in solving the many life problems engendered by the impending surgical experience. Such persons usually can express their fears and will seek assistance provided they believe nurses and other health workers are willing and able to help them.

BEHAVIORAL REACTIONS TO ANXIETY

Much human behavior is motivated by anxiety. The behavioral manifestations of anxiety are varied and depend on the degree of anxiety experienced by the individual and the efficiency of his coping mechanisms.

It is not always easy to infer the existence of anxiety in another human being unless the person is well known to us. For example, some anxious individuals exhibit irritability and anger. The sequence is as follows. Anxiety is experienced whenever there is a threat to need gratification. An individual strives to accomplish a goal, or gratify a need, and perceives a block or barrier to goal accomplishment or need gratification. The object, situation or person blocking the individual becomes the target for hostile feelings and anger is aroused. When caring for an individual exhibiting angry behavior, a nurse who understands that the person has been blocked or thwarted in terms of fulfilling his needs or goals is in a position to help the individual. The nurse begins by eliciting reasons for the anger. It is usually not difficult to discover why an individual is angry—one simply asks the person and proceeds from there. The nurse then structures intervention in such a way as to enable the person to overcome obstacles to goal attainment or to substitute more attainable goals. Needless to say, none of these objectives can be accomplished by a nurse who lacks appreciation of what the individual is experiencing or who reacts to an individual's angry behavior by becoming defensive or punitive.

Depression is another behavioral manifestation of anxiety. Whereas the frustrated individual turns anger outward to the person(s) causing the anger, or "takes his feelings out" on others, the individual who is depressed turns anger inward. In a sense, the depressed person punishes himself, while the angry person tends to punish others or make them feel uncomfortable. The depressed person also makes others uncomfortable, but in a different way. He may try to force others to care for him by exhibiting depressed behavior; looking or acting "miserable" usually calls forth a response from other people. The depressed individual may also try to induce guilt in others by his behavior. Symbolically, depression represents a cry for help. Depression is not necessarily an abnormal state or psychologically pathological condition. This, of course, depends on the severity or intensity of the depressive response. It is normal to feel some degree of depression when threatened by a loss or anticipated loss of a love object, of one's self-esteem or bodily integrity. The losses an individual facing surgery may sustain include loss of life and bodily integrity, and, in some instances, loss of a body part or bodily function. The loss or anticipation of loss of one's self-esteem may be precipitated by the individual's conviction that he will be unable to control his life or destiny.

Many times the nurse can infer the nature of the loss anticipated or experienced by the individual; she then validates this inference with the individual involved. If not, the nurse can elicit from the person the nature of the loss he is experiencing or anticipates experiencing. The nurse then decides what interventive measures can be taken to assist the person. An individual who anticipates the loss of an arm or leg in surgery is bound to experience anticipatory anxiety and depression about the anticipated loss. Even the most skilled and compassionate nurse cannot allay all of an individual's fears, nor can she, by nursing measures, eliminate completely the individual's feelings of depression. She can, however, assist the person to bear, or cope with the reality that must be faced. She can be supportive to the individual undergoing the process of grieving over the loss of a body part. It should be remembered that individuals, under such circumstances, may express anger towards a nurse who coaxes, cajoles, or in any way seems to criticize the individual because he is having difficulty accepting and adjusting to his loss. Actually, it is not possible for a non-disabled person to fully appreciate or understand the mental turmoil and suffering experienced by these individuals. Another person with a similar disability may be better able to assist the individual than the non-disabled nurse. However, by rendering expert physical care, being attentive and supportive, allowing the individual to grieve, refraining from "cheery" pep talks or other "jollying maneuvers," the nurse can be of great assistance to the person disabled by surgery.

There are many variations of depressive and angry behavior. For example, a depressed person may withdraw and appear more quiet, may make derogatory remarks about himself or others, express pessisimism as to his chances for recovery or engage in self-pitying behavior. The individual may act annoyed or irritable, he may complain about the care he receives in the hospital, or he may exhibit his displeasure in some other way. It is important to remember that an individual may be very angry or depressed and still exhibit either a bland facial expression or a smile. *The nurse should never assume she understands how or what an individual is feeling unless, and until, she explores this matter with the individual involved.*

There are many other reactions to anxiety. Some of these include increased preoccupation with fantasy life, usually exhibited in withdrawn behavior. Somatization or increased attention to bodily aches and pains almost to the point of hypochondriacal fixation is another method of coping with anxiety.

Over-valuation of authority may be an attempt to decrease anxiety. Using this maneuver, the individual defends against anxiety by believing in his surgeon's omnipotence and skill. This is exemplified in frequent comments made by individuals facing surgery, as when they say such things as "my surgeon is the best doctor in the world." The surgeon is viewed as an omnipotent figure or magical healer who can do no wrong.

Denial is another reaction to anxiety. In this instance, the individual represses or denies the emotional impact of the experience of surgery. On a cognitive level the individual knows he will undergo surgery; however, he represses or denies the emotional feelings engendered by the impending surgery. The individual who utilizes denial *is* able to discuss his impending surgery in an intelligent, rational manner and seems "adjusted" to the operative procedure. However, one detects a lack of emotional response. The individual gives the impression he is not really worried or concerned about his surgery. Such persons are frequently stereotyped as "good patients" by health workers who do not comprehend the nature of the massive threat experienced by these individuals or the desperate maneuvers these persons have used to ward off unbearable anxiety. At first glance, it may seem that denial is a satisfactory mechanism to use in allaying anxiety. It *is* effective. The danger, however, in using denial, is that it is an unstable mechanism and cannot be maintained over an extended period of time. Sooner or later the individual must cope with the emotional aspects of the surgical experience. The repressed emotional aspects may emerge weeks or months following the traumatic experience, operating in much the same way as a delayed grief reaction. The individual may feel anxious, depressed, angry, irritable or withdrawn, or he may experience feelings of unreality or depersonalization. Because the individual has not coped with his feelings at the time when it was appropriate to do so, he may find that the delayed reaction is very intense and severe. The only preventive measures which can be taken is to provide an opportunity for the individual to discuss his feelings about the surgical experience and to meet the individual's need for cognitive clarity and security.

There are many other possible behavioral responses to anxiety, such as "overdependent" behavior or "exaggerated" independence, being overly solicitous about other individuals on the surgical unit and engaging in clownish behavior, to list a few.

Since anxiety is such a common problem encountered by individuals scheduled for surgery, the nurse should devote her attention to identifying its effects on the individuals and then direct her attention towards intervening in order to diminish the individual's anxiety level.

It should be remembered that not only is anxiety a psychological problem, it is also a physiological problem. Although it has not been proven conclusively, there is some evidence to support the theory that anxiety is physiologically damaging to the individual, especially to the person who experiences a high level of anxiety over a relatively prolonged period of time. It is believed that individuals may die because of a prolonged severe attack of anxiety. It is known that individuals who are extremely anxious and fearful are poor surgical risks and many surgeons will not operate on an individual who believes he will die during surgery.

Although anxiety does not usually cause death, the degree of anxiety experienced by an individual prior to surgery may well have a direct influence on the post-operative period. Individuals who experience a high level of anxiety prior to surgery are more vulnerable to post-operative psychotic reactions than are individuals with a low level of anxiety. Psychotic reactions are also more frequent among individuals undergoing operations on the eyes, genitals and heart. One can only speculate on the degree to which post-operative nausea and vomiting is actually caused by fear and anxiety. To what extent is post-operative pain potentiated by anxiety? To what extent does the amount of anxiety experienced by an individual play a part in determining the length (and turbulence) of the convalescent period? Much research is still needed in order to answer these questions.

The nurse, operating independently and in collaboration with the surgeon and others, can play an important role in assessing the anxiety level of individuals facing surgery and in intervening to reduce anxiety whenever possible.

PART II—PREPARATION OF THE INDIVIDUAL FOR SURGERY

Many articles have been written about the importance of psychologically preparing the individual for surgery. An analysis of the content of many of these articles reveals that "preparation of the patient" focuses on procedures such as teaching the "pre-op" person the importance of coughing, exercising and deep breathing following surgery. Other authors focus on orienting and informing the individual as to the procedures which will be followed as he proceeds through the surgical sequence. The person may be given detailed information as to what will occur during the pre-operative and post-operative period. For example, he will be told that the laboratory technician will draw some blood, the anesthestist will visit, he will be prepped for surgery, etc. The individual will also be informed of the time surgery is scheduled and is told he will be in the recovery room for a time following surgery. He may be told that he will receive blood intravenously, etc. Generally, the purpose of these explanations is to allay anxiety in the individual when he awakens from the anesthesia. It is obvious, however, that much of the orienting information is given in order to enlist the individual's cooperation in order to facilitate the tasks which must be accomplished prior to surgery, rather than to alleviate the person's anxiety per se, although some anxiety may be allayed in the process. "Preparing the patient for surgery" by engaging in the activities mentioned above *are* important. Certainly information given individuals may meet, to some extent, their need for cognitive clarity and security. But more is required than "information-giving" per se. *The individual facing surgery is not a computer to be programmed; he is a human being with feelings, hopes, wishes, dreams and fears.* The individual also needs to experience the personal interest of nurses and others in his welfare, combined with the assurance that the care he will receive will be of a competent, capable and compassionate nature.

THE NURSE'S ROLE

The nurse invariably strives to render expert physical care to individuals and strives to meet the individual's need for cognitive clarity and security throughout the surgical experience.

Using observational and communication skills, the nurse strives to get to know the individual, and be known by him, and begins the data gathering process. Specifically, the nurse strives to accomplish the following goals:

1. Ascertain the way in which the individual perceives the impending surgical experience, i.e., how he feels about undergoing surgery.

2. Assess the individual's anxiety level, or make inferences about the nature of the individual's fears and concerns.

3. Ascertain what the individual knows or has been told by his physician and others about the surgical experience.

4. Identify needs, problems, or gaps in knowledge or information. Ascertain what the individual would like to know about the impending surgical experience.

The purpose of accomplishing these goals is to use the information gained in order to structure nursing intervention and meet the individual's needs for cognitive clarity and security.

How does the nurse ascertain the way in which the individual perceives the impending surgical experience? The nurse can develop many interpretations by listening carefully to the individual's account of what he knows, or has been told, about the surgery. Careful attention should be paid to vocal tone, facial expression, gestures and mannerisms. Often the nurse picks up many clues as to the individual's emotional state through attention paid to the manner in which the individual expresses himself.

The individual may well tell the nurse how he feels about the experience he is to undergo. For example, an individual stated, "I'm not looking forward to it but I know it (the surgery) has to be done. I'll be glad when it's over with." This particular person disliked having to submit to surgery and expressed this dislike on an emotional as well as an intellectual level; however, he was resigned to the reality situation and made an uneventful recovery. Another individual stated, "I'm not worried about the operation . . . it's that spinal (anesthesia)." The focus of this particular person's concern centered about the dreaded spinal. The ill person was reluctant to the tell the surgeon that she feared she would be paralyzed by the spinal anesthesia. The nurse informed the surgeon who then directed that a general anesthesia be given.

The nurse may accomplish the second goal, assessing the individual's anxiety level, while collecting data regarding the way in which the individual perceives the operative experience. In order to assess an individual's anxiety level, however, the nurse must possess a conceptual framework regarding the nature of anxiety as well as the behavioral manifestations exhibited by an individual experiencing a particular level or degree of anxiety. Peplau's work on anxiety is recommended as an excellent theoretical criteria.[1]

No one can "see" anxiety, but the behavioral manifestations are observable. Hence the nurse develops inferences about the probable level of anxiety an individual is experiencing by observing the person's behavior. These inferences are then validated with the person. For example, the nurse can elicit information by saying, "I get the feeling you're worried about your operation." More specifically, if the nurse has inferred a particular focus of concern, she simply asks the individual whether or not her assumption is valid. For example, the nurse might say in a

---

[1] Peplau, Hildegard E.: A working definition of anxiety. Some Clinical Approaches to Psychiatric Nursing. Shirley F. Burd and Margaret A. Marshall (eds.) New York: The Macmillan Company, 1963, pp. 323–327.

questioning way, "You seem worried about how much pain you will have after surgery....?" In summary, the nurse infers the level of anxiety the individual is experiencing and validates this assumption with the individual. Using validated assumptions, the nurse is then able to intervene in such a way as to reduce the individual's anxiety level. The nurse who does not know *why* an individual is anxious simply has no way of helping the person cope with his feelings. The nurse does not strive to relieve the individual facing surgery of *all* anxiety—this is not possible. It is possible, however, to assist the individual to reduce his level of anxiety and strengthen his ability to cope with this feeling.

The third goal, that of ascertaining what the individual knows or has been told by his physician and others about the surgical experience, is attained by asking the individual. For example, the nurse might ask, "what did your doctor tell you about your operation?" "What have you been told about your surgery?" or "What brought you to the hospital?" Such questions sometimes elicit the desired information.

The nurse accomplishes the fourth goal, that of identifying needs, problems or gaps in knowledge or information, by listening and developing and validating inferences. Much of the information the nurse desires can be gained during the admission procedure or orientation process. The nurse introduces herself to the individual and begins the process of orienting the person to the environment and services available. While engaged in the process of orientation the nurse observes the individual, makes inferences as to the individual's anxiety level and develops interpretations. Depending on the data obtained and verified during the assessment process, the nurse acts to supply the information the individual requires in order to understand what is going to happen to him. Generally, most persons facing surgery need detailed information as to what will happen to them during the pre-operative and post-operative periods. Many individuals require information and instruction relative to coughing, deep breathing exercises, etc. The nurse clarifies misconceptions created by inadequate knowledge or information.

Reduction of anxiety is accomplished by supplying needed information and by providing reassurance. The very act of spending time with the individual, discussing with him the impending surgical procedure, may be reassuring. Individuals are usually reassured by a nurse who is sincerely interested in their welfare. The individual's ability to listen to, and comprehend information imparted by the nurse may be affected by the person's anxiety level. It is therefore important for the nurse to ascertain whether or not the individual *has heard* and *does understand*.

Allowing time for the individual to ask questions is essential. Sufficient time is required to perform these important functions. *An unhurried approach is required.* Most hospitalized individuals will not ask questions of health workers who convey, by their behavior, that they are "very busy people."

It cannot be overly emphasized that it is the function of the professional nurse practitioner to orient and psychologically prepare individuals for surgery. Non-professional workers do not have the educational or experiential background to equip them to assess an individual's anxiety level or to identify problems centered around attempts to meet the needs of cognitive clarity and security. If nurses do not assume this responsibility, other health workers will be needed to perform these most necessary functions.

Many problems may emerge during the phases of assessment and intervention. The nurse cannot solve all human problems or meet all of an individual's needs, nor is she expected to accomplish such superhuman feats. The services of other members of the health team are often needed to solve some problems and meet some needs. The nurse assumes the responsibility of consulting with and enlisting the services of members of the other health disciplines as the need arises. There is much that the nurse can accomplish, however, which lies strictly within the realm of nursing practice. If the nurse can reduce an individual's anxiety level, clarify misconceptions, supply needed information or refer the individual to members of other health disciplines (as the need arises) she will have accomplished much.

After the nurse assesses and intervenes to effect changes, she then evaluates the efficacy of the nursing measures taken to relieve distress, supply information and reduce anxiety. The nurse assesses the extent to which the individual was helped by her activities. The nurse knows whether or not she has assisted the individual either by asking him or by noting changes in behavior following nursing intervention.

PART III—SURGERY: THE HUMAN EXPERIENCE

As has been stated, surgery is more than a procedure, it is an experience undergone by a human being. It is sometimes helpful for the nurse to reflect upon what the individual scheduled for surgery must undergo. It is not easy for any human being to submit to surgery. Neither is it easy to submit to such procedures as being prepped, being given enemas, having blood samples taken, etc. These experiences are often distasteful, embarrassing and painful to the individual. Anticipatory anxiety is experienced as the person waits for the hours to pass before the scheduled time of surgery.

An attendant, pushing a stretcher, enters the individual's room and assists him onto the stretcher. Then, strapped to the stretcher, his senses dulled by narcotics, the individual begins the slow long trip to the surgical suite—his visual field restricted to observing the ceiling lights in the corridors until he finally arrives at his destination. Arms move him onto the operating room table where he perceives masked strangers dressed in green, a table of instruments or an overhead light. Perhaps he catches a glimpse of the surgeon before the anesthetists' mask comes over his face. There is then the awakening in the recovery room and with this awakening the experience of the surging thrust of pain or nausea. There is then the return to the nursing unit and the individual begins the long, slow work of recovery.

SECTION SIX

This section includes an Appendix and a Selected Bibliography. The Appendix, "Expanding Empathic Boundaries," includes a consideration of ways and means by which teachers of nursing may assist learners to expand their empathic boundaries. A major belief is that it is the task of the teacher in nursing to assist students in empathizing with ill persons and their families.

The Bibliography is a selected one. Suggested Reading References for each chapter are included in the Bibliography. The Bibliography has been completely revised and updated. References published in the first edition of this text are *not* repeated.

Expanding Empathic Boundaries

Empathy is a phase in the process of achieving relatedness; it is valuable in establishing rapport. It is the third phase in establishing relatedness, the five phases being: the original encounter, emerging identities, empathy, sympathy and rapport. It is believed that the nurse must be able to transcend the empathic phase in order to sympathize with the recipients of her care and eventually to establish relatedness.

It is believed to be the task of the teacher in nursing to assist students in empathizing with ill persons. Since students possess varying degrees of ability to empathize with individuals, it may be necessary for the teacher in nursing to assist learners to expand their empathic boundaries. Some ways and means of assisting students to expand empathic boundaries are discussed in this appendix. (For a complete discussion of the major characteristics of empathy see Chapter X, "The Human-to-Human Relationship.")

PART I

Empathy is dependent upon similarity of experiences between the persons involved; the ability to predict behavior, or comprehend the behavior of another, is limited by one's personal background. According to Halpern and Lesser, "a person's ability to empathize with similar people seems to lie strictly within the bounds of their similarity; and to disappear in personality areas where they differ." [1]

The characteristic of similarity in empathy seems to account, to some extent, for the difficulties that the young student nurse has in trying to develop empathy. Young students may find it difficult to empathize because of a limited reserve of life experiences upon which to draw. Perhaps the student has not lived long enough, or savored a sufficient variety of life experiences; nor has she met, known or encountered people from different walks of life other than her own. This character-

---

[1] Halpern, Howard M., and Lesser, Leona N.: Empathy in infants, adults and psychotherapists. Psychoanal. Rev.47:38, No. 3, 1960.

istic of similarity also seems to account, to some extent, for the apparent innate ability of some older nurses aides, or nursing assistants, to empathize with others. Their years of background enable them to comprehend or understand readily because, in all probability, they know through personal experience many of the experiences and problems confronting the ill person. The student lacks this rich background knowledge which only time brings, through contact and observation.

Nursing educators should be cognizant of the fact that the nature or background of their students will determine, to a large degree, their ability to develop empathy with others. The background of the nursing student of today differs from the background of many of the nursing educators who are trying to understand and empathize with their students. It is erroneous to assume that because we, the nurse educators, were once adolescents, we therefore understand adolescents and young adults of today. The time and manner of living have changed drastically. We cannot expect a young student to empathize or establish rapport with ill persons unless we strive to understand the background of the student, as well as the individual with whom we expect her to develop empathy.

Associating, at an early age, with all types of people from varied backgrounds, occupations, and social classes, it is no wonder the student finds it difficult to empathize with these individuals who are the recipients of her care. She does not speak their language; neither do they speak hers. The student may be repelled by behavior so vastly different from her own. The student who loves humanity in the abstract may find it difficult—if not impossible, to comprehend or understand the ill human being in the flesh. The Hollingshead and Redlich study seems to confirm the fact that social class may serve as a barrier to communication, understanding, or comprehension of the way of life of individuals from different social classes.[2] Social class differences also serve to hinder (or assist) the empathic process.

To what extent would one expect the student nurse, in the following example, to empathize or achieve rapport, bearing in mind that empathy is dependent upon similarity?

Mary Smith, a twenty-one-year-old junior nursing student in a collegiate program, has been assigned to give nursing care to Mr. George Jones, who was admitted to a medical-surgical unit in a large county hospital. Mary's background would be classified as "upper-middle class." Her father manages an insurance company. Her mother is a housewife, a member of the PTA and the Neighborhood Improvement Association and has many other varied interests outside the home. The family has lived in a restricted, suburban residential area for the past fifteen years. Mary has had all of the material advantages, and psychological disadvantages, of this type of upbringing. She is a product of her culture as are all of us. She has never experienced hunger; never lacked for medical attention because her family could not pay the bills; never known pain that was not attended to or alleviated. She is like Margaret Mead's student who had "never seen a seriously sick person . . . a baby under three weeks old . . . never seen a dead person or never seen a serious wound."[3] The boundaries of Mary's world are limited. Her friends too have similar backgrounds, similar interests and similar viewpoints; they even live in similar houses. No one seems very different. Mary attends college and is quite surprised that many students are different from herself, but she

---

[2] Hollingshead, August B., and Redlich, Frederick C.: Social Class and Mental Illness. New York: John Wiley & Sons, 1958, pp. 134–135.

[3] Mead, Margaret: Nursing—primitive and civilized. Amer. J. Nurs. 56:1001, 1956.

soon finds those who are "like" herself and so the pattern is perpetuated. She may be taught by instructors who share a similar background.

Now Mary is in the clinical nursing courses. One day she is assigned to give care to Mr. Jones. Mary wishes to "understand" Mr. Jones in order to ascertain his needs and give him "total nursing care." She wishes to develop empathy and eventually sympathy and rapport with him. What basis of similarity can be used to establish empathy?

Mr. George Jones is a sixty-year-old man admitted to the medical-surgical division. He is recovering from a cardiac infarction. He has suffered from osteoarthritis of both knees for the past ten years. He is a member of the lowest socioeconomic group, comparable to Hollingshead and Redlich's Class V.[4] He is an unskilled laborer who lives in a cold-water flat in a tenement because he cannot afford anything else. He has been on welfare for the past ten years. Poverty, want and hunger are not abstractions to Mr. Jones; he has experienced and lived with them. He has known and lived with the chronic intermittent pain of osteo-arthritis. He is malnourished because of a lack of money with which to buy food, and because he lacks knowledge of the basic foods needed in order to have a proper diet. Even if he had the money he would not spend it on food. His value system differs from that of his nurse, Miss Smith. Mr. Jones is a creature of his culture as is his nurse. The boundaries of his world are limited. His friends have similar backgrounds and similar viewpoints. Mr. Jones completed four years of elementary school. He is sensitive about his lack of schooling and his background; he mistrusts authority figures.

How will Miss Smith be able to empathize with Mr. Jones? What are the similarities? By what process will this student from a suburban upper middle class family, living in a closed experiential circuit and associating only with individuals from the same background as herself, be able to empathize with this person? Will she be motivated to empathize? What similarities can the student draw upon to understand this ill human being.

One similarity is obvious—they are both human beings; but they are different, utterly unique individuals. Each is a one-time-being in this world, like, yet unlike, any other human being who has ever lived or will ever live. Another obvious similarity is that both have the same basic needs; therefore, basic human needs might be the foundation of similarities. Yet basic human needs differ in strength, intensity, and manner of expression. They are modified by the culture from which these two individuals came. There are some life experiences which might be similar, but without a process of exploration it is impossible to guess what these experiences might be. On the surface it would appear that similarity is lacking, as indeed it might be. How then is the gap to be bridged? How can the nurse educator assist this student to understand and develop empathy with this human being?

METHODS

The teacher might assign various pertinent reference readings to enable the student to gain at least a glimpse into a world so different from her own. These readings may be selected from nursing literature, the field of the behavioral

---

[4] Hollingshead and Redlich, *op. cit.,* pp. 114–134.

sciences, and from the humanities. It may be that one can learn more about common human experiences through reading the great classics of literature and poetry than he can learn from reading scientific works. The classics have endured because they have something to say about the human condition: its problems and joys. Assigning reference reading in addition to works commonly used in medicine and nursing presupposes that the nurse educator knows and appreciates these varied sources of information.

It has not been common practice to give students the assignment of reading poetry, plays or selections from the classics during nursing courses—except perhaps in psychiatric nursing—but students can learn much about human behavior through such reading. A sound background in the liberal arts will help both teacher and student to improve their ability to empathize. A liberal education does not guarantee that understanding of others will be a by-product, but it will enrich one's personal background (if even in a vicarious way) and enable one to understand others more easily.

It has been said that no one ever understood anyone else through reading, and the only way an individual can understand or comprehend the mental world of others is by interacting with them. Like many myths this statement has a degree of truth. It is true to the extent that an individual is able to learn through the experience of interacting with others. Repeated interactions will not guarantee understanding of others. If this were true, individuals who have met and mingled with the largest number of people would automatically be individuals most able to empathize and achieve rapport. It is not the number of interactions, but whether or not an individual is able to use the experience of interacting in order to learn and apply that which has been learned. Therefore, neither does the reading of articles or the classics, in and of themselves, imply that students will necessarily learn about people. It simply means that one is given an opportunity to make use of reading experience, in a vicarious way, through attempting to sense the feeling and thinking of a character in a book or a play. One hopes that the knowledge and understanding gained through reading can be transferred and used in a "real life situation." It is the responsibility of the teacher in nursing to assist the transference process.

If assisted, the student may gain intellectual understanding of the mental world of those different from herself; this understanding will be of value in attempting to empathize with others. Intellectual understanding however, is not sufficient. Neither can a student savor all of the possible experiences in life in order to develop empathy and to move beyond empathy towards sympathy. If Miss Smith, the young student nurse, had the creative imagination of a Shakespeare, no problem would be posed, but in reality this does not exist.

The student's empathic boundaries may be expanded by repeated contacts with individuals from varying backgrounds, provided the student is assisted in recognizing similarities between herself and these individuals. Therefore, the student should be assigned to give nursing care to individuals who are vastly different from herself and who come from a different background. These learning experiences should be planned consciously and deliberately by the teacher, for the express purpose of filling in the experiental gaps in the student's background. The learning experiences need to be carefully selected and planned. It is far better for the student to gain depth of understanding in caring for one ill person than to care for masses of people and gain little or no insight. These experiences should begin at the time of the student's first contact with ill persons and continue throughout her education.

The assignment of reference reading and repeated purposeful contacts with individuals from varying backgrounds are not sufficient, unless nurse educators consciously and deliberately aid the empathic process by assisting the student to recognize similarities and dissimilarities between herself and the recipients of her care. This may be accomplished in many different ways and requires creative thinking on the part of the nurse educator as is exemplified in the following:

> A student was striving to establish a relationship with Mrs. Smith, a very depressed woman who was experiencing grief following the recent death of her only child. The ill woman and student were from vastly different social classes and did not "speak the same language." Progress had ceased because the student could not get beyond the phase of emerging identities. The student was able to move into and beyond empathy only when she was helped by the instructor to recall a similar loss that she had suffered. The student had never suffered the loss of a relative, friend, or acquaintance but was finally able to empathize through similarity by recalling her sadness following the death of a much loved pet dog!

Granted that the death of a dog and its meaning to this student were not comparable, in kind or intensity, to the meaning of the death of a child. But it is upon the basis of similarity of some kind that empathy is built.

The instructor in nursing can help the student to consciously explore similarities between herself and the ill human being and thereby develop and go beyond empathy. Role-playing and the group reconstruction approach seem to be most useful in helping students to proceed to the stage of empathy and beyond.

It would be of great practical value, should such a test be valid and reliable, to include an empathy test in the battery of screening devices given in selecting students for schools of nursing. The selection of students and instructors having high empathic ability would be of great assistance, since the foundation will already be present whereby the student can move beyond empathy to achieve eventual rapport.

The ability to increase one's empathic ability could be a major curriculum objective. It may require a change in the school's educational philosophy in order to implement this viewpoint. A change in the educational philosophy would not be needed if the faculty implemented the beliefs already contained in its philosophy.

Careful guidance by the nursing instructor during the empathic phase is essential if the student is to proceed beyond empathy and achieve sympathy, which is the next phase of the relationship. Guidance is necessary, since value judgments made during this phase may determine whether or not the student will be capable of proceeding beyond empathy.

N.B. References used in this chapter are in the footnotes. There are not repeated.

SELECTED BIBLIOGRAPHY

SUGGESTED READING REFERENCES
FOR EACH CHAPTER

Chapter I: The Nature of Nursing

Articles

Anello, Michael: Responsibility for change and innovation in professional nursing. Int. Nurs. Rev. 16:208–221, 1969.

Aydelotte, Myrtle K.: Issues of professional nursing: The need for clinical excellence. Nurs. Forum 7:72–86, 1968.

Baziak, Anna T.: Influencing nursing practice in changing hospital settings. Nurs. Res. 17:146–154, 1968.

————: What constitutes clinical practice? Conflicting views of physicians and nurses. Nurs. Forum 7:98–109, No. 1, 1968.

Bennett, Leland R.: This I believe . . . that nurses may become extinct. Nurs. Outlook 18:28–32, January, 1970.

Berggren, Helen J., and Zagornik, A. Dawn: Teaching nursing process to beginning students. Nurs. Outlook 16:32–35, July, 1968.

Campbell, Emily B.: Not education, not service, but nursing. The process of change. Aust. Nurs. J. 66:8–11, 1968.

Christman, Luther B.: Nursing leadership – style and substance. Amer. J. Nurs. 67:2091–2093, 1967.

Clemence, Sister Madeleine: Existentialism: a philosophy of commitment, Amer. J. Nurs. 66:500–505, 1966.

Conference on the Nature of Science and Nursing. Nurs. Res. 17:484–512, 1968. (Five papers and a panel discussion.)

Covert, Emily C.: Is nursing a profession? Amer. J. Nurs. 18:107–109, 1917.

Darbonne Allen: Crisis: a review of theory, practice and research. Int. J. Psychiat. 6:371–379, No. 5, 1968. (Critical evaluations, pp. 380–384.)

Dickoff, James, and James, Patricia: A theory of theories: a position paper. Nurs. Res. 17:197–203, 1968.

————: James, Patricia: and Wiedenbach, Ernestine: Theory in a practice discipline. Part II. Practice oriented research. Nurs. Res. 17:545–554, 1968.

Ehrlich, Howard J., and Lee, Dorothy: Dogmatism, learning, and resistance to change. A review and a new paradigm. Psychol. Bull. 71:249–260, 1969.

Ellis, Rosemary: The practitioner as theorist. Amer. J. Nurs. 69:1434–1438, 1969.

Farrisey, Ruth M.: Clinic nursing in transition. Amer. J. Nurs. 67:305–309, 1967.

Ferlic, Anne: Existential approach to nursing. Nurs. Outlook 16:30–33, Oct., 1968.

Georgeopoulos, Basil S., and Christman, Luther: The clinical nurse specialist: a role model. Amer. J. Nurs. 70:1030–1039, 1970.

Hadley, Betty Jo: Evolution of a conception of nursing. Nurs. Res. 18:400–405, 1969.

Henderson, Virginia: Excellence in nursing. Amer. J. Nurs. 69:2133–2137, 1969.

Hollander, Edwin P., and Julian, James W.: Contemporary trends in the analysis of leadership processes. Psychol. Bull. 71:387–397, No. 5, 1969.

Jacox, Ada K.: Who defines and controls nursing practice? Amer. J. Nurs. 69:977–982, 1969.

————: Theory in nursing: borrowed and unique. Nurs. Res. 17:206–209, 1968.

Johnson, Dorothy E.: Competence in practice: technical and professional. Nurs. Outlook 14:30–33, Oct., 1966.

Johnson, Dorothy E.; Wilcox, Joan A.; and Moidel, Harriet C.: The clinical specialist as a practitioner. Amer. J. Nurs. 67:2298–2303, 1967.

Lesparre, Michael: The patient as health student. Hospitals 44:75–80, Mar. 16, 1970.

Levine, Eugene: Nurse manpower: yesterday, today, and tomorrow. Amer. J. Nurs. 69:290–296, 1969.

Lewis, Lucile: This I believe . . . about the nursing process – key to care. Nurs. Outlook 16:26–29, May, 1968.

Little, Dolores: The nurse specialist. Amer. J. Nurs. 67:552–556, 1967.

Loomis, Maxine E.: The clinical specialist as a change agent. Nurs. Forum 7:136–145, No. 2, 1968.

Macgregor, Frances C.: Nursing in transition. Challenge for the future. Int. Nurs. Rev. 14:41–43, No. 6, 1967.

Marram, Gwen D.: What is happening to nurses? Int. Nurs. Rev. 16:320–328, No. 4, 1969.

Mayes, Nancy; Shultz, Mary Nell; and Pierce, Chester M.: Commitment to nursing – how is it achieved? Nurs. Outlook 16:29–31, July, 1968.

Millard, Richard Jr.: Liberal and professional nursing education. Nurs. Outlook 16:22–25, July, 1968.

Mussallem, Helen K.: The changing role of the nurse. Canad. Nurse 64:35–37, Nov.,1968.

Nadler, Gerald, and Sahney, Vinod: A descriptive model of nursing care. Amer. J. Nurs. 69:336–341, 1969.

National Commission for the Study of Nursing and Nursing Education. Summary Report and Recommendations. Amer. J. Nurs. 70:279–294, 1970.

Norris, Catherine M.: Direct access to the patient. Amer. J. Nurs. 70:1006–1010, 1970.

Olson, Edith V.: Health manpower. Needed: a shake–up in the status quo. Amer. J. Nurs. 68:1491–1495, 1968.

Paulsen, F. Robert: Nursing goals beyond commitment. Nurs. Outlook, 14:57–58, Dec., 1966.

Piepgras, Ruth: The other dimension: spiritual help. Amer. J. Nurs. 68:2610–2613, 1968.

Quint, Jeanne C.: The case for theories generated from empirical data. Nurs. Res. 16:109–114, 1967.

Riegler, Natalie N.: Is commitment outdated? Canad. Nurse 64:48–50, Feb., 1968.

Rothberg, June: Why nursing diagnosis? Amer. J. Nurs. 67:1040–1042, 1967.

Roy, Sister Callista: Adaptation: a conceptual framework for nursing. Nurs. Outlook 18:42–45, Mar., 1970.

Rubin, Reva: A theory of clinical nursing. Nurs. Res. 17:210–212, 1968.

Sasmor, Jeannette L.: Toward developing theory in nursing. Nurs. Forum 7:191–200, No. 2, 1968.

Sarosi, Grace Mahlum: A critical theory: the nurse as a fully human person. Nurs. Forum 7:349–364, No. 4, 1968.

Shetland, Margaret L.: The responsibility of the professional school for preparing nurses for ethical, moral and humanistic practice. Nurs. Forum 8:17–27, No. 1, 1969.

Smith, Dorothy M.: A discussion of the "into, out of, overall" syndrome in nursing. Int. J. Nurs. Stud. 5:33–39, 1968.

Sullivan, Sister Genevieve: Philosophy of life shapes nursing care. Hosp. Progr. 110–114:119–120, Feb., 1967.

Symposium on Theory Development in Nursing. Nurs. Res. 17:196–227, 1968. (Seven papers and a panel discussion.)

Tayrien, Dorothy, and Lipchak, Amelia: The single-problem approach. Amer. J. Nurs. 67:2523–2527, 1967.

Trites, David K., and Schwartau, Neal W.: Nursing or clerking? Nurs. Outlook 15: 55–56, Jan., 1967.

Vacchiano, Ralph B.; Strauss, Paul S.; and Hochman, Leonard: The open and closed mind: a review of dogmatism. Psychol. Bull. 71:261–273, No. 4, 1969.

Wiedenbach, Ernestine: Nurses' wisdom in nursing theory. Amer. J. Nurs. 70:1057–1062, 1970.

Wolford, Helen: The nurse of the future. Nurs. Outlook. 14:41–42, Apr., 1966.

Books and Reports of Organizations

Bennis, Warren G.; Benne, Kenneth D.; and Chen, Robert: The Planning of Change, ed. 2. New York: Holt, Rinehart and Winston, Inc., 1969.

Brown, Esther Lucile: Nursing and Patient Care. The Nursing Profession: Five Sociological Essays. Fred Davis, editor, New York: John Wiley & Sons, Inc., 1966, pp. 176–203.

————: Nursing Reconsidered. A Study of Change. Part I. The Professional Role in Institutional Nursing. Philadelphia: J.B. Lippincott Company, 1970.

Fuerst, Elinor V., and Wolff, LuVerne: Fundamentals of Nursing. The Humanities and the Sciences in Nursing, ed. 4. Philadelphia: J.B. Lippincott Company, 1969. (See Chapter 1, "Nursing and Its Responsibilities: Prevention-Care-Rehabilitation.")

Henderson, Virginia: The Nature of Nursing. A Definition of Its Implication for Practice, Research, and Education. New York: The Macmillan Company, 1966. (See "The Search for an Official Definition of Nursing," pp. 1–5; "Development of a personal concept," pp. 6–23. See pp. 15–16 for a dicusssion of the unique function of the nurse.)

Kenneth, Hester Young: Community Nursing Service to the "Well Family." ANA Clinical Sessions. ANA, 1968. Dallas. New York: Appleton-Century-Crofts, 1968., pp. 72–79.

Matheney, Ruth V., et. al.: Fundamentals of Patient-Centered Nursing, ed. 2. St. Louis: The C.V. Mosby Company, 1968. (See Chapter 3, "Roles of the Registered Nurse.")

Norris, Catherine M.: Building a useful philosophy of nursing. Developing Behavioral Concepts in Nursing. Loretta T. Zderad and Helen C. Belcher. Report of the Regional Project in Teaching Psychiatric Nursing in Baccalaureate Programs. Atlanta: Southern Regional Education Board, 1968, pp. 104–109.

Redman, Barbara Klug: The Process of Patient Teaching in Nursing. St. Louis: The C.V. Mosby Company, 1968.

Rokeach, Milton: Beliefs, Attitudes and Values. A Theory of Organization and Change. San Francisco: Jossey-Bass, Inc., 1968.

Symposium on Interpersonal Components of Therapeutic Nursing. Luther Christman, Guest Editor. The Nursing Clinics of North America. 1:177–256, No. 2., 1966. (Eight papers.)

Symposium on New Ways of Providing Nursing Service. Laurence E. Souza, Guest Editor. The Nursing Clinics of North America. 4:483–548, No. 3., 1969. (Six papers.)

Symposium on Nursing Practice: Expectations and Reality. Signe S. Cooper, Guest Editor. The Nursing Clinics of North America. 3:95–178, No. 1, 1968. (Nine papers.)

Symposium on the Nurse in the Community. Leah Hoenig, Guest Editor. The Nursing Clinics of North America. 4:301–381, No. 2., 1969. (Eight papers.)

Walker, Virginia H.: Nursing and Ritualistic Practice. New York: The Macmillan Company, 1967.

Watson, Goodwin: The resistance to change. The Planning of Change, ed. 2. Warren G. Bennis; Kenneth D. Benne; and Robert Chen, Editors. New York: Holt, Rinehart and Winston, Inc., 1969, pp. 488–498.

Yura, Helen, and Walsh, Mary B. (ed.): The Nursing Process. Assessing, Planning, Implementing and Evaluation. Washington: The Catholic University of America Press, 1967.

Concept: Health

Articles, Books and Reports of Organizations

Baca, Josephine Elizabeth: Some health beliefs of the Spanish speaking. Amer. J. Nurs. 69:2172–2176, 1969.

Besson, Gerald: The health-illness spectrum. Amer. J. Public Health 57:1901–1905, 1967.

Conceptual Problems in Developing an Index of Health. Vital and Health Statistics: Series 2, Data Evaluation and Methods Research, No. 17. U.S. Department of Health, Education and Welfare. Public Health Service Publication #1000. Office of Health Statistics Analysis. Washington, D.C., May, 1966.

Doxiadis, C.A.: The inhuman city. Health of Mankind. Ciba Foundation. 100th Symposium. Gordon Wolstenholme and Maeve O'Connor, Editors. Boston: Little, Brown and Company, 1967, pp. 178–193. (Discussion, pp. 193–195.)

Health Is a Community Affair. Report of the National Commission on Community Health Services. Cambridge, Mass.: Harvard University Press. 1967.

Kannel, William B.: The Framingham study and chronic disease prevention. Hosp. Pract. 5:78–81; 85–87; 92–94, Mar., 1970.

Levine, David M.: What is health? The New Physician 19:22–27, 1970.

Man's Health and His Environment. A Colloquium. Archives of Environmental Health Preventive, Occupational and Aerospace Medicine. 20:72–140, January, 1970. (Eleven papers.)

Maslow, Abraham H.: Health as transcendence of environment. Pastoral Psychol. 19:45–49, 1968.

McCall, M.G.: Normality. J. Chronic Dis. 19:1127–1132, 1966.

Mechanic, David: Medical Sociology: A Selective View. New York: The Free Press, 1968. (See Chapter 1, "Health, Disease and Deviant Behavior," pp. 15–48; and Chapter 2, "General Perspectives of Health and Disease: Behavioral Science Views," pp. 44–89.)

Mendel, Werner M.: Responsibility in health, illness and treatment. Arch. Gen. Psychiat. 18:697–705, 1968. (See "Responsibility in the Concept of Health," pp. 700–701, and "The Concept of Responsibility in Illness," p. 701.)

Robinette, Tasker K.: What is health planning? Nurs. Outlook 18:33–35, Jan., 1970.

Schuman, Leonard M.: Approaches to primary prevention of disease. Public Health Rep. 85:1–10, 1970.

Suchman, Edward A.: Health attitudes and behavior. Archives of Environmental Health, Preventive, Occupational and Aerospace Medicine. 20:105–110, 1970.

Wylie, Charles M.: The definition and measurement of health and disease. Public Health Rep. 85:100–104, 1970.

Young, Marjorie A.C.: Review of Research and Studies Related to Health Education Practice (1961–1966): What People Know, Believe and Do About Health. Health Education Monograph No. 23. New York: New York Society of Public Health Educators, 1967. (Available from Circulation Service, Meriden, Conn.)

Chapter II: Concept: The Human Being

Articles

Beacher, Abraham I.: Coward, take my coward's hand. Psychotherapy: Theory, Research and Practice 6:243–248, No. 4, 1969.

Beres, Davis: The humanness of human beings. Psychoanalytic considerations. Psychoanal. Quart. 37:487–522, No. 4., 1968.

Bühler, Charlotte: The course of human life as a psychological problem. Hum. Develop. 11:184–200, No. 3., 1968.

Darley, John M., and Latané, Bibb: When will people help in a crisis? Psychol. Today 2:54–57; 70–71, Dec., 1968.

Graubard, Mark: The Frankenstein syndrome: man's ambivalent attitude to knowledge and power. Perspect. Biol. Med. 10:419–443, Spring, 1967.

Khanna, Prabha: A critique of existential guilt. Psychotherapy: Theory, Research and Practice 6:209–211, No. 3, Summer, 1969.

Martin, Alexander Reid: Idle hands and giddy minds: our psychological and emotional unpreparedness for free time. Amer. J. Psychoanal. 29:147–156, No. 2, 1969.

Ostow, Mortimer: The consequences of ambivalence. Psychosomatics 9:255–260, No. 5, 1968.

Schneiderman, Leo: Individualism and the problem of guilt. Psychoanal. Rev. 56: 313–326, No. 2, 1969.

Wolff, Kurt H.: For a sociology of evil. Journal of Social Issues 25:111–126, 1969.

Books and Reports of Organizations

Benne, Kenneth D.: Education for Tragedy: Essays in Disenchanted Hope for Modern Man. Lexington: University of Kentucky Press, 1967.

Blackham, H.J.: Humanism. Baltimore: Penguin Books, 1968.

Boyd, Malcolm: Free To Live. Free to Die. New York: The New American Library, Inc., 1968.

Bühler, Charlotte, and Massarik, Fred (eds.): The Course of Human Life. A Study of Goals in the Humanistic Perspective. New York: Springer Publishing Company, Inc., 1968.

Bychowski, Gustav: Evil in Man. The Anatomy of Hate and Violence. New York: Grune & Stratton, Inc., 1968.

Chapple, Eliot D.: Culture and Biological Man: Explorations in Behavioral Anthropology. New York: Holt, Rinehart and Winston, Inc., 1970.

Comfort, Alex: The Nature of Human Nature. New York: Harper & Row, 1967.

Frankl, Vicktor E.: The Doctor and The Soul. From Psychotherapy to Logotherapy, ed. 2. Richard and Clara Winston (trans.) New York: Alfred A. Knopf, 1965.

Hammarskjöld, Dag: Markings. Leif Sjöberg and W.H. Auden (trans.) New York: Alfred A. Knopf, 1964.

Horosz, William: Escape From Destiny: Self-Directive Theory of Man and Culture. (American Lecture Series. Philosophy. Marvin Farber, Editor.) Springfield, Illinois: Charles C. Thomas, Publisher, 1967.

Kahn, Herman; Wiener, Anthony J., et al.: The Year 2000. A Frame-Work for Speculation on the Next Thirty-Three Years. New York: The Macmillan Company, 1967.

Kemp, Rose: Ambivalence. Behavioral Concepts and Nursing Intervention. Coordinated by Carolyn E. Carlson. Philadelphia: J.B. Lippincott Company, 1970, pp. 207–225.

Knutson, Andie L: The Individual, Society and Health Behavior. New York: Russell Sage Foundation, 1965. (See Chapter 2, "The Unity of Man," pp. 38–43, and Chapter 4, "The Uniqueness of Man," pp. 52–60.)

Latané, Bibb, and Darley, John: The Unresponsive Bystander—Why Doesn't He Help? New York: Appleton-Century-Crofts, 1970.

Lyons, James R. (ed.): The Intellectual Legacy of Paul Tillich. Detroit: Wayne State University Press, 1969.

Lystad, Mary H.: Social Aspects of Alienation. An Annotated Bibliography. Public Health Service Publication No. 1978. Chevy Chase, Maryland, National Institute of Mental Health. Washington D.C., U.S. Government Printing Office, 1969.

May, Rollo: Psychology and the Human Dilemma. Princeton, New Jersey: D. Van Nostrand Company, Inc., 1967. (See "Modern Man's Loss of Significance," pp. 25–39 and "Personal Identity in an Anonymous World," pp. 40–52.)

Morgan, George W.: The Human Predicament. Dissolution and Wholeness. Providence: Brown University Press, 1968.

Muller, Herbert J.: The Children of Frankenstein. A Primer on Modern Technology and Human Values. Bloomington, Indiana: Indiana University Press, 1970.

Powell, Thomas F.: Josiah Royce. New York: Washington Square Press, Inc., 1967. (See Chapter 6, "Identity," pp. 44–54; Chapter 9, "Individualism and Alienation," pp. 81–90, and Chapter 12, "The Problem of Evil," pp. 120–134.)

Rogers, Martha E.: An Introduction to the Theoretical Basis of Nursing. Philadelphia: F.A. Davis Company, 1970. (See Chapter 9, "Life's Pattern and Organization," pp. 61–66, and Chapter 10, "Man: A Sentient Thinking Being," pp. 67–77.)

Scheibe, Karl E.: Beliefs and Values. New York: Holt, Rinehart and Winston, Inc., 1970.

Shaw, Franklin J.: Reconciliation: A Theory of Man Transcending. Sidney M. Jourard and Dan C. Overslade (eds.). Insight Book #35. Princeton: D. Van Nostrand Company, Inc., 1966.

Slater, Philip E.: The Pursuit of Loneliness. American Culture at the Breaking Point. Boston: Beacon Press, 1970.

Taylor, Gordon Rattray: The Biological Time Bomb. (An N.A.L. Book) New York: The World Publishing Company, 1968. (See Chapter 1, "Where Are Biologists Taking Us?" pp. 9–20; Chapter 4, "Is Death Necessary?" pp. 91–124; and Chapter 5, "New Minds For Old," pp. 125–158.)

Chapter III: Concept: The Patient

Articles

Alinsky, Saul D.: The poor and the powerful. Int. J. Psychiat. 4:304–309, No. 4, 1967. (Critical evaluations by Robert Coles, et. al., pp. 309–313; "A Rejoinder" by Saul D. Alinsky, pp. 314–315.)

Auer, Edward T.: The invisible patient. Hosp. Progr. 50:55–59, Dec., 1969.

Bain, Barbara: The special patient. Amer. J. Nurs. 70:1464–1467, 1970.

Brown, Roy E.: Poverty and health in the United States. Some significant considerations. Clin. Pediat. 8:495–498, 1969.

Chafetz, Morris E.: No patient deserves to be patronized. Med. Insight 2:68–75, No. 2, 1970.

Costello, C.G.: It's depressing. Canad. Nurse 65:43–45, Sept., 1969. (Re: Effects of Hospitalization.)

Crichton, Michael: The high cost of cure. How a hospital bill grows 17 feet long. The Atlantic 225:49–57, Mar., 1970.

DeWolfe, Alan S.; Barrell, Robert P.; and Cummings, Jonathan W.: Patient variables in emotional response to hospitalization for physical illness. J. Consult. Psychol. 30:68–72, No. 1., 1966.

Dumas, Rheutaugh G.: This I believe...about nursing and the poor. Nurs. Outlook 17:47–49, Sept., 1969.

Duncan, Mary Lou: The hospital as a primitive society. Amer. J. Nurs. 70:106–107, 1970.

Freemon, Frank R., and Drake, Frank T.: Abnormal emotional reactions to hospitalization jeopardizing medical treatment. Psychosomatics 8:150–155, 1967.

Goldfarb, Charles: Patients nobody wants—skid row alcoholics. Dis. Nerv. Sys. 31:274–281, 1970.

Hutto, Ruth Bishop: Poverty's children. Amer. J. Nurs. 69:2166–2169, 1969.

Jacobson, Leonard I., and Ford, LeRoy H. Jr.: Need for approval, defensive denial and sensitivity to cultural stereotypes. J. Personality 34:596–609, 1966.

Kellner, Robert: Psychiatric ill health following physical illness. Brit. J. Psychiat. 112:71–73, 1966.

Levine, Myra E.: The pursuit of wholeness. Amer. J. Nurs. 69:93–98, 1969.

Linehan, Dorothy T.: What does the patient want to know? Amer. J. Nurs. 66:1066–1070, 1966.

Lipsitt, Don R.: Medical and psychological characteristics of "crocks." Mental Health Digest 2:31–33, July, 1970.

Macgregor, Frances C.: Uncooperative patients: some cultural interpretations. Amer. J. Nurs. 67:88–91, 1967.

McMahon, Arthur W., and Shore, Miles F.: Some psychological reactions to working with the poor. Arch. Gen. Psychiat. 18:562–568, 1968.

Papper, Solomon (ed.): The undesirable patient. J. Chronic Dis. 22:777–779, 1970.

Pavenstedt, Eleanor (ed.): The drifters. Children of disorganized lower-class families. Int. Psychiat. Clin. Vol. 4, No. 4, 1967. (Thirteen papers.)

Scott, Richard; Gaskell, P.G. and Morrell, D.C.: Patients who reside in common lodging-houses. Brit. Med. J. 2:1561–1564, 1966.

Shapiro, Joan H.: Single-room occupancy: community of the alone. Social Work 11:24–33, Oct., 1966.

Smith, Dorothy W.: Patienthood and its threat to privacy. Amer. J. Nurs. 69:509–513, 1969.

Special Supplement: The Sick Poor. Amer. J. Nurs. 69:2423–2454, 1969.

Vincent, Pauline A.: Do we want patients to conform? Nurs. Outlook 18:54–55, Jan., 1970.

Yerby, Alonzo S.: Improving care for the disadvantaged. Amer. J. Nurs. 68:1043–1047, 1968.

Books and Reports of Organizations

Agee, James, and Evans, Walker: Three tenant families. Let Us Now Praise Famous Men. Boston: Houghton Mifflin Company, 1941. (A poignantly beautiful portrayal in words and photographs of the daily life of three tenant families. A classic.)

Becker, Howard S., et. al. (eds.): Institutions and the Person: Essays Presented to Everett C. Hughes. Chicago: Aldine Publishing Company, 1968.

Biddle, Bruce J., and Thomas, Edwin J. (eds.): Role Theory. Concepts and Research. New York: John Wiley & Sons, Inc., 1966.

Deutscher, Irwin, and Thompson, Elizabeth J. (eds.): Among the People: Encounters with the Poor. New York: Basic Books, Inc., 1968.

Downs, Anthony: Who Are the Urban Poor? C.E.D. Supplementary Paper Number 26. New York: Committee For Economic Development, October, 1968.

Field, Minna: Patients Are People. A Medical-Social Approach to Prolonged Illness, ed. 3. New York: Columbia University Press, 1967.

Hunter, David R.: The Slums. Challenge and Response. New York: A Free Press Paperback, The Macmillan Company, 1968.

Kaitz, Edward M.: Pricing Policy and Cost Behavior in the Hospital Industry. New York: Praeger, Publishers, 1968.

Kotz, Nick: Let Them Eat Promises: The Politics of Hunger in America. Englewood, New Jersey: Prentice-Hall, 1969.

Moynihan, Daniel P. (ed.): On Understanding Poverty. Perspectives from the Social Sciences. New York: Basic Books, Inc., 1969.

Murphy, Juanita F.: The patient's plea. Current Concepts in Clinical Nursing, Vol. II, Betty S. Bergersen, et. al. (eds.), St. Louis: The C. V. Mosby Company, 1969., pp. 76–85.

Poverty and Health in the United States. A Bibliography with Abstracts. Semi-Annual Supplement No. 1. New York: Medical and Health Research Association of New York City, 1968. Supplement No. 2, 1968.

Robinson, Lisa: Psychological Aspects of the Care of Hospitalized Patients. Philadelphia: F.A. Davis Co., 1968.

Taylor, Carol: In Horizontal Orbit: Hospitals and the Cult of Efficiency. New York: Holt, Rinehart and Winston, Inc., 1969.

Vail, David J.: Dehumanization and the Institutional Career. Springfield: Charles C. Thomas, Publisher, 1966.

Chapter IV: Concept: The Nurse

Articles, Books and Reports of Organizations

Baruch, Rhoda: The achievement motive in women: implications for career development. J. Personality Soc. Psychol. 5:260–267, No. 3, 1967.

Callaghan, Perquilla: Development of awareness of self for the professional nursing student. Behavioral Concepts and Nursing Intervention. Coordinated by Carolyn E. Carlson. Philadelphia: J.B. Lippincott Company, 1970, pp. 283–301.

Cass, Dorothy E.: Expectations of the staff nurse in nursing practice. The Nursing Clinics of North America, 3:111–115, No. 1, 1968.

Davis, Fred (ed.): The Nursing Profession: Five Sociological Essays. New York: John Wiley & Sons, 1966.

Duff, Raymond S., and Hollingshead, August B.: Sickness and Society. New York: Harper & Row, 1968. (See Chapter 11, "Physicians, Nurses and Patients," pp. 217–247.)

Edwards, Carl N.: Cultural dissonance and dissimulation: a study in role conflict. J. Consult. Clin. Psychol. 32:607–610, No. 5, 1968.

Hadley, Betty Jo, and Dunlap, Marjorie S.: Autocratic versus democratic beliefs of graduate students in nursing. Nurs. Res. 17:19–26, 1968.

Heidgerken, Loretta: Nursing as a career: is it relevant? Amer. J. Nurs. 69:1217–1222, 1969.

Herzberg, Frederick: Work and the Nature of Man. New York: The World Publishing Company, 1966.

Horner, Matina S.: Fail: bright women. Psychol. Today 3:36–38; 62, Nov., 1969.

Kaufmann, Harry: Aggression and Altruism. New York: Holt, Rinehart and Winston, Inc., 1970.

Komisar, Lucy, The new feminism. Saturday Review 27–30; 55. February, 21, 1970.

Lofquist, Lloyd H., and Dawis, Rene V.: Adjustment to Work: A Psychological View of Man's Problems in a Work Oriented Society. New York: Appleton-Century-Crofts, 1969.

Olesen, Virginia L., and Davis, Fred: Baccalaureate students' images of nursing: a follow-up report. Nurs. Res. 15:151–158, 1966.

—————: and Whittaker, Elvi W.: The Silent Dialogue. A Study in the Social Psychology of Professional Socialization. San Francisco: Jossey-Bass, Inc. 1968. (See Chapter 3, "The Nursing World and the Collegiate School," pp. 56–80; Chapter 5, "Themes in the Transmission of Nursing Culture," pp. 110–146; and Chapter 8, "The Cycles of the Inner World," pp. 246–286.)

Olson, Edith V.: Education–for what? Amer. J. Nurs. 70:1508–1510, 1970.

Mereness, Dorothy: Freedom and responsibility for nursing students. Amer. J. Nurs. 67:69–71, 1967.

Reinkemeyer, Sister Agnes M.: It won't be hospital nursing. Amer. J. Nurs. 68:1936–1940, 1968.

Ritvo, Miriam, and Fisk, Claire: Role conflict. Amer. J. Nurs. 66:2248–2251, 1966.

Shopper, Moisy, and Levy, Norman B.: Emotional difficulties in nursing students. Childhood factors: a preliminary report. Arch. Gen. Psychiat. 16:180–184, 1967.

Special Issue: Woman's Place. The Atlantic 225:81–126, March, 1970. (Ten articles.)

Vollmer, Howard M., and Mills, Donald L. (eds.): Professionalization. Englewood Cliffs: Prentice-Hall, Inc., 1966.

The Nurse and the Dying Person

Articles

Abram, Harry S.: The psychiatrist, the treatment of chronic renal failure, and the prolongation of life. II. Amer. J. Psychiat. 126:157–167, 1969.

Adam, Kenneth Stuart: Suicide: a critical review of the literature. Canad. Psychiat. Assoc. J. 12:413–420, Aug., 1967.

Annis, J. W.: The dying patient Psychosomatics 10:289–292, 1969.

Averill, James R.: Grief: its nature and significance. Psychol. Bull. 70:721–748, Part I, No. 6, 1968.

Barckley, Virginia: The crises in cancer. Amer. J. Nurs. 67:278–280, 1967.

Becker, Arthur H., and Weisman, Avery D.: The patient with a fatal illness–to tell or not to tell, J.A.M.A. 201:646–647, Aug. 21, 1967.

Bengtsson, M.; Holmberg, S.; and Jannsson, B.: A psychiatric-psychological investigation of patients who had survived circulatory arrest. Acta Psychia. Scand. 45:327–346, Fasc. 4, 1969.

Birtchnell, John: The possible consequences of early parent death. Brit. J. Med. Psychol. 42:1–12, Part I, 1969.

Bonnie, Gladys N.: Students' reactions to children's deaths. Amer. J. Nurs. 67: 1439–1440, 1967.

Bright, Florence, and France, Sister M. Luciana: The nurse and the terminally ill child. Nurs. Outlook 15:39–42, Sept., 1967.

Browne, Ivor, and Hackett, Thomas P.: Emotional reactions to the threat of impending death: a study of patients on the monitor cardiac pacemaker. Irish J. Med. Sci. Sixth Series, No. 496, 177–187, April, 1967.

Bruhn, John G., and Wolf, Stewart: A psychological study of survivors and nonsurvivors of myocardial infarction. Psychosom. Med. 31:8–19, 1969.

Clayton, Paula; Desmarais, Lynn; and Winokur, George: A study of normal bereavement. Amer. J. Psychiat. 125:168–178, 1968.

Davis, Marcella Zaleski: Patients in limbo. Amer. J. Nurs. 66:746–748, 1966.

Davidson, Ramona Powell: Let's talk about death to give care in terminal illness. Amer. J. Nurs. 66:74–75, 1966.

Dudley, Donald, et al.: Long-term adjustment, prognosis and death in irreversible diffuse obstructive pulmonary syndromes. Psychosom. Med. 31:310–326, 1969.

Durrant, Charles W.: The power of suggestion on the unconscious patient. Canad. Nurse 64:46–48, Oct., 1968.

Farberow, Norman L., et al.: Suicide among patients with cardiorespriatory illnesses. J.A.M.A. 195:422–428, Feb. 7, 1966.

Feifel, Herman: Attitudes toward death: a psychological perspective. J. Consult. Clin. Psychol. 33:292–295, No. 3., 1969.

Francis, Gloria M.: Cancer: the emotional component. Amer. J. Nurs. 69:1677–1681, 1969.

Gartley, Wayne, and Bernasconi, Marion: The concept of death in children. J. Genet. Psychol. 110:71–85, 1967.

Goff, Williard F.: How can a physician prepare his patient for death? J.A.M.A. 201:134, July 24, 1967.

Glaser, Barney: The social loss of aged dying patients. Gerontologist 6:77–80, 1966.

Goldfarb, Charles; Driesen, Jerome; and Cole, Donald: Psychophysiologic aspects of malignancy. Amer. J. Psychiat. 123:1545–1552, 1967.

Grayson, Henry: Grief reactions to the relinquishing of unfulfilled wishes. Amer. J. Psychother. 25:287–295, 1970.

Halley, M. Martin, and Harvey, William F. Jr.: Medical vs. legal definitions of death. J.A.M.A. 204:423–425, May 6, 1968.

Hinton, J.M.: Facing Death. J. Psychosom. Res. 10:22–28, 1966.

Hunter, R.C.A.: On the experience of nearly dying. Amer. J. Psychiat. 124:84–88, 1967.

Johnson, Wayne G.: To die as a man: disease, truth and christian ethics. J. Iowa Med. Soc. 56:813–816, 1966.

Kram, Charles, and Caldwell, John M.: The dying patient. Psychosomatics 10:293–295, 1969.

Kalish, Richard A.: A continuum of subjectively perceived death. Gerontologist 6:73–76, 1966.

Kalish, Richard A.: Social distance and the dying. Community Ment. Health J. 2:152–155, 1966.

Kastenbaum, Robert: Death as a research problem in social gerontology: an overview. Gerontologist 6:67–69; 125, 1966.

Knipe, Mary L.: Serenity for a terminally ill patient. Amer. J. Nurs. 66:2252–2254, 1966.

Koenig, Ronald R.: Fatal illness: a survey of social service needs. Social Work 13: 85–90, Oct., 1968.

Lang, Priscilla A., and Oppenheimer, Jeanette R.: The influence of social work when parents are faced with the fatal illness of a child. Social Casework 49:161–166, No. 3, 1968.

Lazarus, Herbert R., and Kostan, John J., Jr.: Psychogenic hyperventilation and death anxiety. Psychosomatics 10:14–22, 1969.

Lester, David: Experimental and correlational studies of the fear of death. Psychol. Bull. 67:27–36, No. 1, 1967.

Lieberman, Morton A.: Observations on death and dying. Gerontologist 6:70–72; 125, 1966.

Lipman, Aaron, and Marden, Philip W.: Preparation for death in old age. J. Geront. 21:426–431, 1966.

Maddison, David, and Walker, Wendy L.: Factors affecting the outcome of conjugal bereavement. Brit. J. Psychiat. 113:1057–1067, 1967.

Neuringer, Charles: Divergencies between attitudes towards life and death among suicidal, psychosomatic and normal hospitalized patients. J. Consult. Clin. Psychol. 32:59–63, No. 1, 1968.

Noyes, Russell: The dying patient. Dis. Nerv. Syst. 28:790–797, 1967.

Parkes, C. Murray: Effects of bereavement on physical and mental health—a study of the medical records of widows. Brit. Med. J. 2:274–279, 1964.

————: Benjamin, B., and Fitzgerald, R.G.: Broken heart: a statistical study of increased mortality among widowers. Brit. Med. J. 1:740–743, 1969.

Pattison, E. Mansell: The experience of dying. Amer. J. Psychother. 21:32–43, 1967.

Payne, Edmund C., Jr., and Krant, Melvin J.: The psychosocial aspects of advanced cancer, J.A.M.A. 210:1238–1242, Nov., 1969.

Pearlman, Joel; Stotsky, Bernard A.; and Dominick, Joan R.: Attitudes towards death among nursing home personnel. J. Genet. Psychol. 114:63–75, 1969.

Quint, Jeanne C.: Obstacles to helping the dying. Amer. J. Nurs. 66:1568–1571, 1966.

Roose, Lawrence J.: To Die alone. Ment. Hyg. 53:321–326, 1969.

Silverman, Phyllis Rolfe: Services to the widowed: first steps in a program of preventive intervention. Community Ment. Health J. 3:37–44, No. 1, 1967.

Stavraky, Kathleen M., et al.: Psychological factors in the outcome of human cancer. J. Psychosom. Res. 12:251–259, 1968.

Vanden Bergh, Richard L.: Let's talk about death. To overcome inhibiting emotions. Amer. J. Nurs. 66:71–73, 1966.

Verwoerdt, Adriaan: Euthanasia: a growing concern for physicians. Geriatrics, 22:44; 48; 52; 56; 60, Aug., 1967.

Verwoerdt, Adriaan, and Wilson, Ruby: Communication with fatally ill patients—tacit or explicit? Amer. J. Nurs. 67:2307–2309, 1967.

Wagner, Frederick F.: The psychiatrist and the dying hospital patient. Ment. Hyg. 51:486–488, 1967.

Walker, J.V.: Attitudes to death. Geront. Clin. 10:304–308, 1968.

Wallace, Elspeth, and Townes, Brenda D.: The dual role of comforter and bereaved. Ment. Hyg. 53:327–332, 1969.

Weisman, Avery D.: Misgivings and misconceptions in the psychiatric care of terminal patients. Psychiatry 33:67–81, 1970.

White, Laurens P. (Consulting editor and conference chairman): Care of patients with fatal illness. Ann. N.Y. Acad. Sci. 164:635–896. Art. 3, Dec. 19, 1969 (twenty-one papers).

Wolff, Kurt: Personality type and reaction toward aging and death. Geriatrics, 21:189–192, Aug., 1966.

————: Helping elderly patients face the fear of death. Hosp. Community Psychiat. 18:142–144, 1967.

Wygant, W.E., Jr.: Dying, but not alone. Amer. J. Nurs. 67:574–577, 1967.

Young, Michael; Benjamin, Bernard; and Wallis, Chris: The mortality of widowers. Lancet 2:454–456, 1963.

Zinker, J.C., and Fink, S.L.: The possibility for psychological growth in a dying person. J. Gen. Psychol. 74:185–199, 1966.

Books and Reports of Organizations

Aguilera, Donna Conant: Crisis: death and dying. ANA Clinical Sessions. ANA, 1968, Dallas. New York: Appleton-Century-Crofts, 1968, pp. 269–278.

Drummond, Eleanor E.: Communication and comfort for the dying patient. The Nursing Clinics of North America. 5:55–63, 1970.

Duff, Raymond S., and Hollingshead, August B.: Sickness and Society. New York: Harper & Row, 1968. (See Chapter 15, "Dying and Death," pp. 306–330.)

Farberow, Norman L.: Bibliography on Suicide and Suicide Prevention. 1897–1957; 1958–1967. Chevy Chase, Maryland: National Institute of Mental Health. Public Health Service Publication #1979, Washington D.C., U.S. Government Printing Office, 1969.

Frankl, Viktor E.: The Doctor and the Soul. From Psychotherapy to Logotherapy, ed. 2. Richard and Clara Winston (trans.) New York: Alfred A. Knopf. 1965. (See "On the Meaning of Life," pp. 26–62, and "On the Meaning of Death," pp. 63–92.)

Garner, H.H.: Psychosomatic Management of the Patient with Malignancy. Springfield, Illinois: Charles C. Thomas, Publisher, 1966.

Glaser, Barney G., and Strauss, Anselm L.: Time for Dying. Chicago: Aldine Publishing Company, 1968. (Sequel to Awareness of Dying by Glaser and Strauss.)

Hinton, John: Dying. Baltimore: Penguin Books, 1967.

Jackson, Nancy A.: A child's preoccupation with death. ANA Clinical Sessions. ANA, 1968, Dallas. New York: Appleton-Century-Crofts, 1968, pp. 172–179.

Kalish, Richard: Experiences of persons reprieved from death. Death and Bereavement. Austin H. Kutscher (ed.) Springfield: Charles C. Thomas, Publisher, 1969, pp. 84–96.

Kubler-Ross, Elizabeth: On Death and Dying. New York: The Macmillan Company, 1969.

Kutscher, Austin H. (ed.): Death and Bereavement. Springfield: Charles C. Thomas, Publisher, 1969.

Lippincott, Richard C.: The physician's approach to the patient with cancer. The Surgical Clinics of North America. 47:559–564, 1967.

Mangen, Sister Frances Xavier: Psychological aspects of nursing the advanced cancer patient. The Nursing Clinics of North America 2:649–658, Dec., 1967.

Moriarity, David M. (ed. and compiler): The Loss of Loved Ones: The Effects of a Death in the Family on Personality Development. Springfield, Illinois: Charles C. Thomas, Publisher, 1967.

Olsen, Emily: Effect of nurse-patient interaction on a terminal patient. ANA Clinical Sessions. ANA, 1968, Dallas. New York: Appleton-Century-Crofts, 1968, pp. 90–94.

Pearson, Leonard (ed.): Death and Dying. Current Issues in the Treatment of the Dying Person. Cleveland: The Press of Case Western Reserve University, 1969. (See "Selected Bibliography on Death and Dying," pp. 133–235.)

Quint, Jeanne C.: The dying patient: a difficult nursing problem. The Nursing Clinics of North America 2:763–773, Dec., 1967.
————: The Nurse and the Dying Patient. New York: The Macmillan Company, 1967.

Schoenberg, Bernard: The nurse's education for death. Death and Bereavement. Austin H. Kutscher (ed.) Springfield, Illinois: Charles C. Thomas, Publisher, 1969, pp. 55–74.

Schwab, Sister M. Loyola: The nurse's role in assisting families of dying geriatric patients to manage grief and guilt. ANA Clinical Sessions. ANA, 1968, Dallas. New York: Appleton-Century-Crofts, 1968, pp. 110–116.

Simmons, Leo W., and Jaeger, Dorothea: Aged Dying Patients. Their Nursing Care. New York: Appleton-Century-Crofts, 1968.

Toynbee, Arnold, et al.: Man's Concern with Death. New York: McGraw-Hill Book Company, 1968.

Verwoerdt, Adriaan: Communication with the Fatally Ill. Springfield, Illinois: Charles C. Thomas, Publisher, 1966.

Winter, Arthur (ed.): The Moment of Death; A Symposium. Springfield, Charles C. Thomas, Publisher, 1969.

Chapter V: Concept: Illness

Articles

Abrams, Harry S.: Psychological responses to illness and hospitalization. Psychosomatics 10:218–224, 1969.

Anthony, E. James: The impact of mental and physical illness on family life. Amer. J. Psychiat. 127:138–146, 1970.

Beard, Bruce H.: Fear of death and fear of life. The dilemma in chronic renal failure, hemodialysis and kidney transplantation. Arch. Gen. Psychiat. 21:373–380, 1969.

Bishop, Louis F., and Reichert, Philip: The psychological impact of the coronary care unit. Psychosomatics 10:189–192, 1969.

Briggs, R.F.: The emotional needs of children in hospital. Canad. Med. Assoc. J. 94:485–487, Mar. 5, 1966.

Callahan, Eileen M., et al.: The sick role in chronic illness: some reactions. J. Chronic Dis. 19:883–897, 1966.

Cardone, Samuel S., and Olson, Ronald: Psychophysical studies of body–image. IV. Disturbances in a hemiplegic sample. Arch. Gen. Psychiat. 21:464–469, 1969.

Carnes, G. Derwood: Personality abnormalities among patients on a physical medicine and rehabilitation service. Arch. Phys. Med. 48:180–184, 1967.

Christopherson, Victor A.: Role modifications of the disabled male. Amer. J. Nurs. 68:290–293, 1968.

Croog, Sydney H., and Levine, Sol: Social status and subjective perceptions of 250 men after myocardial infarction. Public Health Rep. 84:989–997, 1969.

Dominian, J., and Dobson, M.: Study of patients' psychological attitudes to a coronary care unit, Brit. Med. J. 4:795–798, 1969.

Feder, Samuel L.: Psychological considerations in the care of patients with cancer. Ann. N. Y. Acad. Sci. 125: 1020–1027, Jan. 21, 1966.

Fineberg, M. Herbert; Lange, Daniel J., and Cruser, Robert W.: Why long–term patients won't leave the hospital. Mod. Hosp. 109:124;126;128;166, Aug., 1967.

Fowler, Roy S.; Fordyce, Wilbert E.; and Berni, Rosemarian: Operant conditioning in chronic illness. Amer. J. Nurs. 69:1226–1228, 1969.

Freemon, Frank R., and Drake, Frank T.: Abnormal emotional reactions to hospitalization jeopardizing medical treatment. Psychosomatics 8:150–155, 1967.

Garner, H.H.: Chronic disability and the sick role, Illinois Med. J. 132:293–298, 1967.

Gillespie, Irene, and Johnston, Betty Jane: The disabled college woman and her use of time. Rehab. Lit. 28:379–382, 1967.

Gochman, David S.: Children's perceptions of vulnerability to illness and accidents. An exploratory study. Public Health Rep. 85:69–73, No. 1., 1970.

Hackett, Thomas P., and Cassem, N.H.: How do patients react to heart disease? Med. Insight 2:78–91, No. 3, 1970.

Janicki, Matthew P.: Attitudes of health professionals toward twelve disabilities.

Percept, Motor Skills 30:77–78, No. 1, 1970.

Jenkins, C. David: The semantic differential for health: a technique for measuring beliefs about diseases. Public Health Rep. 81:549–558, 1966.

Jenney, E. Ross: The case against promotion of health. Lancet 2:1245–1246, 1966.

Kasl, Stanislav V., and Cobb Sidney: Health behavior, illness behavior and sick role behavior. I. Health and illness behavior. Archives of Environmental Health, Preventive, Occupational and Aereospace Medicine. 12:246–266, 1966. II. Sick–role behavior, *Ibid.*, 12:531-541, 1966.

Klein, Robert F.; Dean, Alfred; and Bogdonoff, Morton D.: The impact of illness upon the spouse, J. Chronic Dis. 20:241–248, 1967.

Ludwig, Edward G., and Collette, John: Disability, dependency and conjugal roles. Journal of Marriage and the Family 31:736–739, 1969.

MacDonald, A.P., Jr., and Hall, Janet: Perception of disability by the nondisabled. J. Consult. Clin. Psychol. 33:654–660, No. 6, 1969.

Martin, Helen L.: The significance of discussions with patients about their diagnosis and its implications. Brit. J. Med. Psychol. 40:233–242, 1967.

Mendeloff, Albert I., et al.: Illness experience and life stresses in irritable colon and ulcerative colitis. New Eng. J. Med. 282:14–17, 1970.

Mordkoff, Arnold M,. and Rand, Melvin A.: Personality and adaptation to coronary artery disease. J. Consult. Clin. Psychol. 32:648–653, 1968.

Moses, Rafael, and Cividali, Nizza: Differential levels of awareness of illness: Their relation to some salient features in cancer patients. Ann. N. Y. Acad. Sci. 125:984–994, Jan. 21, 1966.

Nicholas, James R.: The chains of illness as an old friend. G. P. 37:112–116, Apr., 1968.

Norris, Catherine M.: The work of getting well. Amer. J. Nurs. 69:2118–2121, 1969.

Olin, Ronald: Diseases of medical progress. J. Lancet 87:390–392, 1967.

Rahe, Richard H.; McKean, Joseph D., Jr.; and Arthur, Ransom J.: A longitudinal study of life–change and illness patterns. J. Psychosom. Res. 10:355–366, 1967.

Reed, Dixie L.: Social disengagement in chronically ill patients. Nurs. Res. 19:109–115, 1970.

Reed, Julian W.: Rehabilitating the chronically ill: a 5 year follow–up of 341 chronically ill ambulatory medical outpatients. J. Chronic Dis. 20:457–468, 1967.

Robinson, David: Mothers' fear, their children's well–being in hospital, and the study of illness behavior. Brit. J. Prev. Soc. Med. 22:228–233, 1968.

Rosen, Jacqueline L., and Bibring, Grete L.: Psychological reactions of hospitalized male patients to a heart attack. Age and social–class differences. Psychosom. Med. 28:808–821, No. 6, 1966.

Rosillo, Ronald H., and Fogel, Max L.: Correlation of psychologic variables and progress in physical rehabilitation: 1. Degree of disability and denial of illness. Arch. Phys. Med. 51:227–233, 1970.

Rusalem, Herbert: Penetrating the narrow circle. A review of the literature concerning the vocational rehabilitation of homebound persons. Rehab. Lit. 28:202–217, 1967.

Schwab, John J., et al.: Evaluating Anxiety of medical patients. J. Chronic Dis. 19:1049–1057, 1966.

————, et al.: Anxiety, severity of illness and other medical variables. J. Psychosom. Res. 10:297–303, 1966.

————, and Harmeling, James D.: Body image and medical illness. Psychosom. Med. 30:51–61, 1968.

Sheldon, Alan, and Hooper, Douglas: An enquiry into health and ill–health and adjustment in early marriage. J. Psychosom. Res. 13:95–101, 1969.

Sorenson, Karen M., and Amis, Dorothy Bruner: Understanding the world of the chronically ' ill. Amer. J. Nurs. 67:811–817, 1967.

Starkey, Pearl Davidoff: Sick–role retention as a factor in non–rehabilitation. J. Counseling Psychol. 15:75–79, 1968.

Tagliacozzo, Daisy M., and Ima, Kenji: Knowledge of illness as a predictor of patient behaviour. J. Chronic Dis. 22:765–775, 1970.

Titley, R.W., et al.: Expression of aggression toward the physically handicapped. Percept. Motor Skills 29:51–56, Aug., 1969.

Waxenbert, Sheldon E.: The importance of the communication of feelings about cancer. Ann. N. Y. Acad. Sci. 125: 1000–1005, Jan., 1966.

Weinstein, Morton R.: The illness process. Psychosocial hazards of disability program. J.A.M.A. 204:209–213, Apr. 15, 1968.

Books and Reports of Organizations

Duff, Raymond S., and Hollingshead, August B.: Sickness and Society. New York: Harper & Row, 1968. (See Chapter 9, "The Physical Illness," pp. 151–178; Chapter 13, "Reactions to Hospitalization," pp. 268–287; and Chapter 14, "The Patient Views His Illness," pp. 291–305.)

Dumas, Rhetaugh Graves: Utilization of the concept of stress as a basis for nursing practice. ANA Clinical Sessions. ANA, 1966, San Francisco. New York: Appleton-Century-Crofts, 1967, pp. 193–201 (discussion pp. 201–212).

Freedman, J.L., and Doob, A.N.: Deviancy: The Psychology of Being Different. New York: Academic Press, 1968.

Gaspard, Nancy J.: The family of the patient with long–term illness. The Nursing Clinics of North America 5:77–84, 1970.

Gordon, Gerald: Role Theory and Illness. A Sociological Perspective. New Haven: College and University Press, 1966. (See "The Sick Role," pp. 35-44; and "Behavioral Expectations Relevant to Illness," pp. 71-96.)

————: et al.: Disease. The Individual and Society. Social–Psychological Aspects of Disease: A Summary and Analysis of a Decade of Research. New Haven: College and University Press, 1968.

Holland, Bernard C., and Ward, Richard S.: Homeostasis and Psychosomatic Medicine. American Handbook of Psychiatry, Vol. 3, Silvano Arieti (ed.) New York: Basic Books, Inc., pp. 341-361. (See esp. "Physical Illness with Psychological Reactions," pp. 358–360.)

Kiening, Sister Mary Martha: Denial of illness. Behavioral Concepts and Nursing Intervention. Coordinated by Carolyn E. Carlson. Philadelphia: J.B. Lippincott Company, 1970, pp. 9–28.

Mechanic, David: Medical Sociology. A Selective View. New York: The Free Press, 1968. (See Chapter 4, "The Patient's Perspective of His Illness: The Study of Illness Behavior," pp. 115–157.)

Moser, Robert H.: Diseases of Medical Progress: A study of Iatrogenic Disease: A Contemporary Analysis of Illnesses Produced by Drugs and Other Therapeutic Procedures, ed. 3. Springfield, Illinois, Charles C. Thomas, Publisher, 1969.

Silverman, Samuel: Psychological Aspects of Physical Symptoms. A Dynamic Study of Forty–Five Hospitalized Medical Patients. New York: Appleton–Century–Crofts, 1968.

Sussman, Marvin B.; Caplan, Eleanor K; Haug, Marie R.; and Stern, Marjorie: The Walking Patient. A Study of Outpatient Care. Cleveland: The Press of Western Reserve University, 1967.

Symposium on Chronic Disease and Rehabilitation. June S. Rothberg, Guest Editor, The Nursing Clinics of North America 1:352–519, September, 1966. (Seventeen papers.)

Symposium on Nursing in Long–Term Illness. Irene S. Palmer, Guest Editor. The Nursing Clinics of North America 5:1-84, March, 1970. (Eight papers.)

Van Den Berg. J.H.: The Psychology of the Sickbed. Pittsburgh: Duquesne University Press, 1967.

Illness and the Elderly Person

Articles, Books and Reports of Organizations

Arje, Frances B.: Disengagement. A Review of the Theory and Its Implications for Rehabilitation Nursing With Geriatric Patients. The Nursing Clinics of North America 1:235–244, June, 1966.

Bell, Tony: The relationships between social involvement and feeling old among residents in homes for the aged, J. Geront. 22:17–22, 1967.

Berwick, Keith: The "senior citizen" in America: a study of unplanned obsolescence. Gerontologist 7:257–260, 1967.

Burnside, Irene Mortenson: Clocks and calendars. Amer. J. of Nurs. 70:117–119, 1970.

Calnan, Mary E.: Helping the nurse to meet the challenge of the geriatric patient. The Nursing Clinics of North America 3:717–727, December, 1968.

Cameron, Paul: Ego strength and happiness of the aged, J. Geront. 22:199–202, 1967.

Cumming, Elaine: New thoughts on the theory of disengagement. Int. J. Psychiat. 6:53–67, 1968. (Critical evaluations, pp. 67–76.)

Davis, Robert W.: Psychologic aspects of geriatric nursing. Amer. J. Nurs. 68:802–804, 1968.

Elizabeth, Sister Regina: The dignity of aging: reminders for nursing service. Hosp. Progr. 48:110–116, Mar., 1967.

Evangela, Sister M.: The influence of family relationships on the geriatric patient . . . the nurse's role. The Nursing Clinics of

North America 3:653–662, December, 1968.

Field, Minna: Aging with Honor and Dignity. Springfield, Illinois: Charles C. Thomas, Publisher, 1968.

————(ed.): Depth and Extent of the Geriatric Problem: Authoritative Original Contributions. Springfield, Illinois: Charles C. Thomas, Publisher, 1969.

Giffin, Kim: Personal trust and the interpersonal problems of the aged person. Gerontologist 9:286–292, Part I, 1969.

Harrison, Cherie: The institutionally–deprived elderly. A challenge for nurses to change their role. The Nursing Clinics of North America 3:697–707, December, 1968.

Hoffman, Adeline M. (ed. and compiler): The Daily Needs and Interests of Older People. Springfield, Illinois: Charles C. Thomas, Publisher, 1969.

Hodkinson, Mary A.: Some clinical problems of geriatric nursing. The Nursing Clinics of North America 3:675;686, December, 1968.

Miller, Michael B., and Harris, Audrey P.: The chronically ill aged: paradoxical patient–family behavior. J. Amer. Geriat. Soc. 15:480–495, 1967.

More, Sister Mary Thomas: What went wrong? ANA Clinical Sessions. ANA, 1968, Dallas. New York: Appleton–Century–Crofts, 1968, pp. 83–89.

Moses, Dorothy V.: The older patient in the general hospital. The Nursing Clinics of North America 2:705–714, December, 1967.

————: Reality orientation in the aging person. Behavioral Concepts and Nursing Intervention. Coordinated by Carolyn E. Carlson, Philadelphia: J.B. Lippincott Company, 1970, pp. 171–186.

Rehabilitation Issue. Geriatrics 25:99–172, Mar., 1970 (eight papers).

Sloane, R. Bruce, and Frank, Diana: The mentally affected old person, Geriatrics 25:125–132, Mar., 1970.

Special Section: Geriatrics. Amer. J. Psychiat. 123:1226–1259, 1967 (five papers).

Stotsky, Bernard: Nursing homes: a review, Amer. J. Psychiat. 123:249–258, 1966.

Symposium on Care of the Elderly Patient. Harriet C. Lane, Guest Editor. The Nursing Clinics of North America 3:649–748, December 1968 (nine papers).

Symposium: The Problems of Aging. Psychosomatics 8:2–73, Section 2, 1967. (seventeen papers).

Symposium on Ecology of Aging and of the Aging Process. Gerontologist 8:76–119 and 134. No. 2, 1968 (ten papers).

Tanenbaum, David E.: Loneliness in the aged, Ment. Hyg. 51:91–99, 1967.

Verwoerdt, Adriaan, and Eisdorfer, Carl: Geropsychiatry – the psychiatry of senescence. Geriatrics 22:139–149, July, 1967.

Walton, Margaret: An old person living alone in the community. Geront. Clin. 10:358–368, 1968.

Wang, H. Shan; Obrist, Walter D; and Busse, Ewald W.: Neurophysiological correlates of the intellectual function of elderly persons living in the community. Amer. J. Psychiat. 126:1205–1212, 1970.

Weinstock, Comilda, and Bennett, Ruth, Problems in communication to nurses among residents of a racially heterogenous nursing home. Gerontologist 8:72–75, 1968.

Weymouth, Lilyan T.: The nursing care of the so–called confused patient. The Nursing Clinics of North America 3:709–715, December, 1968.

Chapter VI: Concept: Suffering

Articles

Arlow, Jacob A.: Fantasy, memory and reality testing. Psychoanal. Quart. 38:28–51, 1969.

Berblinger, Klaus W.: A psychiatrist looks at loneliness. Psychosomatics 9:96–102, 1968.

Best, Gary A.: The minority status of the physically disabled. Cereb. Palsy J. 28:3–4 and 8, May-June, 1967.

Brawley, Peter, and Pos, Robert: The informational underload (sensory deprivation) Model in contemporary psychiatry, Canad. Psychiat, Assoc. J. 12:105–124, Apr., 1967.

Carnes, G. Derwood: Personality abnormalities among patients on a physical medicine and rehabilitation service. Arch. Phys. Med. 48:180–184, 1967.

Davitz, Lois Jean, et al.: Nurses' inferences of suffering. Nurs. Res. 18:100–107, 1969.

Fitzgerald, Roy G.: Reactions to blindness. An exploratory study of adults with recent loss of sight. Arch. Gen. Psychiat. 22:370–379, 1970.

Gardner, Richard A.: The guilt reaction of parents of children with severe physical illness. Amer. J. Psychiat. 126:636–644, 1969.

Kahn, Marvin W., and Kirk, William E.: The concepts of aggression: a review and reformulation. The Psychological Record 18:559–573, 1968.

Kendall, Robert E.: Relationship between aggression and depression. Epidemiological implications of a hypothesis. Arch. Gen. Psychiat. 22:308–318, 1970.

Lerner, Melvin J., and Matthews, Gail: Reactions to suffering of others under conditions of indirect responsibility. J. Personality Soc. Psychol. 5:319–325, 1967.

Lesse, Stanley: The nultivariant masks of depression. Amer. J. Psychiat. 124: Suppl. 35–40, 1968.

O'Connor, Daniel: The phenomenon of boredom. J. Exist. 7:380–399, 1967.

Rosekrans, Frank M.: Choosing to suffer as a consequence of expecting to suffer. A replication. J. Personality Soc. Psychol. 7:419–423, 1967.

Rosenthal, Saul H., and Gudeman, Jon E.: The self-pitying constellation in depression. Brit. J. Psychiat. 113:485–489, 1967.

Schecter, Nathan: Psychological aspects of chronic cardiac disease. Psychosomatics 8:166–169, 1967.

Schwab, John J., et al.: Sociocultural aspects of depression in medical inpatients. I. Frequency and social variables. Arch. Gen. Psychiat. 17:533–538, 1967. II. Symptomatology and class. Ibid., 17:539–543, 1967.

Siggins, Lorraine D.: Mourning: a critical review of the literature. Int. J. Psycho–Anal. 47:14–25, 1966.

Swift, Charles R.; Seidman, Frances, and Stein, Harry: Adjustment problems in juvenile diabetes. Psychosom. Med. 29:555-571, 1967.

Tanenbaum, David E.: Loneliness in the aged. Ment. Hyg. 51:91–99, 1967.

Taylor, Dalmas A., et al.: Personality factors related to response to social isolation and confinement. J. Consult. Clin. Psychol. 33:411–419, 1969.

Weinstein, Sidney, et al.: Bibliography of sensory and perceptual deprivation, isolation and related areas. Percept. Motor Skills 26:1119–1163, 1968. Monograph Suppl. 4–v26, 1968 (item 1199 bibliography re: sensory and perceptual deprivation).

Zubek, John P., and MacNeill, M.: Perceptual deprivation phenomena: role of the recumbent position. J. Abnorm. Psychol. 72:147–150, 1967.

Books and Reports of Organizations

Bakan, David: Disease, Pain and Sacrifice. Toward a Psychology of Suffering. Chicago: The University of Chicago Press, 1968.

Bowker, John: Problems of Suffering in the Religions of the World. London: Cambridge University Press, 1970.

Chauchard, Paul: Teilhard de Chardin on Love and Suffering. Marie Chene (trans.) New York: Paulist Press. Deus Books, 1966.

Clark, Eloise: Aspects of loneliness: toward a framework of nursing intervention. Conference on Teaching Psychiatric Nursing in Baccalaureate Programs. Atlanta: Southern Regional Education Board, 1967, pp. 18–39.

Epstein, Seymour: Toward a unified theory of anxiety. Progress in Experimental Personality Research. Brendan A. Maher (ed.) 4:1–89, 1968.

Frankl, Viktor E.: The Doctor and The Soul. From Psychotherapy to Logotherapy, ed. 2. Richard and Clara Winston, (trans.) New York: Alfred A. Knopf, 1965. (See "On the Meaning of Suffering," pp. 105–116.)

————: Psychotherapy and Existentialism. New York: Simon and Schuster. A Clarion Book, 1967. (See "Logotherapy and the Challenge of Suffering," pp. 87– 94.)

McGee, C. Douglas: The Recovery of Meaning. New York: Random House, 1966. (See Chapter IV, "The Uses of Suffering," pp. 139–176.)

Parets, Albert D.: Emotional reactions of chronic physical illness. Implications for the internist. The Medical Clinics of North America 51:1399–1408, 1967.

Petri, Asenath: Individuality in Pain and Suffering. Chicago: University of Chicago Press, 1967.

Ruff, George E.: Isolation and Sensory Deprivation. American Handbook of Psychiatry. Vol. 3, Silvano Arieti (ed.) New York: Basic Books Inc., 1966, pp. 362–376.

Zubek, John P.: Sensory Deprivation: Fifteen Years of Research. New York: Appleton–Century–Crofts, 1969.

Concept: Pain

*Articles, Books and Reports of
Organizations*

Baer, Eva; Davitz, Lois Jean; and Lieb, Renee: Inferences of physical pain and psychological distress. I. In relation to verbal and non-verbal communication. Nurs. Res. 19:388–392, 1970.

Bakan, David: Disease, Pain and Sacrifice. Toward a Psychology of Suffering. Chicago: The University of Chicago Press, 1968. (See II. "Pain and the Functions of the Ego," pp. 57–91.)

Bandler, Richard J., Jr.; Madaros, George R.; and Bem, Daryl J.: Self–observation as a source of pain perception. J. Personality Soc. Psychol. 9:205–209, 1968.

Blitz, Bernard W., and Lowenthal, Milton: The role of sensory restriction in problems with chronic pain. (editorial) J. Chronic Dis. 19:1119–1125, 1966.

Bond, M.R., and Pearson, I.B.: Psychological aspects of pain in women with advanced cancer of the cervix. J. Psychosom. Res. 13:13–19, 1969.

Bond, M.R. and Pilowsky, I.: Subjective assessment of pain and its relationship to the administration of analgesics in patients with advanced cancer. J. Psychosom. Res. 10:203–208, 1966.

Bowers, Kenneth S.: Pain, anxiety, and perceived control. J. Consult. Clin. Psychol. 32:596–602, 1968.

Casey, Kenneth L.: Toward a neurophysiology of pain. Headache 8:141–153, 1969.

Chambers, Wilda G., and Price, Geraldine G.: Influence of nurse upon effects of analgesics administered. Nurs. Res. 16:228–233, 1967.

Davidson, P.O., and McDougall, C. Evalyne A.: The generality of pain tolerance. J. Psychosom. Res. 13:83–89, 1969.

Dinnerstein, Albert J.; Lowenthal, Milton, and Blitz, Bernard: The interaction of drugs with placebos in the control of pain and anxiety. Perspect. Biol. Med. 10:103–117, Autumn, 1966.

Eckenhoff, James E., Guest Editor: Pain and its clinical management. The Medical Clinics of North America 52:1–244, 1968 (twenty-two papers).

Fisher, Albert L.: The role of pain and its variations in effecting change. Headache 6:55–65, 1966.

Fitzgerald, M.J.T.: Pain mechanisms. J. Irish Med. Assoc. 63:252–256, 1970 (re: the neurology of pain).

Gallemore, J.L., Jr., and Wilson, W.P.: Complaint of pain in the clinical setting of affective disorders. Southern Med. J. 62:551–555, 1969.

Gonda, Thomas A.: Pain, relief, addiction and the dying patient. Death and Bereavement. Austin H. Kutscher (ed.) Springfield Illinois: Charles C. Thomas, Publisher, 1969, pp. 10–13.

Hackett, Thomas P.: The surgeon and the difficult pain problem. Int. Psychiat. Clin. 4:179–188, 1967.

Hightower, P.R.: The control of pain. Amer. J. Clin. Hypn. 9:67–70, 1966.

Hunger, Raymond A.: Fear, guilt, anxiety, and depression in the painful man. Arizona Med. 26:1030–1031, 1969.

Klein, Robert F., and Brown, Walter: Pain descriptions in the medical setting. J. Psychosom, Res. 10:367–372, 1967.

Lenburg, Carrie Byrd; Glass, Helen P.; and Davitz, Lois Jean: Inferences of physical pain and psychological distress. II. In relation to the stage of the patient's illness and occupation of the perceiver. Nurs. Res. 19:392–398, 1970. III. In relation to length of time in the nursing education program. *Ibid.,* 19:399–401. 1970.

Lewis, Muriel Rees; Skolnik, Michele; and Parkhouse, James: How do you measure pain? Nurs. Times 62:792–794, 1966.

Lowinger, Paul, and Dobie, Shirley: What makes the placebo work? A study of placebo response rates. Arch. Gen. Psychiat. 20:84–88, 1969.

McCaffery, Margo: Nursing Practice Theories Related to Cognition, Bodily Pain and Man-Environment Interactions. Los Angeles, University of California School of Nursing, Center for the Health Sciences, 1968.

————, and Moss, Fay: Nursing intervention for bodily pain. Amer, J. Nurs. 67:1224–1227, 1967.

McBride, Mary Angela B.: Nursing approach, pain and relief: an exploratory experiment. Nurs. Res. 16:337–341, 1967.

————: The additive to the analgesic. Amer. J. Nurs. 69:974–976, 1969.

Merskey, H., and Spear, F.G.: The concept of pain. J. Psychosom. Res. 11:59–67, 1967.

————: Pain: Psychological and Psychiatric Aspects. London: Bailliere, Tindall and Cassell, 1967.

Moldofsky, H., and Chester, W.: Pain and mood patterns in patients with rheumatoid arthritis: a prospective study. Psychosom. Med. 32:309–318, 1970.

Ownes, Guy: Control of pain in patients with cancer. J. Lancet 87–287–290, 1967.

Prior, Jerilynn C.: Some aspects of the clinical communication of pain. J. Amer. Med. Wom. Assoc. 22:725–731, 1967.

Programmed Instruction: Pain–Part I. Basic concepts and assessment. Amer. J. Nurs. 66:1085–1108, 1966. Part II, Rationale for intervention. *Ibid.*, 66:1345–1368, 1966.

Rogers, Ada: Pain and the cancer patient. The Nursing Clinics of North America 2:671–682, Dec., 1967.

Sternbach, Richard A.: Pain: A psychophysical analysis. New York: Academic Press, Inc., 1968.

Stravino, Vincent D.: The nature of pain. Arch. Phys. Med. 51:37–44, 1970.

Symposium on Pain. Practitioner 198:759–803, 1967 (five papers).

Szasz, Thomas S.: The painful person. J. Lancet 88:18–22, 1967.

Wilson, W.P., and Nashold, B.S., Jr.: Pain and emotion. Postgrad. Med. 47:183–187, 1970.

Zborowski, Mark: People in Pain. San Francisco: Jossey-Bass Inc., 1969. (See Chapter 1, "The Cultural Dimensions of Pain," pp. 14-48; Chapter 3, "The Patient Knows Best," pp. 97–135; and Chapter 5, "They Suffer Alone," pp. 187–235.)

Chapter VII: Concept: Hope

Articles, Books and Reports of Organizations

Frank, Jerome: The role of hope in psychotherapy. Int. J. Psychiat. 5:383–395, 1968. (Critical evaluations pp. 396–412.)

Fromm, Erich: The Revolution of Hope. Toward a Humanized Technology. New York: Harper & Row, 1968. (See Chapter II, "Hope." pp. 6–24.)

Goldsborough, Judith: Involvement. Amer. J. Nurs. 69: 66–68, 1969.

Harper, Ralph: Nostalgia. An Existential Exploration of Longing and Fulfillment in the Modern Age. Cleveland: Press of Western Reserve University, 1966.

Korner, Ija N.: Hope as a method of coping. J. Consult. Clin. Psychol. 34:134–139, 1970.

Laney, M. Louise; Hope as a healer. Nurs. Outlook 17:45–46, Jan., 1969.

Lynch, William F.: Images of Hope: Imagination as Healer of the Hopeless. New York: The New American Library. A Mentor-

Omega Book. 1965. (See "On Hope," pp. 23–37; "On Hopelessness," pp. 37–51; and "On Wishing and Hoping," pp. 109–122.)

O'Connor, Daniel: The phenomena of boredom. J. Exist. 7:381–399, 1967.

Schmale, Arthur H., Jr., and Iker, Howard P.: The affect of hopelessness and the development of cancer. I. Identification of uterine cervical cancer in women with atypical cytology. Psychosom. Med. 28:714–721, 1966.

Singer, Jerome L.: Daydreaming. An Introduction to the Experimental Study of Inner Experience. New York: Random House, 1966.

Stotland, Ezra: The Psychology of Hope. San Francisco: Jossey–Bass, Inc., 1969. (See Chapter 2, "Hope and Action," pp. 14–27; Chapter 3, "Hope and Anxiety," pp. 28–36; Chapter 9, "Help from Other People," pp. 133–151; and Chapter 12, "The Therapy of Hope," pp. 206–230.)

Supplement: Depression. Amer. J. Psychiat. 124:1–64, 1968 (seven papers).

Tesser, Abraham; Gatewood, Robert; and Driver, Michael: Some determinants of gratitude. J. Personality Soc. Psychol. 9:233–236, No. 3., 1968.

Vaillot, Sister Madeleine Clemence: Hope: the restoration of being. Amer. J. Nurs. 70:268; 270–273, 1970.

Wasli, Evelyn: Hope–a basic nursing concept. Conference on Teaching Psychiatric Nursing in Baccalaureate Programs. Atlanta: Southern Regional Education Board, 1967, pp. 121–136.

Wilson, Warner: Correlates of avowed happiness. Psychol. Bull. 67:294–306, No. 4, 1967.

Wright, Beatrice A., and Shontz, Franklin C.: Process and tasks in hoping. Rehab. Lit. 29:322–331, 1968.

Chapter VIII: Illness and Suffering as Human Experience

Articles, Books and Reports of Organizations

Bartemeier, Leo L.: An Introspective Account of Meniere's Syndrome. Bull. Menninger Clin. 31:193–196, 1967.

Bell, Milton A.: Pheochromocytoma. A personal experience. J. Albert Einstein Medical Center 8:45–48, 1960.

Bevan, P. Gilroy: Cholecystectomy in a surgeon. Lancet 1:214–215, 1964.

Bourke–White, Margaret: Portrait of Myself. New York: Simon & Schuster, Inc., 1963. (Famous photographer and journalist is afflicted with Parkinson's disease.)

Brown, Helen: Ignorance is not always bliss. Nursing Mirror and Midwives Journal 122:516, Aug. 26, 1966. (Student nurse undergoes appendectomy)

Chaput, Richard: Not to Doubt. New York: Pageant Press, Inc., 1964. (Victim of poliomyelitis relates his experiences.)

Crawford, John: Living without a balancing mechanism. Brit. J. Ophthal. 48:357–360, 1964.

Dunbar, Roxanne: Maternity. (Excerpt from an autobiographical essay.) No More Fun and Games. A Journal of Female Liberation. Issue 2, 88–96, February, 1969.

Frankel, Esther C.: I spoke with the dead. Amer. J. Nurs. 69:105–107, 1969. (Teacher, stricken with encephalitis, relates her experiences.)

Gargan, William: Why Me? An Autobiography. New York: Doubleday & Co., 1969. (Actor, suffering from cancer of the larynx, relates his experiences.)

Heath, Millard J.: Myocardial infarction: a personal account. J. Rehab. 32:46–47, 1966.

Howarth, Winifred: Living at home as a totally disabled person. Int. Nurs. Rev. 17:238–253, No. 3, 1970. (Victim of automobile accident, almost totally paralyzed, relates her experiences.)

Hunt, Paul (ed.): Stigma. The Experience of Disability. Englewood Cliffs, New Jersey: Prentice–Hall, Inc., 1966. (A collection of essays by physically handicapped individuals.)

Impressions of a Steriod Taker. By a Urological Guinea–Pig. Practitioner 198: 549–551, 1967.

Jones, William R.: Living with emphysema. Nurs. Outlook 15:53–57, Sept., 1967.

Judy, Frederick R.: A doctor has a heart attack. G. P. 34:201–205, Sept., 1966.

Kay, Claire: Living with angina. Nursing Mirror and Midwives Journal 121:xi and xvi, Feb. 25, 1966.

Kesten, Yehuda: Diary of a Heart Patient, Twice Operated on by Dr. Debakey. A Patient Tells of His Experience. New York: McGraw–Hill Book Company, 1968.

Knicely, Kathryn H.: The world of distorted perception. Amer. J. Nurs. 67:998–1002, 1967. (Nurse author undergoes surgery and relates her distorted perceptions while under the influence of drugs.)

La Baw, Wallace L.: A subjective report by a physician who suffered a cerebral concussion with concomitant acute brain syndrome. Resident Physician 13:149–160, 1967.

————: Denial inside out: subjective experience with anosognosia in closed head injury. Psychiatry 32:174–188, 1969. (Comment on "Denial Inside Out," by Edwin A. Weinstein, pp. 189–191.) (Child psychiatrist involved in an automobile accident. Suffers amnesia and loss of memory for 25 days.)

Levin, Max: Delerium: an experience and some reflections. Amer. J. Psychiat. 124:1120-1123, 1968.

Macginniss, Oscia: Rheumatoid arthritis–My tutor. Amer. J. Nurs 68:1699–1701, 1968.

Miers, Earl Schneck: The Trouble Bush. Chicago: Rand McNally & Company, 1966. (Individual with cerebral palsy recounts his experiences.)

Page, Irving H.: One out of every five. (editorial.) Modern Medicine 35:23–24, Sept. 11, 1967. (Physician suffers a heart attack.)

Perkins, Faith: My fight with arthritis. New York: Random House, Inc., 1964.

Poole, Lynn: I Am a Chronic Cardiac. New York: Dodd, Mead & Company, 1964.

Robinson, Charles R.: What the doctor saw was dirt and disorganization. Mod. Hosp. 107:76–77, Aug., 1966. (A physician feigns low back pain to get admitted to the hospital.)

Ryle, John A., The sense of dying–a postscript. Guy Hosp. Rep. 99:224–229, 1950. (Author relates his perception of living with angina.)

————: Angor animi, or the sense of dying. Guy Hosp. Rep. 99:230–235, 1950.

Smittkamp, James: Paraplegia: As seen by a paraplegic. The New Physician 13:37–39, 1964. (Individual with paraplegia relates his experiences with illness over a period of nineteen years.)

Stuart, Mrs. Grace: Private World of Pain. London: Allen and Unwin, 1953. (Author, afflicted with rheumatoid arthritis for thirty years, relates her experiences.)

Whatley, Dr. Elizabeth: Record of an illness. Develop. Med. Child Neurol. Supplement No. 19, 1969. (See entire issue.) (Psychiatrist who had a left craniotomy, followed by radiotherapy, relates her experiences.)

Wint, Guy: The Third Killer: Meditations on a Stroke. London: Chatto & Windus, Ltd., 1965.

Chapter IX: Concept: Communication

Articles

Alpert, Murray; Frosch, William A., and Fisher, Saul H.: Teaching the perception of expressive aspects of vocal communication. Amer. J. Psychiat. 124:202–209, 1967.

Brodsky, Stanley L., and Dixon, James C.: Impersonal and personal language patterns of repressors and sensitizers. J. Gen. Psychol. 78:27–33, 1968.

Berscheid, Ellen; Boye, David; and Walster, Elaine: Retaliation as a means of restoring equity. J. Personality Soc. Psychol. 10:370–376, 1968.

Craytor, Josephine K.: Talking with persons who have cancer. Amer. J. Nurs. 69:744–748, 1969.

Dean, Edward S.: The meaning of nagging. Mind 1:203–206; 211–212, 1963.

Dittmann, Allen T., and Llewellyn, Lynn G.: Relationship between vocalizations and head nods as listener responses. J. Personality Soc. Psychol. 9:79–84, No. 1, 1968.

Dodge, Joan S.: Factors related to patients' perceptions of their cognitive needs. Nurs. Res. 18:502–513, 1969.

Goldin, Phyllis, and Russell, Barbara: Therapeutic communication. Amer. J. Nurs. 69:1928–1930, 1969.

Giffin, Kim: The contribution of studies of source credibility to a theory of interpersonal trust in the communication process. Psychol. Bull. 68:104–120, No. 2, 1967.

Hays, Joyce Samhammer: Analysis of nurse–patient communications. Nurs. Outlook 14:32–35, Sept., 1966.

Horowitz, Milton, and Berkowitz, Alan: Listening and reading, speaking and writing: an experimental investigation of differential acquisition and reproduction of memory. Percept. Motor Skills 24:204–215, 1967.

Lindauer, Martin S.: The nature and use of the cliche. J. Gen Psychol. 78:133–143, 1968.

Mahl, George F.: Some clinical observations on nonverbal behavior in interviews. J. Nerv. Ment. Dis. 144:492–505, 1967.

Manthey, Marie E.: A guide for interviewing. Amer. J. Nurs. 67:2088–2090, 1967.

Maselli, Mary D., and Altrocchi, John: Attribution of intent. Psychol. Bull. 71:445–454, No. 6, 1969.

McGuire, Michael T., and Lorch, Stephen: Natural language conversation modes. J. Nerv. Ment. Dis. 146:239–248, 1968.

Mehrabian, Albert: Attitudes in relation to the forms of communicator-object relationship in spoken communications. J. Personality 34:80–93, 1966.

————: Attitudes inferred from neutral verbal communications. J. Consult. Psychol. 31:414–417, 1967.

————: Communication without words. Psychol. Today 2:52–55, Sept., 1968.

————: Inference of attitudes from the posture, orientation, and distance of a communicator. J. Consult. Clin. Psychol. 32:296–308, 1968.

————: Significance of posture and position in the communication of attitude and status relationships. Psychol. Bull. 71:359–372, 1969.

————, and Ferris, Susan R.: Inference of attitudes from nonverbal communication in two channels. J. Consult. Psychol. 31:248–252, 1967.

————, and Friar, John T.: Encoding of attitudes by a seated communicator via posture and position cues. J. Consult. Clin. Psychol. 33:330–336, No. 3, 1969.

————, and Wiener, Morton: Decoding of inconsistent communications. J. Personality Soc. Psychol. 6:109–114, 1967.

Molde, Donald A., and Wiens, Arthur N.: Interview interaction behavior of nurses with task versus person orientation. Nurs. Res. 17:45–51, 1968.

Orlinsky, David E., and Howard, Kenneth I.: Communication rapport and patient progress. Psychotherapy: Theory, Research and Practice 5:131–136, 1968.

Pilisuk, Marc, et al.: Honesty, deceit and timing in the display of intentions. Behav. Sci. 12:205–215, 1967.

Polansky, Norman A.: On duplicity in the interview. Amer. J. Orthopsychiat. 37:568–579, 1967.

Pope, Benjamin, and Siegman, Aron W.: Interviewer warmth in relation to interviewee verbal behavior. J. Consult. Clin. Psychol. 32:588–595, No. 5, 1968.

Rice, F. Edward, and Ratner, Stanley C.: Toward a description of language behavior: II. The listening action. Psychological Record 17:493–502, 1967.

Rous, Peyton: The fly in the social ointment. Perspect. Biol. Med. 11:1–8, Autumn, 1967. (An article on tactless persons.)

Slap, Joseph William: On sarcasm. Psychoanal. Quart. 35:98–107, 1966.

Spiegel, John P.: Classification of body messages. Arch. Gen. Psychiat. 17:298–305, 1967.

Books and Reports of Organizations

Barbara, Dominick: The Art of Listening. Springfield, Illinois: Charles C. Thomas, Publisher, 1966.

Bermosk, Loretta Sue: Interviewing: A key to therapeutic communication in nursing practice. The Nursing Clinics of North America, 1:205–214, June, 1966. (See pp. 206–214 for "Principles of Interviewing in Nursing.")

Black, Max (ed.): The Importance of Language. Ithaca: Cornell University Press, 1969.

Budd, Richard W.; Thorp, Robert K., and Donohew, Lewis: Content Analysis of Communications. New York: The Macmillan Company, 1967.

Cherry, Colin: On Human Communication: A Review, a Survey, and a Criticism, ed. 2. Cambridge, Mass.: M.I.T. Press, 1966.

Dance, Frank E.X. (ed.): Human Communication Theory: Original Essays. New York: Holt, Rinehart and Winston, Inc., 1967.

Deese, James: The Structure of Associations in Language and Thought. Baltimore: The Johns Hopkins Press, 1966.

De Cecco, John P.: The Psychology of Language, Thought and Instruction: Readings. New York: Holt, Rinehart and Winston, Inc., 1967.

Dixon, Theodore R., and Horton, David L. (ed.): Verbal Behavior and General Behavior Theory. Englewood Cliffs, New Jersey: Prentice–Hall, Inc., 1968.

Erway, Ella A.: Listening: A Programmed Approach. New York: McGraw–Hill Book Company, 1969. (Set of tapes for "Listening: A Programmed Approach," McGraw–Hill Book Company, 1969.)

Goffman, Erving: Interaction Ritual: Essays on Face–to–Face Behavior. Chicago: Aldine Publishing Company, 1967.

Ichheiser, Gustav: Appearances and Realities. Misunderstanding in Human Relations. San Francisco: Jossey–Bass, Inc., 1970.

Kuiper, Pieter C.: On Being Genuine and Other Essays. New York: Basic Books Inc., 1968.

Matson, Floyd W., and Montagu, Ashley, (eds.): The Human Dialogue. Perspectives on Communication. New York: The Free Press, 1967.

Miller, George A.: The Psychology of Communication. Seven Essays. New York: Basic Books, Inc., 1967.

Murphy, Gardner: The communications continuum. Communication: Concepts and Perspectives. Lee Thayer (ed.) Washington, D. C.: Spartan Books, 1967, pp. 241–257.

Parry, John: The Psychology of Human Communication. New York: American Elsevier Publishing Co., Inc., 1968.

Ramphal, Marjorie, et al.: Clinical decision-making. Current Concepts in Clinical Nursing. Betty S. Bergersen, et al. (eds.) St. Louis: The C.V. Mosby Company, 1969, pp.1-13.

Sorenson, Robert C.: Effective communications and personal values: a theory. Communication: Concepts and Perspectives. Lee Thayer (ed.) Washington, D.C.: Spartan Books, 1967, pp. 207–225.

Smith, Alfred G. (ed): Communication and Culture: Readings in the Codes of Human Interaction. New York: Holt, Rinehart and Winston, Inc., 1966.

Solomon, Arthur: Interpersonal Communication: A Cross-Disciplinary Approach. Springfield, Illinois: Charles C. Thomas, Publisher, 1969.

Toch, Hans, and Smith, Henry Clay (eds.): Social Perception. Princeton, New Jersey: D. Van Nostrand Company, Inc., 1968.

Travelbee, Joyce: Intervention in Psychiatric Nursing. Process in the One–to–One Relationship. Philadelphia: F.A. Davis Company, 1969. (See Chapter V, "Communicating With Patients," esp. pp. 67–84 and pp. 91–104.)

Wiener, Morton, and Mehrabian, Albert: Language Within Language: Immediacy, A Channel in Verbal Communication. New York: Appleton–Century–Crofts, 1968.

Wilson, Lucille: Listening. Behavioral Concepts and Nursing Intervention. Philadelphia: J.B. Lippincott Company, 1970, pp. 153–170.

Concepts: Perception and Observation

Articles, Books and Reports of Organizations

Aarson, Doris: Temporal factors in perception and short-term memory. Psychol. Bull. 67:130–144, No. 2., 1967.

Bakan, Paul: Attention. Insight Book No. 34. Princeton: D. Van Nostrand, Inc., 1966.

Forgus, Ronald H.: Perception. The Basic Process in Cognitive Development. New York: McGraw–Hill Book Company, 1966.

————: The hierarchial organization of perception. Int. J. Neurol. 6:138–146, No. 2, 1967.

Garner, W.R.: To perceive is to know. Amer. Psychol. 21:11–19, 1966.

Gibson, Eleanor J.: The development of perception as an adaptive process. Amer. Sci. 58:98–107, 1970.

Haber, Ralph Norman (ed): Contemporary Theory and Research in Visual Perception. New York: Holt, Rinehart and Winston, Inc., 1968.

————: Eidetic images. Sci. Amer. 220:36–44, Apr., 1969.

Macrae J. H.H.: A general theory of perception, Develop. Med. Child Neurol. 11:654–662, 1969.

Natsoulas, Thomas: What are perceptual reports about? Psychol. Bull. 67:249–272, 1967.

Peterson, Linda Whitney: Operant approach to observation and recording. Nurs. Outlook 15:28–32, Mar., 1967.

Piaget, Jean: The Mechanisms of Perception. G.N. Seagrin (trans.) New York: Basic Books Inc., 1969.

Richards, I.A.: The secrets of "feedforward." Saturday Review 14–17, February 3, 1968

Travelbee, Joyce: The concept of observation. Communication in the Helping Process in Nursing. Proceedings of a Nursing Conference. Sponsored by Louisiana State Board of Health, Louisiana State Department of Hospitals and the National Institute of Mental Health. New Orleans, February, 1965, pp. 17–22.

————: Intervention in Psychiatric Nursing. Process in the One–to–One Relationship. Philadelphia: F.A. Davis Company, 1969. (See, "Observation," pp. 28–35; "Interpretation," pp. 35–41; and "Appraisal of Nursing Action," pp. 44–45.)

Weintraub, Daniel J., and Walker, Edward I.: Perception. Belmont, California: Brooks Cole, 1966.

Wyatt, Frederick: How objective is objectivity? Reflections on scope and limitations of a basic tenet in the study of personality. J. Project. Techn. 31:3–19, Oct., 1967.

Concepts: Decision-Making and Clinical Judgement

Articles, Books and Reports of Organizations

Anthony, Nicholas: The use of facts and cues in clinical judgements from interviews. J. Clin. Psychol. 24:37–39, 1968.

Atta, Ralph E. Van: Concepts employed by accurate and inaccurate clinicians. J. Counseling Psychol. 15:338–345, July, 1968.

Bailey, Daniel E.: Clinical inference in nursing: analysis of nursing action patterns. Nurs. Res. 16:154–160, 1967.

Chalk, David N.: The decision making process in leadership. Amer. Assoc. Industr. Nurses J. 15:10–12, 1967.

Feinstein, Alvan R.: Clinical Judgement. Baltimore: The Williams & Wilkins Company, 1967.

Gerard, Harold B.: Choice difficulty, dissonance and the decision sequence. J. Personality 35:91–108, 1967.

Hansen, Ann C., and Thomas, Donald B.: A conceptualization of decision-making: its application to a study of role–and situation-related differences in priority decisions. Nurs. Res. 17:436–443, 1968.

Hammond, Kenneth R., et al.: Clinical inference in nursing: analyzing cognitive tasks representative of nursing problems. Nurs. Res. 15:134–138, 1966.

————, et al.: Clinical inference in nursing: use of information-seeking strategies by nurses. Nurs. Res. 15:330–336, 1966.

————, et al.: Clinical inference in nursing: revising judgments. Nurs. Res 16:38–45, 1967.

O'Neill, Audrey Myerson: The bases of clinical inference. J. Clin. Psychol. 24:366–372, 1968.

Olson, Marian: Social influence on decision–making. J. Nurs. Educ. 7:11–16, 1968.

Pepitone, Albert: Motivations in decision making. Trans. Acad. Sci. Ser. II, No. 7, pp. 920–934, 1967.

Pribyl, Mark K.; Hunt, William A.; and Walker, Ronald E.: Judgment as a function of manifest anxiety and social conditions. Percept. Motor Skills 21:759–765, 1965.

————: Some learning variables in clinical judgment. J. Clin. Psychol. 24:32–36, 1968.

Singer, Estelle, and Roby, Thornton B.: Dimensions of decision–Making behavior.

Percept. Motor Skills 24:571–595, 1967. (Monograph Supplement 3–V20.)

Stevens, S.S.: On the operation known as judgment, Amer. Sci. 54:385–401, 1966.

Travelbee, Joyce: Intervention in Psychiatric Nursing. Process in the One–to–One Relationship. Philadelphia: F.A. Davis Company, 1969. (See "Decision-Making and Nursing Action," pp. 41–43.)

Chapter X: The Human-to-Human Relationship

Articles

Briscoe, May E.; Woodyard, Howard D.; and Shaw, Marvin E.: Personality impression change as a function of the favorableness of first impressions. J. Personality 35: 343–357, 1967.

Burnand, G.: The nature of emotional support. Brit. J. Psychiat. 115:139–147, 1969.

Byrne, Donn; Griffitt, William; and Stefaniak, Daniel: Attraction and similarity of personality characteristics. J. Personality Soc. Psychol. 5:82–90, No. 1, 1967.

Dreyfus, Edward A.: Openness: an examination and formulation. J. Exist. 7:309–317, No. 27, 1967.

Efran, Jay S.: Looking for approval: effects on visual behavior of approbation from persons differing in importance. J. Personality Soc. Psychol. 10:21–25, 1968.

Hayter, Jean: What does caring really mean? Canad. Nurse 62:29–32, Oct., 1966.

Jorgensen, E. Clay, and Howell, Robert J.: Judging unposed emotional behavior. Psychotherapy: Theory, Research and Practice 6:161–165, No. 3, 1969.

Krebs, Dennis L.: Altruism—an examination of the concept and a review of the literature. Psychol. Bull. 73:258–302, 1970.

Mascaro, Guillermo: Interpersonal attraction and uncertainty reduction as functions of judgmental similarity. Percept. Motor Skills. 30:71–75, 1970.

McDowell, Wanda: Gifts to give. Amer. J. Nurs. 67:1016–1017, 1967.

Novak, David W., and Lerner, Melvin J.: Rejection as a consequence of perceived similarity. J. Personality Soc. Psychol. 9:147–152, 1968.

Ohnmacht, Fred W., and Muro, James J.: Self–acceptance: some anxiety and cognitive style relationships. J. Psychol. 67: 235–259, 1967.

Perk, David, Commitment. S. Afr. Med. J. 40:31–34, Jan. 8, 1966.

Peterson, Donald I.: Developing the difficult patient. Amer. J. Nurs. 67:522–525, 1967.

Rentz, R. Robert, and White, William F.: Congruence of the dimensions of self– as–object and self–as–process. J. Psychol. 67:277–285, 1967.

Schutt, Barbard G. (ed): Authentic humans or automatons? Amer. J. Nurs. 67:521, 1967. 1967.

Simmons, Carolyn H. and Lerner, Melvin J.: Altruism as a search for justice. J. Personality Soc. Psychol. 9:216–225, No. 3, 1968.

Ujhely, Gertrud E.: What is realistic emotional support? Amer. J. Nurs. 68:758–762, 1968.

Walker, Daphne: Reassure the patient? Yes, but how? Canad. Nurse 64:27, Dec., 1968.

Ziller, Robert C., et al.: Self–esteem: a self–social construct. J. Consult. Clin. Psychol. 33:84–95, No. 1, 1969.

Books and Reports of Organizations

Coopersmith, Stanley: The Antecedents of Self-Esteem. San Francisco: W.H. Freeman and Company, 1967.

Epstein, Cynthia F.: Woman's Place. Berkeley: University of California Press, 1970.

Frankl, Viktor E.: The Doctor and The Soul. From Psychotherapy to Logotherapy, ed. 2. Richard and Clare Winston. (trans.) New York: Alfred A. Knopf, 1965. (See "On the Meaning of Love," pp. 132–175.)

Gould, Grace T.: The nurse–patient relationship: a monologue. The Nursing Clinics of North America. 3:129–134, Mar., 1968.

Hagerman, Zerita: The concept of love as it relates to nursing intervention. Conference on Teaching Psychiatric Nursing in Baccalaureate Programs, Atlanta: Southern Regional Education Board, 1967, pp. 64–83.

————: The patient who is unable to love. The Nursing Clinics of North America, 4:691–699, Dec., 1969.

Halmos, Paul: The Faith of the Counsellors. A Study in the Theory and Practice of Social Case Work and Psychotherapy. New York: Schocken Books, 1966. (See Chapter 3, "The Counsellor's Love as Therapeutic Skill," pp. 49–74.)

Harper, Ralph: Human Love–Existential and Mystical. Baltimore: The Johns Hopkins Press, 1966.

Hoffmann, Georgianna S.: The concept of love. The Nursing Clinics of North America, 4:663–672, December 1969.

Huether, Sue E., and Acquaviva, Roberta A.: The physically disabled patient in the general hospital, The Nursing Clinics of North America, 2:785–796, December, 1967.

Lamper, Neil: Compassion. New York: Appleton–Century–Crofts, Inc., 1970.

Rohweder, Anne W.: Can love, compassion and involvement be scientific? The Nursing Clinics of North America, 4:701–707, December, 1969.

Smith, Henry Clay: Sensitivity to People. New York: McGraw–Hill Book Company, 1966.

Symposium on Compassion and Communication in Nursing. Grace Theresa Gould, Guest Editor, The Nursing Clinics of North America. 4:651–707, December, 1969.

Wallace, Caroline Ogilvie: Acceptance. Conference on Teaching Psychiatric Nursing in Baccalaureate Programs. Atlanta: Southern Regional Education Board, pp. 10–17.

Concepts: Empathy and Sympathy

Articles, Books and Reports of Organizations

Aderman, David, and Berkowitz, Leonard: Observational set, empathy and helping. J. Personality Soc. Psychol. 14:141–148, 1970.

Astin, Helen S.: Assessment of empathic ability by means of a situational test. Journal of Counseling Psychology, 14:57–60, No. 1, 1967.

Bachrach, Henry: Adaptive Regression, empathy and psychotherapy: theory and research study. Psychotherapy: Theory, Research and Practice 5:203–209, No. 4.

Bergin, Allen C., and Jasper, Lawrence G.: Correlates of empathy in psychotherapy: a replication. J. Abnorm. Psychol. 74:477–481, 1969.

Boyd, Harry: Love versus omnipotence: the narcissistic dilemma. Psychotherapy: Theory, Research and Practice 5:272–277, 1968.

Browne, Kevin, and Freeling, Paul: Doctor–patient relationship. The role of sympathy. Part I. Practitioner 196:454–458, 1966. The role of sympathy, Part II. *Ibid.*, 196:593–596, 1966.

Brunclik, Helen; Thurston, John R.; and Feldhusen, John: The empathy inventory. Nurs. Outlook 15:42–45, June, 1967.

Freund, Hedi: Listening with any ear at all. Amer. J. Nurs. 69:1650–1653, 1969.

Guerney, Bernard, Jr.; Stover, Lillian; and DeMerritt, Stephen: A measurement of empathy in parent-child interaction. J. Genet. Psychol. 112:49–55, 1968.

Hogan, Robert: Development of an empathy scale. J. Consult. and Clin. Psychol. 33:307–316, No. 3, 1969.

Holmes, David S.: Dimensions of projection. Psychol. Bull. 69:248–268, No. 4, 1968.

Hunsdahl, Jorgen B.: Concerning Einfühlung (empathy): a concept analysis of its origin and early development. Journal of the History of the Behavioral Sciences 3:180–191, 1967.

Korson, Selig M., and Hayes, Winifred L.: Empathic relationship therapy utilizing student nurses: a five year pilot study. Amer. J. Psychiat. 123:213–216, 1966. (Discussion by Paul F. Haun, pp. 217–218.)

Kjos, Karen: Listening with sympathy. Amer. J. Nurs. 66:2471–2473, 1966.

Laughlin, Henry P.: The Neuroses in Clinical Practice. Philadelphia: W.B. Saunders, Co., 1956. (See "Identification," pp. 96–101, and "Projection," pp. 109–116.)

Lide, Pauline D.: Dynamic mental representations: an analysis of the empathic process. Social Casework 47:146–151, Mar., 1966.

Meerloo, Joost A.M.: Why do we sympathize with each other? Arch. Gen. Psychiat. 15:390–397, 1966.

Paul, Norman L.: The use of empathy in the resolution of grief. Perspect. Biol. Med. 11:153–169, Autumn, 1967.

Pierce, William, and Mosher, Donald L.: Perceived empathy, interviewer behavior and interviewee anxiety. J. Consult. Psychol. 31:101, No. 1, 1967.

Schonbar, Rosalea Ann: Identification and the search for identity. Contemporary Psychoanalysis 3–4:75–95, 1966–68.

Shapiro, Jeffrey G.; Foster, Charles P.; and Powell, Tom: Facial and bodily cues of genuineness, empathy and warmth. J. Clin. Psychol. 24:233–236, 1968.

Stewart, David A.: Empathy–a revised concept. J. Exist. 6:215–221, No. 22, 1965–1966.

Taft, Ronald: Accuracy of empathic judgments of acquaintances and strangers. J. Personality Soc. Psychol. 3:600–604, 1966.

Travelbee, Joyce: What do we mean by rapport? Amer. J. Nurs. 63:70–72, 1963.

————: What's wrong with sympathy? Amer. J. Nurs. 64:68–71, 1964.

Triplett, June L.: Empathy is . . . The Nursing Clinics of North America. 4:673–681, Dec., 1969.

Truax, Charles C.: Therapist empathy, warmth and genuineness and patient personality change in group psychotherapy. J. Clin. Psychol. 22:225–229, 1966.

Walstedt, Joyce J.: Teaching empathy. Ment. Hyg. 52:600–611, 1968.

Yufit, Robert I.: Variations of intimacy and isolation. J. Project. Techn. 33:49–58, 1969.

Zanger, Allyn: A study of factors related to clinical empathy. Smith College Studies in Social Work, 38:116–132, 1967.

Zderad, Loretta: Empathic nursing: realization of a human capacity. The Nursing Clinics of North America 4:655–662, Dec., 1969

Zimmer, Jules M., and Anderson, Susan: Dimensions of positive regard and empathy. Journal of Counseling Psychology 15:417–426, No. 5, 1968.

Chapter XI: Nursing Intervention

Articles, Books and Reports of Organizations

Bühler, Charlotte, and Massarik, Fred (eds.): The Course of Human Life. A study of Goals in the Humanistic Perspective. New York: Springer Publishing, Inc., 1968.

Burnside, Irene Mortenson: The patient I didn't want. Amer. J. Nurs. 68:1666–1669, 1968.

Burton, Arthur: The authentic person in existential psychology. Pastoral psychology 20:17–26, 1969.

Clemence, Sister Madeleine: Existentialism: a philsosphy of commitment. Amer. J. Nurs. 66:500–505, 1966.

Fabrey, Joseph B.: The Pursuit of Meaning. Logotherapy Applied to Life. Boston: Beacon Press, 1968.

Frankl, Viktor E.: What is meant by meaning? J. Exist. 7:21–28, No. 25, 1966.

————: Psychotherapy and Existentialism. New York: Simon & Schuster, A Clarion Book, 1967. (See "The Philosophical Foundations of Logotherapy," pp. 1–18; "Logotherapy and Existence," pp. 53–55; "Psychiatry and Man's Quest for Meaning," pp. 71–86; and "Logotherapy and the Channenge of Suffering," pp. 87–94.)

————: The Will To Meaning. Foundations and Applications of Logotherapy. New York: The World Publishing Company. An N.A.L. Book, 1969.

Gaspar, Nancy J.: The family of the patient with long-term illness. The Nursing Clinics of North America, 5:77–84, Mar., 1970.

Giovacchini, Peter L.: Characterological problems: the need to be helped. Arch. Gen. Psychiat. 22:245–251, 1970.

Hilliard, Mary E.: One dimension of nursing. Amer. J. Nurs. 67:756–759, 1967.

Kaczanowski, Godfrey: Logotherapy—a new psychotherapeutic tool. Psychosomatics 8:158–161, 1967.

Levin, Sidney: Toward a classification of external factors capable of inducing psychological stress. Int. J. Psychoanal. 47:546–551, 1966.

Lipp, Leland, et al.: Denial of disability and internal control of reinforcement: a study using a perceptual defense paradigm. Journal of Consulting and Clinical Psychology 32:72–75, No. 1, 1968.

Meinhart, Noreen T., and Aspinall, Mary Jo: Nursing intervention in hypovigilance. Amer J. Nurs. 69:994-998, 1969.

Minckley, Barbara Blake: Space and place in patient care. Amer. J. Nurs. 68:510–516, 1968.

Minton, Henry L.: Power as a personality construct. Progress in Experimental Personality Research 4:229–267, New York: Academic Press, 1967.

Poole, Pamela E.: Nurse, please show me that you care! Canad. Nurse 66:25–27, Feb., 1970.

Robinson, Vera M.: Humor in nursing. Amer. J. Nurs. 70:1065–1069, 1970.

Rosenthal, S.H., and Gudeman, J.E.: The self-pitying constellation in depression. Brit. J. Psychiat. 113:485–489, 1967.

Schoen, Eugenia A.: Clinical problem: the demanding, complaining patient. The Nursing Clinics of North America, 2:715–724, Dec., 1967.

Schwartz, Barry: The social psychology of privacy. Amer. J. Sociol. 73:741–752, 1968.

Social isolation: an under rated aspect of disability. Rehab. Rec. 7:24–35, 1966 (four papers).

Stein, Leonard I.: The doctor—nurse game. Amer. J. Nursing 68:101–105, 1968.

Symposium on Chronic Disease and Rehabilitation. June S. Rothberg, Guest Editor, The Nursing Clinics of North America 1:352–519, Sept., 1966 (sixteen papers).

Symposium on the Difficult Patient. Vera M. Rubenstein, Guest Editor, The Nursing Clinics of North America 2:691–796, Dec., 1967 (nine papers).

Thomas, Mary Durand: Anger in nurse—patient interactions. The Nursing Clinics of North America 2:737–745, Dec., 1967.

Ujhely, Gertrud B.: When adult patients cry. The Nursing Clinics of North America 2:725–735, Dec., 1967.

Tripodi, Tony, and Miller, Henry: The clinical judgment process: a review of the literature. Social Work 11:63–69, July, 1966.

Wald, Florence: Emerging nursing practice. Amer. J. Public Health 56:1252–1260, 1966.

Watts, William A.: Commitment under conditions of risk. J. Personality Soc. Psychol. 3:507–515, No. 5, 1966.

Weisskopf-Joelson, Edith: Meaning as an integrating factor. The Course of Human Life. A Study of Goals in the Humanistic Perspective. Charlotte Bühler and Fred Massarik (eds.). New York: Springer Publishing Company, Inc., 1968, pp. 359–383.

Westcott, Malcolm R.: Toward a Contemporary Psychology of Intuition. A Historical, Theoretical and Empirical Inquiry. New York: Holt, Rinehart and Winston, Inc., 1968.

Chapter XII: Surgery—A Human Experience

Articles

Baxter, Carol R.: Three days with Mrs. M. Amer. J. Nurs. 67:774–778, 1967.

Abram, Harry S.: Adaptation to open heart surgery: a psychiatric study of response to the threat of death. Amer. J. Psychiat. 122:659–667, 1965. (Discussion by Thomas P. Hackett, pp. 659–667.)

————: The Van Gogh syndrome: an unusual case of polysurgical addiction. Amer. J. Psychiat. 123:478–481, 1966.

————(ed.): Psychological aspects of surgery. Int. Psychiat. Clin. 4:3–204, No. 2, 1967 (twelve papers).

Blacher, Richard S., and Basch, Samuel H.: Psychological aspects of pacemaker implanation. Arch. Gen. Psychiat. 22:319–323, 1970.

Blachly, Paul H.: Open–heart surgery: physiological variables of mental functioning. Int. Psychiat. Clin. 4:133–155, 1967.

Brown, J.: The theory and the practice: patients' reactions to amputation of the lower limb. Nurs. Times 62:639–640, May 13, 1966.

Clarkson, Patrick W.: Appearance, cosmetic surgery and mental health. Nursing Mirror and Midwives Journal 122:x–xiii, May 20, 1966; and 122:vi–viii, May 27, 1966.

Cramond, W. A.: Renal homotransplantation—some observations on recipients and donors. Brit. J. Psychiat. 113:1223–1230, 1967.

————: Knight, P.R.; and Lawrence, J.R.: The psychiatric contribution to a renal unit undertaking chronic haemodialysis and renal homotransplantation. Brit. J. Psychiat. 113:1201–1212, 1967.

————, et al.: Psychological screening of potential donors in a renal homotransplantation programme. Brit. J. Psychiat. 113:1213–1221, 1967.

Darbonne, Allen R.: Crisis: a review of theory, practice and research. Psychotherapy: Theory, Research and Practice 4:49–56, 1967.

Dlin, Barney M.; Fischer, H. Keith; and Huddell, Benjamin: Psychologic adaptation to pacemaker and open heart surgery. Arch. Gen. Psychiat. 19:599–610, 1968.

Dorfman, Wilfred: Hypochondriasis as a defense against depression. Psychosomatics 9:248–251 1968.

Druss, Richard, and Kornfeld, Donald S.: The survivors of cardiac arrest – a psychiatric study. J.A.M.A. 201:291–296, 1967.

Eisendrath, Robert M.: The role of grief and fear in the death of kidney transplant patients. Amer. J. Psychiat. 126:381–387, 1969.

Ferber, Andrew S., et al.: Men with vasectomies: a study of medical, sexual and psychosocial changes. Psychosom. Med. 29:354–366, 1967.

Fleck, Stephen: Some psychiatric aspects of abortion. J. Nerv. Ment. Dis. 151:42–50, 1970.

Gardner, William H.: Adjustment problems of laryngectomized Women. Arch. Otolaryng. 83:31–42, 1966.

Gershon, Elliot S.; Cromer, Marjorie; and Klerman, Gerald: Hostility and Depression. Psychiatry 31:224–235, 1968.

Gould, Roger L., and Nahum, Alan M.: Psychological motivation in stapes surgery. Trans. Amer. Acad. Opthal. Otolaryng. 70:398–403, 1966.

Greene, William A., and Moss, Arthur J.: Psychosocial factors in the adjustment of patients with permanently implanted cardiac pacemakers. Ann. Intern. Med. 70:897–902, 1969.

Havens, Leston L.: Dependence: definitions and strategies. Rehab. Rec. 8:23–28, 1967.

Healy, Kathryn M.: Does prooperative instruction make a difference? Amer. J. Nurs. 68:62–67. 1968.

Jarvis, John H., Post–mastectomy breast phantom, J. Nerv. Ment. Dis. 144:266–272, 1967.

Johnson, Jean E.; Dabbs, James M. Jr; and Leventhal, Howard: Psychosocial factors in the welfare of surgical patients. Nurs. Res. 19:18–29, 1970.

Johnstone, F.R.C.; Holubitsky, I.B.; and Debas, H.T.: Post–gastrectomy problems in patients with personality defects: the "albatross" syndrome. Canad. Med. Assoc. J. 96:1559–1564, 1967.

Katz, Jack L., et al.: Stress, distress and ego defenses. Psychoendocrine response to impending breast tumor biopsy. Arch. Gen. Psychiat. 23:131–142, 1970.

Kemph, John P.: Renal failure, artificial kidney and kidney transplant. Amer. J. Psychiat. 122:1270–1274, 1966.

————: Psychotherapy with patients receiving kidney transplant. Amer. J. Psychiat. 124:623–629, 1967.

————; Bermann, Eric A; and Coppolillo, Henry P.: Kidney Transplant and shifts in family dynamics. Amer. J. Psychiat. 125:1485–1490, 1969.

Kennedy, Janet, and Bakst, Hyman: Influence of emotions on outcome of cardiac surgery: predictive study. Bull. N. Y. Acad. Med. 42:811–845, 1966.

Kennedy, Mary Jane: An exploratory study of the responses of the patients to the cancellation of his surgery. Int. J. Nurs. Stud. 6:121–132, 1969.

Kimball, Chase Patterson: Psychological responses to the experience of open heart surgery I. Amer. J. Psychiat. 126:348–359, 1969.

Kolouch, Fred T.: Indications for psychiatric evaluation of the surgical patient. J. Lancet 88:87–90, 1968.

Kornfeld, Donald S.: Psychiatric view of the intensive care unit. Brit. Med. J. 1:108–110, 1969.

Kuromaru, S., et al.: The effect of LSD on the phantom limb phenomenon. J. Lancet 87:22–27, 1967.

Lazarus, Herbert R., and Hagens, Jerome H.: Prevention of psychosis following open–heart surgery. Amer. J. Psychiat. 124:1190–1195, 1968.

Levine, Dale C., and Fiedler, June P.: Fears, facts and fantasies about pre– and postoperative care, Nurs. Outlook 18:26–28, Feb., 1970.

Lorr, Maurice; Sonn, Thomas M.; and Katz, Martin M.: Toward a definition of depression. Arch. Gen. Psychiat. 17:183–186, 1967.

Lunde, Donald T.: Psychiatric complications of heart transplants. Amer. J. Psychiat. 126:369–373, 1969.

McKegney, F. Patrick: Intensive care syndrome: the definition treatment and prevention of a new "disease of medical progress," Conn. Med. 30:633–636, 1966.

Mefferd, Roy B., Jr., and Wieland, Betty A.: Comparison of responses to anticipated stress and stress. Psychosom. Med. 28:795–807, No. 6, 1966.

Mezzanotte, Elizabeth Jane: Group instruction in preparation for surgery. Amer. J. Nurs. 70:89–91, 1970.

Morse, Robert M. and Litin, Edward M.: Postoperative delerium: a study of etiologic factors. Amer. J. Psychiat. 126: 388–395, 1969.

Robertiello, Richard C.: The role of infantile omnipotence in the dynamics of depression. Psychotherapy: Theory, Research and Practice 6:37–38, 1969.

Russek, Allen S.: Pre and postoperative management of the potential diabetic amputee. New York J. Med. 66:1659–1662, 1966.

Simpson, Elaine B., and Albronda, Henry F.: Psychologic aspects of amputation of a lower limb. J. Lancet 87:429–431, 1967.

Special Section: Psychiatric complications of surgical procedures. Amer. J. Psychiat. 126:348–395, 1969 (six papers).

Symposium: Some aspects of anxiety and depression. H. J. Walton, Guest editor. Brit. J. Clin. Pract. 24:53–84, 1970 (five papers).

Weiler, Sister M. Cashel: Postoperative patients evaluate preoperative instruction. Amer. J. Nurs. 68:1465–1467, 1968.

Weiss, Stephen M.: Psychosomatic aspects of symptom patterns among major surgery patients. J. Psychosom. Res. 13:109–112, 1969.

Woodforde, J.M.: Intensive care – a crisis situation. Australian Nurses Journal 65:50–54, 1967.

Wolf, Sanford R.: Emotional reactions to hysterectomy. Postgrad. Med. 47:165–169, 1970.

Ziegler, Frederick J.; Rogers, David A.; and Prentiss, Robert J.: Psychosocial response to vasectomy. Arch. Gen. Psychiat. 21:46–54, 1969.

Books and Reports of Organizations

Brady, Eugenia: Grief and amputation. ANA Clinical sessions. American Nurses Association, 1968, Dallas. New York: Appleton–Century–Crofts, 1968, pp. 297-301.

Care of the Surgical Patient. Ina Love Williams, Guest Editor. The Nursing Clinics of

North America. 3:489–541, September, 1968 (seven papers).

Katona, Elizabeth A.: A patient–centered living–oriented approach to the patient with an artificial anus or bladder. The Nursing Clinics of North America 2:6 23–634, Dec., 1967.

Kolb, Laurence C.: Distrubances of the body image. American Handbook of Psychiatry, Vol. 1, Silvano Arieti, Editor, New York: Basic Books Inc., 1959., pp. 749–769.

Kornfeld, Donald S.; Maxwell, Teresita; and Momrow, Dawn: Psychological hazards of the intensive care unit. The Nursing Clinics of North America. 3:41–51, Mar., 1968.

Laughlin, Henry P.: The Neuroses. Washington, D.C.: Butterworths, 1967. (See Chapter 1, "The Nature and Origins of Anxiety," pp. 1-54.)

Lazarus, Richard S.: Psychological Stress and the Coping Process. New York: McGraw–Hill Book Company, 1966.

Norris, Catherine M.: The professional nurse and body image. Behavioral Concepts and Nursing Intervention. Coordinated by Carolyn E. Carlson. Philadelphia: J.B. Lippincott Company, 1970. pp. 39–65.

Symposium on Intensive Care Nursing. Hattie Mildred McIntyre, Guest editor, The Nursing Clinics of North America, 3:1-93, Mar., 1968.

*

Concept: Anxiety

Articles, Books and Reports of Organizations

Appley, Mortimer H., and Trumbull, Richard (eds.): Psychological Stress: Issues in Research. The Century Psychology Series. New York: Appleton–Century–Crofts, 1967.

Bridges, P.K.; Jones, M.T.; and Leak D.: A comparative study of four physiological concomitants of anxiety. Arch. Gen. Psychiat. 19:141–145, 1968.

Burkhardt, Marti: Response to anxiety. Amer. J. Nurs. 69:2153–2154, 1969.

Carnevali, Doris: Preoperative anxiety. Amer. J. Nurs. 66:1536–1538, 1966.

Cottle, Thomas J.: Temporal correlates of the achievement value and manifest anxiety, J. Consult. Clin. Psychol. 33:541–550, 1969.

Day, Merle E.: An eye–movement indicator of type and level of anxiety: some clinical observations. J. Clin. Psychol. 23:438–441, 1967.

Drew, Frances L.; Moriarity, Richard W.; and Shapiro, Alvin P.: An approach to the measurement of pain and anxiety responses of surgical patients. Psychosom. Med. 30:826–836. 1968.

Epstein, Seymour: Toward a unified theory of anxiety. Progr. Exp. Personality Res. Vol. 4, Academic Press, New York, 1968, pp. 1–89.

Gottschalk, Louise A., and Frank, Edward C.: Estimating the magnitude of anxiety from speech. Behav. Sci. 12:289–295, 1967.

Hendrix, Harville: The ontological character of anxiety. Journal of Religion and Health 6:46–65, 1967.

Hulbeck, Charles R.: The irrational and the nature of basic anxiety. Amer. J. Psychoanal. 30:3–12, No. 1, 1970.

Jacobson, Gerald F.: Crisis theory and treatment strategy: some sociocultural and psychodynamic considerations. J. Nerv. Ment. Dis. 141:209–218, 1965.

Jones, Warren L.: The A–B–C method of crisis management. Ment. Hyg. 52:87–89, 1968.

Kaplan, David M.: Observations on crisis theory and practice. Social Casework 49:151–155, Mar., 1968.

Kelly, Desmond, and Walter, C.J.S.: A clinical and physiological relationship between anxiety and depression. Brit. J. Psychiat. 115:401–406, 1969.

Kilpatrick, Helen M.: The frightened patient in the emergency room. Amer. J. Nurs. 66:1031–1032, 1966.

Krauss, Herbert H.: Anxiety: the dread of a future event. J. Individ. Psychol. 23:88–93, 1967.

Laughlin, Henry P.: The Neuroses. Washington: Butterworths, 1967. (See Chapter 1, "The Nature and Origins of anxiety ... Fear in the Absence of a Known Cause," pp. 1–54.)

Magill, Kathleen A.: How one patient handled fear. Amer. J. Nurs. 67:1248–1249, 1967.

May, Rollo: Psychology and the Human Dilemma. Princeton, New Jersey: D. Van Nostrand Company, Inc., 1967. (See Chapter 4, "Historical Roots of Modern Anxiety Theories," pp. 55–71; and Chapter 5, "Anxiety and Values," pp. 72–83.)

McGee, Thomas F.: Some basic considerations in crisis intervention. Community Ment. Health J. 4:319–325, 1968.

Pitts, Ferris N., Jr.: The biochemistry of anxiety. Sci. Amer. 220:69–75, Feb., 1969.

Powers, Maryann E., and Storlie, Frances: The apprehensive patient. Amer. J. Nurs. 67:58–63, 1967.

Prick, J.J.G.: Sketch of anxiety and fear in its normal and pathological appearance. Psychiat. Neurol. Neurochir. 71:155–168, 1968.

Programmed Instruction. Anxiety and Intervention. Prepared by Basic Systems Inc. under the supervision of Journal editors, Amer. J. Nurs. 65:130–152, 1965.

Rangell, Leo: A further attempt to resolve the "problem of anxiety." J. Psychoanal. Assoc. 16:371–404, 1968.

Schumacher, A.S.; Wright, J.M.; and Wiesen, A.E.: The self as a source of anxiety. J. Consult. Clin. Psychol. 32:30–34, No. 1, 1968.

Schwab, John J., et al.: Evaluating anxiety in medical patients. J. Chronic Dis. 19:1049–1057, 1966.

Spielberger, Charles D. (ed): Anxiety and Behavior. New York: Academic Press, 1966.

Williams, James G.L.; Jones, John R.; and Williams, Barbara: A physiological measure of preoperative anxiety. Psychosom. Med. 31:522–527, 1969.

Wolf, Stewart, and Goddell, Helen: Harold G. Wolff's Stress and Disease. Second revised edition, edited by Stewart Wolf. Springfield, Illinois: Charles C. Thomas, 1968.

INDEX